ENT Essentials

To Temple
Otolaryngology –
Head & Neck Surgery
with best wishes
and thanks!

[signature]

ENT Essentials

Editors

Elina M Toskala MD PhD MBA
Professor
Department of Otolaryngology—
Head and Neck Surgery
Thomas Jefferson University
Philadelphia, Pennsylvania, USA

David W Kennedy MD FACS FRCSI
Professor
Department of Otorhinolaryngology—
Head and Neck Surgery
Perelman School of Medicine
University of Pennsylvania
Philadelphia, Pennsylvania, USA

Foreword

Michael J Ruckenstein MD MSc FACS

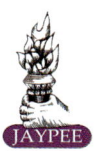

JAYPEE BROTHERS MEDICAL PUBLISHERS
The Health Sciences Publisher
New Delhi | London

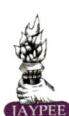 **Jaypee Brothers Medical Publishers (P) Ltd**

Headquarters
Jaypee Brothers Medical Publishers (P) Ltd
4838/24, Ansari Road, Daryaganj
New Delhi 110 002, India
Phone: +91-11-43574357
Fax: +91-11-43574314
E-mail: jaypee@jaypeebrothers.com

Overseas Office
JP Medical Ltd
83 Victoria Street, London
SW1H 0HW (UK)
Phone: +44 20 3170 8910
Fax: +44 (0)20 3008 6180
E-mail: info@jpmedpub.com

Website: www.jaypeebrothers.com
Website: www.jaypeedigital.com

© 2020, Jaypee Brothers Medical Publishers

Inquiries for bulk sales may be solicited at: jaypee@jaypeebrothers.com

ENT Essentials

First Edition: **2020**

ISBN: 978-93-5152-947-7

Printed at: Samrat Offset Pvt. Ltd.

Dedicated to

Garrett, Kirin, Paavali and Aurora

Contributors

Sidrah M Ahmad MD
Assistant Professor of Surgery
Division of Otolaryngology—
Head and Neck Surgery
Stony Brook University Hospital
Stony Brook, New York, USA

Kamil Amer MD
Lewis Katz School of Medicine
Temple University
Philadelphia, Pennsylvania, USA

Samir Ketan Bhandutia DO
Coney Island Hospital
Brooklyn, New York, USA

Anthony E Brissett MD
Associate Professor of
Otolaryngology—
Head and Neck Surgery
Baylor College of Medicine
Houston, Texas, USA

Norman Chan MD
ENT-Otolaryngologist
Mount Sinai School of Medicine
New York City, New York, USA

Michael S Cohen MD
Assistant Professor of
Otolaryngology
Harvard Medical School
Boston, Massachusetts, USA

Jennifer R Cracchiolo MD
Assistant Attending Surgeon
Head and Neck Surgery
Memorial Sloan Kettering
Cancer Center
New York City, New York
USA

Gillian R Diercks MD MPH
Division of Pediatric
Otolaryngology
Massachusetts Eye and Ear
Infirmary
Wellesley, Massachusetts, USA

Barbara Ebersole MA
Speech-Language Pathologist
Philadelphia, Pennsylvania, USA

Christopher E Fundakowski
MD FACS
Attending Surgeon
Head and Neck Oncology
Fox Chase Cancer Center
Assistant Professor of
Otolaryngology—
Head and Neck Surgery
Temple University School of
Medicine
Philadelphia, Pennsylvania, USA

Sarah A Gitomer MD
Department of Otolaryngology
(Ear, Nose and Throat)
Baylor College of Medicine
Houston, Taxes, USA

Purva Gumaste MD
Infectious Diseases
Wagoner Medical Group
CHI Health Saint Francis
Grand Island, Nebraska, USA

Samuel Hahn MD
Maryland Center for Facial
Plastic Surgery
Baltimore, Maryland, USA

George Harris IV MD
Director of Pediatric
Otolaryngology
Summerville Pediatric
Specialists
Summerville Medical Center
Summerville, South Carolina
USA

Kristen Hurst MD
ENT-Otolaryngologist
University of Iowa Hospitals
and Clinics
Iowa City, Iowa, USA

Glenn Isaacson MD FAAP
Professor
Otolaryngology— Head and
Neck
Surgery and Pediatrics
Lewis Katz School of Medicine
Temple University
Philadelphia, Pennsylvania, USA

Fredric Jaffe DO FCCP FAASM
Diplomate of the American
Board of Sleep Medicine
Associate Professor of Clinical
Medicine
Department of Thoracic
Medicine and Surgery
Temple University Hospital
Philadelphia, Pennsylvania, USA

Nausheen Jamal MD
Residency Program Director
and Clerkship Director
Co-Director of ENT Curriculum
PA Program
Assistant Professor
Department of
Otolaryngology—
Head and Neck Surgery
Assistant Professor
Department of Surgical
Oncology
Fox Chase Cancer Center
Temple Head and Neck Institute
Lewis Katz School of Medicine
Temple University
Philadelphia, Pennsylvania, USA

Douglas R Johnston MD
Assistant Professor
Otolaryngology and Pediatrics
Ann and Robert Lurie
Hospital for Children
Northwestern University
Chicago, Illinois, USA

Deborah S F Kacmarynski
MD MS
Paul N Johnson Associate
Professor in Craniofacial
Abnormalities
Pediatric Otolaryngology
Clinical Associate Professor
Co-Director of Cleft and
Craniofacial Team
Department of
Otolaryngology—
Head and Neck Surgery
Pediatrics and Biomedical
Engineering
University of Iowa
Iowa City, Iowa, USA

Jarrod Keeler MD
ENT-Otolaryngologist
University of Pennsylvania
Philadelphia, Pennsylvania, USA

Lori A Lemonnier MD
Assistant Professor and
Program Director
Director of Rhinology and
Skull Base Surgery
Department of
Otolaryngology—
Head and Neck Surgery
Louisiana State University
Health Sciences Center
Shreveport
Shreveport, Louisiana, USA

Gary Linkov MD
ENT-Otolaryngologist
Philadelphia, Pennsylvania, USA

Jeffrey C Liu MD FACS
Associate Professor of
Otolaryngology—Head and
Neck Surgery
Lewis Katz School of Medicine
Temple University
Associate Professor
Head and Neck Surgery
Fox Chase Cancer Center
Philadelphia, Pennsylvania, USA

Yuan F Liu MD
ENT-Otolaryngologist
David Geffen School of
Medicine at UCLA
Los Angeles, California, USA

Benjamin Marcus MD
ENT-Otolaryngologist
University of Wisconsin
Hospitals
Middleton, Wisconsin, USA

Katherine M McKee-Cole MD
Physician, Colorado West
Health Care System
Adjunct Faculty Member
University of Utah
Division of Otolaryngology
Salt Lake City, Utah, USA

Sam P Most MD
Chief, Division of Facial Plastic
and Reconstructive Surgery
Professor
Departments of
Otolaryngology—Head and
Neck Surgery (Plastic)
Stanford University School of
Medicine
Stanford, California, USA

Taha Ahmad Mur MD
Department of
Otolaryngology—
Head and Neck Surgery
Boston Medical Center
Massachusetts, New England
USA

Scott R Owen MD
Director Facial Plastic and
Reconstructive Surgery
Department of
Otolaryngology—
Head and Neck Surgery
University of Iowa Hospitals
and Clinics
Iowa City, Iowa, USA

Robert C O'Reilly MD
Physician in the Division of
Otolaryngology
Director of the Balance and
Vestibular Program at
Children's Hospital
Philadelphia, Pennsylvania, USA

Mariah Pate MD
Ear, Nose and Throat Associates
Clearwater, Florida, USA

Natasha Pollak MD MS
Associate Professor
Department of
Otolaryngology—
Head and Neck Surgery
Lewis Katz School of Medicine
Temple University
Philadelphia, Pennsylvania, USA

Pamela C Roehm MD PhD
Director
Division of Otology and
Neurotology
Professor of Otolaryngology
Department of
Otolaryngology—
Head and Neck Surgery
Lewis Katz School of Medicine
Temple University
Philadelphia, Pennsylvania, USA

Paul Sabini MD FACS
Private Practice
Newark, Delaware, USA

Rafik Samuel MD
Infectious Disease Specialist
Fox Chase Cancer Center
American Oncologic Hospital
Philadelphia, Pennsylvania, USA

Joseph Sciarrino MD
Otolaryngologist
South Carolina ENT Allergy and
Sleep Medicine
Lugoff, South Carolina, USA

Ahmed M S Soliman MD
Professor and Interim Chair
Director, Head and Neck
Institute
Director, Voice, Airway, and
Swallowing Center
Department of
Otolaryngology—
Head and Neck Surgery
Lewis Katz School of Medicine
Temple University
Philadelphia, Pennsylvania, USA

Donald Solomon MD
Assistant Professor of Surgery
Cooper Rowan Medical School
Attending Otolaryngologist
Cooper Health Systems
Specialty: Pediatric
Otolaryngology
Camden, New Jersey, USA

Resha S Soni MD
Department of
Otolaryngology—
Head and Neck Surgery
Lewis Katz School of Medicine
Temple University
Philadelphia, Pennsylvania, USA

Carly J Stewart MD
Department of Otolaryngology
University of Colorado School of
Medicine
Aurora, Colorado, USA

Michael Teixido MD
Otolaryngologist and Otologist/
Neurotologist
Department of
Otolaryngology—Head
and Neck Surgery with Jefferson
Medical College
Director at Balance and
Mobility Center
of Christiana Care and the
Delaware
Otology Medicine and Surgery
Fellowship
Wilmington, Delaware, USA

Gabriela Timoney MD
General Surgeon
Temple University
Philadelphia, Pennsylvania, USA

Derrick Tint MD
Temple Head and Neck Institute
Philadelphia, Pennsylvania, USA

Elina M Toskala MD PhD MBA
Professor
Department of
Otolaryngology—
Head and Neck Surgery
Thomas Jefferson University
Philadelphia, Pennsylvania, USA

Maria Elena Vega MD
Assistant Professor of Medicine
Department of Thoracic
Medicine and Surgery
Lewis Katz School of Medicine
Temple University
Philadelphia, Pennsylvania, USA

Andrew A Winkler MD
Otolaryngology, Plastic
Surgery—
Head and Neck
Assistant Professor
Facial Plastic and
Reconstructive Surgery
and Director, Visage Center
Lone Tree, Colorado, USA

Charles Woodard MD
ENT-Otolaryngologist
Duke Raleigh Hospital
Durham, North Carolina, USA

Helen Xu MD
Associate Professor
Department of
Otolaryngology—
Head and Neck Surgery
Loma Linda University
School of Medicine
Loma Linda, California, USA

Foreword

Why should I read this book?

Otolaryngology is a confusing medical specialty. Even its name is confusing! Officially, it goes by the long and somewhat convoluted names of Otolaryngology—Head and Neck Surgery or the even longer Otorhinolaryngology—Head and Neck Surgery. Colloquially, we are known as Ear, Nose and Throat doctors or ENTs for short. Because we are a regional subspecialty, we are involved in the treatment of disease processes in multiple different organ systems. Although we are surgeons, we treat many medical disorders. In order to do this, we use a variety of tools, including small, subspecialized endoscopes to access areas of the body not normally accessible on physical exam. Is it any wonder that our colleagues are often a bit mystified about what we do and how we do it?

Conservative estimates indicate that 10–20% of visits to a primary care physician result from ear, nose, and throat disorders. Yet medical students typically obtain a maximum of a 1 week of exposure to otolaryngology during their medical training. Many medical schools do not even offer that level of experience. Residency training programs for primary care physicians most often do not include any formal rotations in otolaryngology. For those students who do rotate on our services, and for Physician Assistant and Nurse Practitioners who work in our clinics, a concise, up-to-date, practical text on our specialty, has, until now, been lacking.

The editors have assembled an outstanding team of authors to create this symptom-based text. This approach provides a very readable and practical book that can be read cover to cover or referred to for help with specific clinical complaints. It is appropriate reading for medical students, junior residents, and mid-level providers who are seeking more in-depth knowledge typically provided in more basic, introductory texts. It should also serve as a valuable, readily available online reference that can be accessed from the clinic. The format of this text allows for rapid acquisition of material that is directly of interest to targeted readers. Particularly exciting are the case examples that are provided in the accompanying 'app' that offer an excellent interactive case review in the specified topics. I applaud the editors for providing all of us interested in medical education with a text that we can refer our students to with great enthusiasm!

Michael J Ruckenstein MD MSc FACS
Professor and Vice Chairman
Residency Program Director
Department of Otorhinolaryngology—
Head and Neck Surgery
University of Pennsylvania
Philadelphia, Pennsylvania, USA

Preface

The goal for this book is to create a symptom-based up-to-date text which can be easily referenced either electronically or in hard copy by students performing an elective in the specialty and residents at an early point in their residency, and mid-level providers who are specializing in otolaryngology. Further, the book aims to provide an easy symptom-based reference for those familiar with the specialty, but faced with a problem outside of their usual field of practice. Using a symptom-based format, the book significantly builds upon what is available as a basic text from the Academy, Primary Care Otolaryngology. *ENT Essentials*, available both in print and electronically, incorporates an interactive case-based app, and utilizes this wherever appropriate. This book is divided into sections based upon on regional anatomy; The Ear, The Face, The Nose, The Larynx, The Head and Neck, with additional section on Sleep Medicine and Pediatric ENT.

The chapters themselves are based on patient symptomatology and take the reader through the relevant physical examination, diagnosis and treatment utilizing these symptoms. The book incorporates images, cases and apps. Written by a broad spectrum of subspecialty academic authors each of whom are well recognized within their respective fields the text provides a wealth of basic knowledge. To ensure that the chapters are truly relevant to problems faced by students and residents, many senior authors also worked with residents closer to this point of their training. We believe that this first edition will fulfill an important niche within the otolaryngology educational pathway and sincerely hope that it will be helpful to those pursuing a career within the specialty.

Elina M Toskala MD PhD MBA
David W Kennedy MD FACS FRCSI

Acknowledgments

We would like to take this opportunity to thank all the authors for their untiring work on this project. Like most books the creation took more time than anticipated and they have worked with us to create a book that we believe should be truly beneficial to medical students and residents starting within the field. We would also like to thank Mr Jitendar P Vij (Group Chairman), Mr Ankit Vij (Group President), Ms Chetna Malhotra Vohra (Associate Director–Content Strategy) and Kritika Dua (Senior Development Editor) of M/s Jaypee Brothers Medical Publishers, New Delhi, India for their work, especially for creating the app for the different illustrative cases.

Contents

Section 3: Sleep Medicine

***Section Editor:** Fredric Jaffe*

Section 4: The Larynx

***Section Editor:** Ahmed M S Soliman*

Section 5: The Head and Neck

Section Editor: *Jeffrey C Liu*

Section 6: The Nose

Section Editor: *Elina M Toskala*

Section 7: Pediatric ENT

Section Editor: Donald Solomon

Section

1

The Ear

Section Editor: *Natasha Pollak*

Chapter 1

Ear Infections

Pamela C Roehm, Taha Ahmad Mur

> ***Chief Complaint***
> *"I have an earache". "My ear is draining".*

DEFINITIONS

External otitis: Inflammation or infection of the outer ear, including the external auditory canal and/or auricle.

Acute otitis media: The rapid onset of signs and symptoms of acute inflammation in the middle ear.

Acute mastoiditis: The rapid onset of signs and symptoms of acute inflammation in the mastoid air cells inside the temporal bone, frequently associated with acute otitis media.

Chronic draining ear: Infection of the middle ear with a perforated tympanic membrane and persistent otorrhea from the middle ear.

Cholesteatoma: Keratinized squamous epithelium that has become trapped within the middle ear or mastoid, often associated with a chronic infection.

ANATOMY AND PHYSIOLOGY OF THE EAR

Experiencing normal sound conduction requires:[1]

1. *Sound production*: An object vibrating in matter moves the air particles surrounding it, disseminating a pulse of vibration through the air.
2. *Pinna*: The pinna (auricle) serves to collect these sound waves and direct them into the external auditory canal.
3. *External auditory canal*: Disturbance of air flow passing through the unimpeded ear canal will reach the tympanic membrane.
4. *Tympanic membrane*: In order for air pressures to be transmitted further, the tympanic membrane amplifies air vibration and converts it into a vibration of the ossicles.
5. *Ossicles*: Include three bones, the malleus, incus, and stapes located within the middle ear, which transmit the mechanical vibration energy into the inner ear.

The body's defense against infections and inflammation within the ear requires:

1. *Tragus and antitragus*: Form a partial barrier to the entrance of the ear, preventing entry of large foreign bodies.
2. *Isthmus of the external auditory canal*: A narrowed section of the ear canal at the junction of the bony and cartilaginous portions; blocks entry of larger foreign bodies.
3. *Hair*: Located in the lateral portion of the external ear canal; help prevent entry of foreign particles deeper into the external auditory canal.
4. *Apopilosebaceous unit*: Consists of the hair follicle, erector pili muscle, and its associated apocrine and sebaceous glands. Sloughed squamous epithelium combines with glandular secretions to produce cerumen, which contains saturated fatty acids and lysozyme. Cerumen is also acidic. These properties help in the formation of a primary barrier to infection of the canal.
5. *Eustachian tube*: Connects the middle ear to the nasopharynx. Functions to ventilate the middle ear space.

6. *Immune system*: A competent immune system is required to prevent bacterial, viral, and fungal infections.

Infection or inflammation of the ear can result in obstruction of one or more parts of the pathway. Signs to watch for are: "I have a fever and earache" and "This is not the first time."

EAR INFECTIONS

Physiologic Predisposition[1-6]

Otitis media is the main reason for medical visits of preschool-aged children. This is due to the shorter and more horizontal angle of their eustachian tube, which increases susceptibility to bacterial infiltration of the middle ear.

Older patients tend to have a weaker immune system and are thus more susceptible to infection, particularly otitis externa.

Congenital Predisposition[5-7]

This includes congenital craniofacial anomalies caused by diseases such as cleft palate, Down's syndrome, choanal atresia, Cri-du-chat syndrome, DiGeorge's syndrome, and microcephaly. Such abnormalities often lead to eustachian tube dysfunction, which increases the likelihood of middle ear infections (otitis media), cholesteatoma, and chronic otitis media, even after craniofacial deformities are surgically corrected.

Acute Otitis Externa[2-4]

An infection of the external auditory canal: Common symptoms include pruritus, fullness, pain, and loss of hearing. Commonly referred to as swimmer's ear, this is caused by anything that removes the protective lipid barrier from the canal, allowing room for microorganisms to invade the environment. Pathogens most commonly associated with acute otitis externa (AOE) include *Pseudomonas aeruginosa* and *Staphylococcus aureus*. Initial symptoms include itching in the canal that may be followed by scratching, leading to proliferation of bacteria. Ultimately, purulent discharge develops and infection may progress to, and involve, the auricle. Hallmark signs of AOE include tenderness of the tragus and/or the pinna. Furthermore, patients may present with lymphadenitis, cellulitis, or fever. Symptoms should have been present for <6 weeks. On otoscopy, the ear canal is edematous and erythematous, and purulent otorrhea or skin debris may be present. The tympanic membrane is usually intact and mobile.

Treatment[2,3,4,8]

1. If pain is present, use of an analgesic is recommended.
2. Aural toilet should be performed.
3. Clinician should prescribe topical preparation for therapy.
   a. Systemic antimicrobials should not be prescribed as part of the initial therapy for uncomplicated AOE, unless the infection progresses outside the ear canal.
   b. Topical therapies include antibiotic ear drops (cortisporin otic, ofloxacin, ciprofloxacin–dexamethasone) or acidifying agents (acetic acid).
4. Patients with an infection that does not resolve with initial therapy within a few weeks should be reassessed to confirm the diagnosis of AOE.[8]

Chronic Otitis Externa

Chronic pruritus and scaling of the auditory canal predisposes the patient to recurrent episodes of AOE.[2] Over time, the ear canal may become scaly and a marked thickening may be observed. A potential complication is that the ear canal may ultimately become obliterated.

Treatment

1. Thorough and frequent cleaning of the external ear, removing any macroscopic objects and debris.
2. Medications
   - Topical antibiotics or antifungals, if bacterial involvement is suspected.

- Analgesics as needed.
- Acetic acid ear drops or boric acid ear powder to reestablish acidity of the ear environment, which can be efficacious for treating both fungal and bacterial colonization.
- Occasional use of anti-inflammatory agents and oral steroids can be helpful to control chronic pruritus that leads to repeated self-inflicted ear canal trauma for some patients.

3. Educating patients on how to avoid future episodes.

Fungal Otitis Externa

Mycotic infections of the external ear are usually opportunistic and superimpose on an underlying chronic condition, such as a bacterial infection.[2] The most common causative organisms in mycotic infections are the *Aspergillus* species, with the *Candida* spp. following as a close second. Typical presentation includes white, black, or gray colonies, sometimes with visible hyphae.

Treatment

The first step involves thorough removal and cleaning of fungal debris. This is followed by acidifying the external ear with topical agents such as acetic acid to make the environment less inhabitable for the invading organism. Ototopical antifungals such as clotrimazole are used adjunctively to ensure resolution.

Viral Otitis Externa

Herpes zoster (or varicella-zoster) and herpes simplex are two examples of direct viral mediators of otitis externa. In the case of both herpes strains, the patient may experience symptoms of burning, itching, pain, or a localized headache.[2] With herpes zoster, vesicles form, persist for some time, rupture, then dry and form a thin yellowish crust. Signs of herpes zoster oticus (Ramsay Hunt syndrome) include unilateral dermatopic distribution of vesicles, cranial nerve VII palsy, sensorineural hearing loss, and unilateral peripheral vestibulopathy.

Human immunodeficiency virus (HIV) involves a more indirect effect on outer ear infections by causing systemic immunodeficiency, thereby increasing the susceptibility of patients to ear infections.

Treatment

Appropriate antiviral therapy is indicated.[2] Topical antibiotics should be applied to the lesion only to prevent or treat a bacterial superinfection.

Necrotizing Otitis Externa (NOE; Malignant Otitis Externa or Skull Base Osteomyelitis)

A rare, potentially life-threatening condition that presents in patients of advanced age or in patients who are immunodeficient due to poorly controlled diabetes mellitus.[2,4] NOE usually begins as an unresolved AOE. Progression of the infection leads to spread from the external auditory canal to the bone of the base of the skull and temporomandibular joint, resulting in osteomyelitis. Associated symptoms may include otalgia lasting over a month, trismus, purulent otorrhea despite adequate treatment for a typical otitis externa, and symptoms related to lower cranial nerve involvement. One hallmark symptom is a deep, boring pain at night. Signs of NOE include purulent otorrhea associated with granulation tissue and exposed bone within the external auditory canal, and cranial nerve (CN) involvement, particularly of CN VII, IX, X, and XI. The most common pathogen associated with NOE is *P. aeruginosa*. However, *S. aureus*, particularly methicillin-resistant strains (MRSA), is also a frequent cause of this condition. If untreated, the infection may progress to meningitis, brain abscess, and death. Prognosis is poor if treated late in the course of the infection. Classically, NOE was initially imaged and followed with radionuclide scans. Initial imaging was performed with a technetium Tc-99 bone scan of the skull base. Follow-up imaging was conventionally performed using red cells tagged with gallium. More recently, investigators have reported the use of computed tomography (CT) or magnetic resonance imaging (MRI) to provide initial diagnostic and follow-up imaging.[4] Noncontrast CT of the temporal bone provides detailed information of the bony structures. Intracranial involvement can be visualized using MRI with contrast. Response to treatment can also be monitored by erythrocyte sedimentation rate (ESR), which can be drawn at initial diagnosis and then followed weekly or biweekly thereafter until it normalizes.

Treatment[2,4]

Granulation biopsies and culture swabs should be obtained, if possible.

1. If *P. aeruginosa* or MRSA is present, treat with appropriate antibiotics. If not, the patient should be presumptively treated for *P. aeruginosa*. Modern treatment of NOE has been revolutionized by the use of oral fluoroquinolone antibiotics, which may allow outpatient treatment for this condition.
2. The ear should be debrided carefully while visualized under a microscope.
3. The immunocompromised state should be treated. If the patient is diabetic, glycemic status should be tightly controlled.
4. Surgery is needed in only a minority of cases. The objective is not to remove all affected tissue; rather, it is to address a specific symptom that is refractory to medical therapy, such as pain or facial nerve palsy, and to reduce disease burden.
   a. The primary surgical goal is to remove the underlying necrotic tissue and to allow vascularized tissue to replace it.
   b. The onset of facial weakness may be alleviated by removal of granulation tissue, thus decompressing the facial nerve.

Acute Otitis Media (AOM)

An extremely common bacterial infection of the middle ear, especially among children; 85% of children will experience at least one episode of AOM.[5] Acute, in this sense, refers to an infection that occurs de novo in a previously normal, uninfected ear. Factors that may be associated with AOM include upper respiratory tract infections, eustachian tube dysfunction, and impaired immunological status. Typical presentation includes fever, an edematous and erythematous tympanic membrane, exudative fluid in the middle ear cleft, white blood cell infiltration (suppuration), and pain in the middle ear. Complications associated with AOM, although uncommon, involve bacterial infiltration of surrounding regions, leading to mastoiditis, facial nerve palsy, meningitis, brain abscesses, or chronic otitis media. Otoscopy should be used to confirm the infection. If the tympanic membrane is intact, there should be purulent material present within the middle ear, with moderate to severe bulging of the tympanic membrane. If the tympanic membrane has ruptured, there will be purulent material within the external auditory canal and a perforation in the tympanic membrane. Tympanocentesis can be used to obtain bacterial samples for culture if the tympanic membrane is intact; however, this may not be necessary, except in very young infants or patients with severe immunosuppression. If the tympanic membrane has ruptured, cultures can be readily taken from the external auditory canal with a calcium alginate swab. Prognosis is often good.

Treatment[5]

1. If otalgia is present, use of analgesics is indicated.
2. Appropriate antibiotics should be prescribed in children with severe AOM.
   a. In cases of non-severe infection in older infants, children, and adults who are not immunosuppressed, the clinician should offer observation with close follow-up versus antibiotic therapy.
3. Myringotomy and tube placement may be indicated for acute otitis media, particularly in situations where the better or only-hearing ear is affected, where there is facial nerve palsy associated with the infection, or where vestibular function has been substantially impaired.[5,7]

Acute Mastoiditis

A common complication of AOM in which the infection has spread from the middle ear to the mastoid air cells of the temporal bone.[7] The presence of AOM, mastoid findings, and radiological findings is highly indicative of acute mastoiditis. The patient may develop a fever with pain behind and deep to the ear that is typically worse at night. On physical examination, the patient often has proptosis of the ipsilateral auricle, erythema, and tenderness to slight palpation of the mastoid, and may have fluctuance beneath the skin of the mastoid. Noncontrast CT of the temporal bones reveals fluid or soft tissue density within the ipsilateral mastoid air cells and middle ear. Severe acute mastoiditis may lead to erosion of the bone within the mastoid, breaking down the bony trabeculae between the mastoid air cells (coalescent mastoiditis) and eroding through the bone of the tegmen mastoideum, tegmen tympani, cerebellar plate, and the bone overlying the sigmoid sinus.

Treatment[6,7]

1. Antibiotics may resolve mastoiditis if caught early and in a noncoalescent state.
2. Myringotomy and tube placement, in addition to antibiotic therapy, is indicated for noncoalescent mastoiditis that is not associated with complications such as meningitis or brain abscess.
3. Mastoidectomy, in addition to antibiotic therapy and myringotomy and tube placement, is indicated for patients with coalescent mastoiditis, or patients with complications of mastoiditis such as otitic meningitis and subdural or brain abscess. The timing of this surgery in patients with central complications of mastoiditis needs to be coordinated closely with the patient's neurosurgical and neurological care teams.

Chronic Draining Ear

This is also referred to as chronic suppurative otitis media.[6] Infection of the middle ear usually starts with an acute episode of otitis media, which results in the perforation of the tympanic membrane. Further inflammation and infection develops as a result of bacterial infiltration and colonization of the middle ear via the perforation, leading to a chronic infection. Typical presentation includes draining ear (otorrhea), sudden hearing loss in the affected ear, fever, vertigo, and pain. The discharge may range from fetid and purulent to clear and serous. Granulation tissue may develop in the inner portion of the ear canal or the middle ear space. Chronic suppurative otitis media may also be associated with cholesteatoma (see further). The bacterial species typically responsible for these infections is *P. aeruginosa*.

Cerebrospinal fluid (CSF) otorrhea is a rare intracranial complication of chronic otitis media.[6,7] Computed tomography imaging with fine, sub-millimeter cuts should be utilized to assess for erosive changes within the mastoid air cells and the surrounding bony structures, consistent with erosion of the bony tegmen by chronic infection. Fluid collected from the ear may also be sent to test for β-2-transferrin for confirmation of CSF otorrhea. However, this test is often not useful, as samples must be fairly large (often requiring 0.5–1 mL of fluid) and cannot have any red blood cells present within the fluid. Typically, it is very difficult to collect this volume of fluid, even with a definite CSF leak.

Treatment[7]

1. Aspiration and cleaning of debris within the ear.
2. Ototopical antibiotic agents such as topical quinolones are the first-line treatment.
3. Oral antibiotics are also an effective means of treatment, but should be avoided as first-line therapy, given their systemic side effects and the epidemiological concerns with regard to the generation of resistant bacteria.
4. *Surgery*: Mastoidectomy
   a. Utilized when chronic otitis media fails to resolve after medical therapy.

Cholesteatoma

Non-cancerous cyst lined by stratified squamous epithelium that contains desquamated keratin.[6] Most commonly, cholesteatomas infiltrate the middle ear and mastoid, but they may also involve other portions of the temporal bone. This accumulation of keratin can cause infection, otorrhea, hearing loss, and bone resorption leading to ossicular erosion, erosion of the bony external auditory canal wall, erosion of the bone separating the mastoid and middle ear from the brain, and erosion into the semicircular canals.[6,7] Palsy of CN VII can occur as well. The most common symptoms of cholesteatoma are painless otorrhea that is unresponsive to antibiotics and a tympanic retraction perforation in the pars flaccida. Noncontrast CT of the temporal bones is the diagnostic method of choice, and is used to assess for bone erosion. MRI should be performed if cranial or dural involvement is suspected. Prognosis is favorable, with the majority of cases resolving postoperatively. The postoperative recidivism rate is high (up to 30% over the course of 10 years); therefore, patients should be followed long term for the recurrence of cholesteatomas and related signs and symptoms.

Treatment

All cholesteatomas should be excised surgically. Patients in whom surgery is not an option should regularly have their ears cleaned, although this neither completely treats nor prevents cholesteatomas.

Immunocompromised Patients

Patients with congenital or acquired immunocompromised states are likelier to develop ear infections.[2-7] Isolated, superficial infections of the external and middle ear may progress to catastrophic variations of perichondritis, cellulitis, and erysipelas. These patients are also much more susceptible to necrotizing otitis externa.

DIAGNOSTIC WORKUP (FLOWCHART 1.1)

Flowchart 1.1: Evaluation of otologic pain or otorrhea.

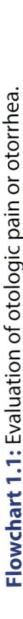

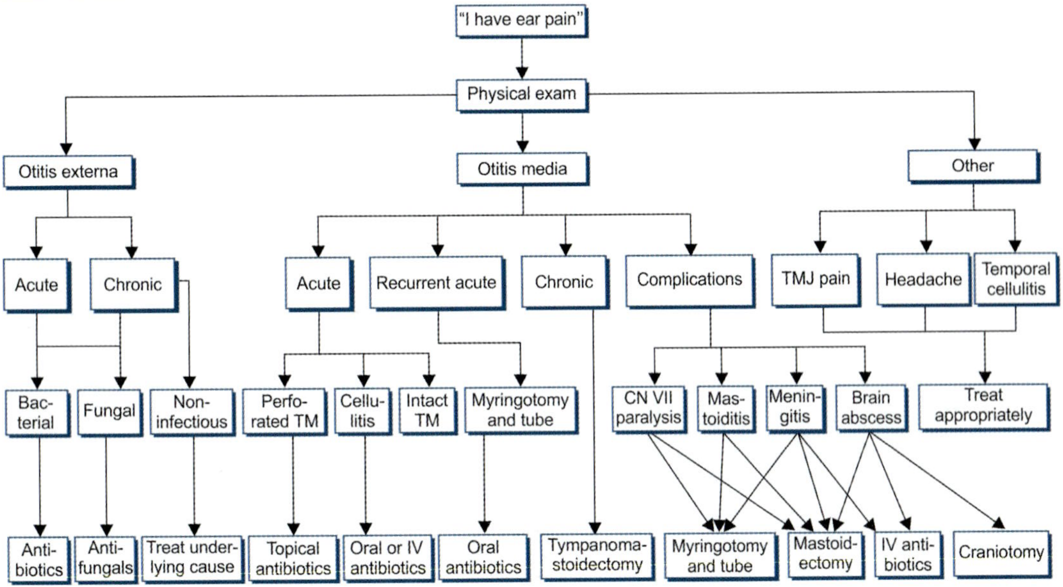

(TMJ: Temporomandibular joint; TM: Tympanic membrane).

History

"Do you have pain in your ear? When did it start? Does it go away and then return? Does your ear drain intermittently?"

"Have you experienced any itching, burning, or painful sensations inside the ear?"

"Is your hearing normal?"

"Are you dizzy?"

"Have you noticed any popping, ringing, or fullness in your ears?"

"Do you have a headache, fever, runny or stuffy nose, or cough?"

"Does your infant has problems feeding, sleeping, or is fussy, irritable, or vomiting?"

"Have you ever had problems with ear infections? Have you ever had ear surgery?"

"Do you have diabetes, rheumatoid arthritis, or an organ transplant? Are you on steroids on a long-term basis?"

Physical Examination

1. *Assessment of the external ear*: Tenderness, erythema, and swelling.
2. *Otoscopic investigation*: Look for signs of infection, macroscopic objects, inflamed ear canal, and colonies of bacteria or fungus. Assess the tympanic membrane for erythema, bulging, or perforation.

Audiology

An audiogram should be performed to determine whether the infection has impacted auditory function. Unless there is a perforation with purulent material within the external auditory canal, a tympanogram should also be performed to assess the tympanic membrane and middle ear.

REFERENCES

1. Francis WH. Anatomy of the temporal bone, external ear and middle ear. In: Flint PW, Haughey BH, Lund VJ, et al. (Eds).

Cummings Otolaryngology—Head & Neck Surgery, 5th edition. Philadelphia, PA: Mosby/Elsevier; 2010. pp. 1821-30.

2. Guss J, Ruckenstein, MJ. Infections of the external ear. In: Flint PW, Haughey BH, Lund VJ, et al. (Eds). Cummings Otolaryngology—Head & Neck Surgery, 5th edition. Philadelphia, PA: Mosby/Elsevier; 2010. pp. 1944-9.

3. Rosenfeld RM, Schwartz SR, Cannon CR, et al. Clinical practice guideline: acute otitis externa. Otolaryngol Head Neck Surg. 2014;150(1 Suppl):S1-24.

4. Peleg U, Perez R, Raveh D, et al. Stratification for malignant external otitis. Otolaryngol Head Neck Surg. 2007;137(2):301-5.

5. Grainger J, Siddiq S, Prentice P. The diagnosis and management of acute otitis media: American Academy of Pediatrics Guidelines 2013. Arch Dis Child Educ Pract Ed. 2015;100(4):193-7.

6. Chole RA, Sudhoff HH. Chronic otitis media, mastoiditis, and petrositis. In: Flint PW, Haughey BH, Lund VJ, et al (Eds). Cummings Otolaryngology—Head & Neck Surgery, 5th edition. Philadelphia, PA: Mosby/Elsevier; 2010. pp. 1963-78.

7. El-Kashlan HK, Harker LA, Shelton C, et al. Complications of temporal bone infections. In: Flint PW, Haughey BH, Lund VJ, et al. (Eds). Cummings Otolaryngology—Head & Neck Surgery, 5th edition. Philadelphia, PA: Mosby/Elsevier; 2010:1979-98.

8. Farrior J, Lee KJ. Noninfectious disorders of the ear. In: Lee KJ (Ed). Essential Otolaryngology: Head and Neck Surgery, 10th edition. New York, NY: McGraw-Hill; 2012. pp. 338-63.

SUGGESTED READING

1. Linstrom JC, Lucente EF. Diseases of the external ear. In: Rosen CA, Johnson JT (Eds). Bailey's Head and Neck Surgery—Otolaryngology, 5th edition. Philadelphia, PA: Wolters Kluwer Health/Lippincott Williams & Wilkins; 2014. pp. 2333-57.

2. Meyer AT, Strunk Jr CL, Lambert RP. Cholesteatoma. In: Rosen CA, Johnson JT (Eds). Bailey's Head and Neck Surgery—Otolaryngology, 5th edition. Philadelphia, PA: Wolters Kluwer Health/Lippincott Williams & Wilkins; 2014. pp. 2433-66.

3. Pulcini C, Mahdyoun P, Cua E, et al. Antibiotic therapy in necrotising external otitis: case series of 32 patients and review of the literature. Eur J Clin Microbiol Infect Dis. 2012;31(12):3287-94.

Chapter 2

Hearing Loss

Kamil Amer, Pamela C Roehm

> ***Chief Complaint***
> *"I can't hear/I can't hear as well as I did before".*
> *"My child is not speaking yet/My child is not paying attention".*
> *"My child/parent is turning up the volume too high on the television".*
> *"My parent does not seem to be engaged with others and often seems isolated".*

DEFINITIONS

Conductive hearing loss: Conductive hearing loss (CHL) occurs when sound is not conducted efficiently through the external ear canal, the tympanic membrane, or the bones (ossicles) of the middle ear. CHL usually involves a reduction in the ability to hear faint sounds, although sound clarity is maintained.

Sensorineural hearing loss: Sensorineural hearing loss (SNHL) occurs when there is damage to the inner ear (or cochlea) or to the nerve pathways from the inner ear to the brain. This is the most common type of permanent hearing loss. The SNHL reduces the ability to hear faint sounds. Even when speech is loud enough to be heard, it may still be unclear.

Mixed hearing loss: Mixed hearing loss is a combination of CHL and SNHL.

Sudden sensorineural hearing loss: A subset of patients with SNHL develop a unilateral hearing loss rapidly, frequently awakening with it in the morning or developing a rapidly progressive loss over 72 hours or less.

ANATOMY AND PHYSIOLOGY OF HEARING

Experiencing normal hearing requires the following:[1-3]

1. *Adequate stimulus (sound)*: Sound waves generated by a vibrating object move the air particles surrounding the object, which is transmitted through air and water.
2. *An opening through the pinna and external auditory canal*: The outer ear consists of the pinna (auricle) and the ear canal external auditory meatus. The pinna helps to collect sound vibrations and guides the vibrations into the external auditory canal. The disturbance of airflow passing through the unimpeded external auditory canal will reach the tympanic membrane.
3. *A normal middle ear*: In its transition through the middle ear, the sound wave is changed to a mechanical vibration. The middle ear begins with the tympanic membrane at the lateral end of the external auditory canal. The middle ear contains three small bones, or ossicles (the malleus, incus, and stapes). In order for air pressure to be transmitted to the inner ear, the tympanic membrane converts air vibration into vibration of the ossicles. The ossicles make a connection from the tympanic membrane to the inner ear.
4. *A normal cochlea*: The inner ear contains the sensory organs for hearing (the cochlea) and balance. The cochlea is a bony structure filled with two fluids—endolymph and perilymph—and the mechanoreceptors for hearing, which are the inner ear hair cells (IHCs). Transmitted mechanical energy displaces the stapes footplate into the cochlea. This force compresses perilymph within the cochlea. Transmission of the energy of this fluid wave moves the basilar membrane of the cochlea, which vibrates in specific areas based on the frequency of the sound. The movement of the basilar membrane deflects sterocilia on IHCs in those areas of vibration of the basilar membrane.

5. *A normal auditory nerve, auditory brainstem, and auditory cortex*: Deflection of the sterocilia on IHCs leads to the generation of action potentials within that cell. The IHC then signals across the synapse to its corresponding cochlear nerve cell. Firing of multiple cochlear nerve cells is then converted into impulses of the cochlear or auditory nerve. The cochlear nerve carries impulses from the cochlea to the cochlear nuclei, where signals cross in the trapezoid body and then, via the lateral lemniscus, reach the superior olive in the brainstem. Sound information is then transferred to the inferior colliculus in the midbrain and through the medial geniculate body in the thalamus before reaching the cortex in the auditory cortex (superior temporal gyrus).

HUMAN HEARING DYSFUNCTION

Physiological Hearing Loss

More than 40% of patients over the age of 65 tend to suffer from hearing loss that decreases their quality of life.[2,4] Although hearing loss in the geriatric population is often due to presbycusis, other causes should also be considered.

There are many factors that determine the auditory system's durability. In any individual person, it can be difficult to determine which components of the hearing loss are due to genetic factors and which are the result of acoustic trauma, viral infections, otologic diseases, vascular diseases, or ototoxic medications. Several anatomic changes that affect hearing and balance occur due to physiologic aging.

1. Modified apocrine sweat glands atrophy with age and causes cerumen to become drier, harder, and less likely to be moved out of the external auditory canal by the canal's normal transport and cleansing mechanism.
2. Tragal hairs in adult males become coarser, larger, and more prominent with age. Their presence can prevent the natural cleaning of cerumen from the external auditory

canal, contributing to the increased incidence of cerumen impaction in the elderly male.

3. Histopathological changes associated with presbycusis:
   a. *Sensory*: Epithelial atrophy with loss of sensory cells and the supporting cells of the organ of Corti. Progressive IHC reduction begins at age 40.
   b. *Neural*: A reduction in the number of functioning cochlear neurons. Of the 35,500 cochlea neurons present at birth, up to 2, 100 neurons are lost each decade. When neuronal reduction reaches 50%, hearing loss develops.
   c. *Strial*: Atrophy of the stria vascularis. A loss of 30% or more of strial tissue can result in hearing loss.
   d. *Conductive*: Basilar membrane alterations typically produce stiffening of this structure. The precise nature of these changes is not fully understood; however, these changes appear to result in hearing loss.

Pathological Hearing Loss

Autoimmune Diseases

A number of systemic autoimmune diseases cause hearing loss by damaging the inner ear and the eighth cranial nerve, including systemic lupus erythematosis (SLE), Wegener's granulomatosis, ulcerative colitis, Cogan's syndrome, and multiple sclerosis.[2,5] Treatment for hearing loss in these conditions is achieved through appropriate treatment of the underlying disorder.

Autoimmune inner ear disease: Autoimmune inner ear disease (AIED) is a rare, idiopathic, rapidly progressing (weeks to months) disorder that ultimately leads to bilateral SNHL.[5] Often, one ear is affected, followed by the other; however, both may be affected simultaneously. Typically, hearing loss is accompanied by imbalance or vertigo (seen in 50% of affected patients). Twenty percent of patients have vertigo and other symptoms consistent with Ménière's disease. The exact immunologic mechanism of damage is unclear. Despite the lack of a definite etiology, this disease represents one of the few medically reversible causes of SNHL and is sometimes responsive to immunosuppressive agents. If improved hearing thresholds are noted after a course of high-dose steroids, patients are referred to a rheumatologist for a trial of other immunosuppressive medication.

Primary AIED is a very rare disease. Secondary AIED is also rare and typically involves multisystemic, organ nonspecific autoimmune diseases that may affect the inner ear. Cogan's disease, a classic form of secondary AIED, is defined by the presence of labyrinthine and ocular pathology. Wegener's granulomatosis, which can have multiple upper airway and kidney manifestations, can cause CHL in 30–50% of affected patients. In addition, SLE has been shown to have a strong association with secondary AIED.

Treatment: Treatment of AIED is not urgent, as it has been shown that there is a 6- to 12-month period wherein significant recovery can be achieved through the administration of high-dose corticosteroids.[5] Initial therapy is 60 mg of prednisone per day for 4 weeks. The response varies significantly and the treatment must be personalized per patient.

Cerumen Impaction or Foreign Body in the Ear Canal

Conditions that block the external auditory canal can lead to CHL.[6] Appropriate management includes removal of the blockage, either by irrigation or instrumentation.

Hereditary Hearing Loss

Mutations in hundreds of individual genes can lead to hearing loss. Inheritance can be autosomal recessive (most common), autosomal dominant, X-linked, or mitochondrial.[3,7] Hereditary hearing loss may be present at birth, worsen after birth, or have onset later in life. Different mutations in the same genes can be responsible for hearing loss with different inheritance patterns. Congenital hearing disorders fall into two main categories—syndromic and nonsyndromic. Syndromic hearing disorders involve hearing loss that is also associated with other organ systems and parts of the body. In contrast, nonsyndromic hearing disorders are not associated with other signs and symptoms.

Mutations in connexin-26 (gap junction protein 2, GJB2) are the most common genetic defects leading to hereditary hearing loss. The Hereditary Hearing Loss Homepage (http://hereditaryhearingloss.org/main.aspx?c=.HHH&n=86162) includes an up-to-date list of syndromes and mutations leading to hearing loss.

Otitis Media—Infection of the Middle Ear

This can lead to both acute and chronic changes in hearing.[2] Acute changes occur due to filling of the middle ear space with fluid and acute damage to the tympanic membrane. Chronic changes occur due to erosive effects of cholesteatoma, chronic tympanic membrane perforation, and recurrent infection on ossicles. Management of these conditions is discussed in Chapter 1.

Otosclerosis

This is an autosomal dominant osteodystrophy that exclusively affects the otic capsule.[8] It has a variable penetrance and expression. Otosclerosis usually affects the stapes, which is located at the oval window. Abnormal deposits of new bone fix the stapes, decreasing its ability to move and, thereby, decreasing its ability to transfer sound energy to the inner ear, leading to CHL. The most common area for stapes fixation is at the anterior edge of the stapes footplate (the fistula ante fenestrum). Sensorineural hearing loss can result from otosclerotic lesions on the otic capsule near the cochlea.

Otosclerosis is most common in whites (1%), followed by Asians and then blacks. Age at onset of hearing loss is typically the 20s. Up to 70% of patients will present with bilateral hearing loss. Otosclerosis is more prevalent in women, with a 2:1 ratio female:male distribution. Hearing loss resulting from otosclerosis is often accelerated during pregnancy.

Examination and Treatment[2,8]

1. *Physical examination including otoscopy*: Pneumo-otoscopy is important to rule out middle ear serous fluid or a small perforation that could be the cause of CHL.

2. *Weber test*: Strike a 512-Hz tuning fork and place the tip of the fork on the center of the forehead, the bridge of the nose or the anterior incisors. The sound will lateralize to the ear with the greater CHL if significant SNHL is not present.

3. *Rinne test*: Strike a 512-Hz tuning fork and place the tip of the fork firmly on the mastoid. Ask the patient to compare the loudness of that sound to the loudness when the tuning fork is next held beside the patient's ipsilateral pinna. If a significant CHL is present, the sound will be perceived as louder when the tuning fork tip is on the mastoid.

4. *Audiometric evaluations* such as air conduction, bone conduction, and speech audiometry should be performed. In addition, acoustic reflexes, which are sensitive measures of the movement of the stapes, are absent in patients with otosclerosis. If acoustic reflexes are present in a patient with a CHL or air–bone gap, then superior semicircular canal dehiscence should be suspected.

5. *Surgery*: Stapes surgery options include total stapedectomy, partial stapedectomy, or stapedotomy. Footplate fenestration can be performed with a laser or microdrill. Complications of surgery include SNHL, vertigo, perilymphatic fistula, infection, and tympanic membrane perforation.

   Alternative treatments include hearing aids.

Ototoxic Exposures

A number of medications are damaging to hearing, or ototoxic, including aminoglycoside antibiotics and chemotherapeutic agents.[2] Moreover, exposure to loud sounds—either chronically or sudden very loud sounds—can damage hearing. The majority of these agents damage the inner ear, leading to IHC damage and death. Treatment includes limitation of further exposure, hearing aids, or cochlear implantation.

Perilymphatic Fistula

This is an abnormal communication between the inner ear and middle ear. The inner ear is normally covered by dense bone.[2] This bone may be disrupted by a number of conditions, including trauma, acute otitis media, and cholesteatoma. Inner ear fistulae present with hearing loss, vertigo, and imbalance. Clinical presentations range in severity. There is typically associated SNHL that can vary from an isolated high-frequency loss to a low-frequency SNHL or flat losses. Vestibular symptoms are also variable and include episodic incapacitating vertigo, positional vertigo, motion intolerance, or occasional disequilibrium.

Evaluation and Treatment[2]

1. The following tests should be conducted if a perilymphatic fistula is suspected: a fistula test, Valsalva test, and pure tone and speech audiometry. Occasionally, electrocochleography and electronystatograms may be helpful. Following a traumatic injury, high-resolution temporal bone computed tomography can help identify the site of the fistula and other associated traumatic injury to the surrounding bone.
2. For a definite perilymphatic fistula, patching the defect with a tissue graft can preserve hearing and minimize vertigo.
3. Following head trauma, initial management of suspected fistula is bed rest and stool softeners. Some post-traumatic fistulae seal spontaneously. The time course of observation is typically several weeks.
4. Surgery should be considered if symptoms are progressive and dizziness is debilitating.

Temporal Bone Trauma

Traumatic injuries to the temporal bone can cause both SNHL and CHL.[2] These injuries can be mediated either through direct injury from fracture line through critical structures (tympanic membrane, ossicles, or cochlea) or through indirect injury leading to delayed onset of hearing loss (post-concussive hydrops). Appropriate management depends on the mechanism of injury.

Serous Otitis Media

Fluid within the middle ear space that can affect hearing by dampening sound transmission through the ossicular chain.[2] This can be either acute or chronic and often follows acute otitis media. Management includes watchful waiting or myringotomy and tube placement.

Sudden Sensorineural Hearing Loss

A subset of patients with SNHL develop hearing loss over the course of 3 days or less.[2,9] This is defined as a sudden SNHL if hearing loss is greater than 30 dB HL in three consecutive frequencies. There are over a hundred potential causes of sudden SNHL, but most often this condition is idiopathic.

The incidence of sudden SNHL is 5–20 per 100,000. Any age group can be affected, with peak incidence in the sixth decade. Males and females are affected equally. Bilateral involvement is extremely rare. Tinnitus is often present in the affected ear. Sudden SNHL is accompanied by vertigo or disequilibrium in approximately 40% of patients.

Sudden hearing loss may result from the following etiologies:
1. Infectious disorders (viral infection, meningitis, syphilis, Lyme disease, HIV)
2. Neoplasms (acoustic neuroma, other neoplasms)
3. Traumatic membrane rupture (head injury, perilymphatic fistula)
4. Pharmacologic or noise toxicity
5. Immunologic disorders
6. Vascular disorders
7. Developmental abnormalities
8. Idiopathic but otherwise described disorders (Ménière's disease, multiple sclerosis, sarcoidosis)

9. Psychogenic disorders
10. Idiopathic sudden SNHL.

Therefore, a thorough search for potentially treatable causes of sudden SNHL must be undertaken with an exhaustive history, thorough physical examination, audiological evaluation, and carefully selected laboratory and radiographic studies. Four factors affect the prognosis of idiopathic sudden SNHL: severity of hearing loss, audiographic pattern of the hearing loss, presence of vertigo/imbalance, and age at onset.

Treatment

1. Sudden SNHL is regarded as an otological emergency and treatment is based on its etiology.[2,9] If a defined cause can be found, then the patient should be treated appropriately in an expedited fashion; 32–65% of cases of sudden SNHL recover spontaneously. High-dose steroids are the most common accepted treatment option for idiopathic sudden SNHL. A gadolinium-enhanced MRI of the internal auditory canal and the cerebellopontine angle is obtained to rule out vestibular schwannoma or other central causes of sudden SNHL. A 10-day course of prednisone (1 mg/kg PO OD for 7 days) is prescribed, followed by a steroid taper. If a partial recovery is noted at the end of the 10 days, the full dose may be extended (http://oto.sagepub.com/content/146/3_suppl/S1.long).

2. Idiopathic sudden SNHL can also be treated with intratympanic (IT) steroid injections if the hearing loss is less than 70 dB HL or if the patient is unable to tolerate oral steroid therapy.

3. After failure of initial management, IT steroid treatment can occasionally improve hearing in patients initially treated with oral steroids who had incomplete recovery. Clinicians should obtain follow-up audiometric evaluation within 6 months of diagnosis for patients with idiopathic sudden SNHL.

4. Long-term follow-up is recommended, especially for patients in whom an underlying cause was not evident at

initial presentation. In addition, the patient with partial or no hearing recovery, or persistent tinnitus, will require ongoing management from otolaryngological, audiological, and psychological perspectives.

5. Clinicians should counsel patients with incomplete recovery of hearing about the possible benefits of hearing aids, hearing-assistive technology, cochlear implantation, and other supportive measures.

Vestibular Schwannoma (Previously Acoustic Neuroma)

Benign schwannomas of the eighth cranial nerve are slow-growing neoplasms that originate in the nerve sheath.[10,11] They constitute 2% of intracranial tumors and are the most common skull base neoplasms affecting the posterior fossa. They arise principally from the vestibular division of the nerve; 95% of cases are unilateral and sporadic, whereas the remaining 5% are due to inherited disorders. The differential diagnosis for these tumors includes meningiomas, epidermoids (cholesteatomas of the internal auditory canal and petrous apex), facial nerve schwannomas, and, very rarely, metastatic tumors.

Bilateral vestibular schwannomas are pathognomonic for neurofibromatosis type 2 (NF2). This condition has nearly 100% penetrance and originates from deletions of portions of the NF-2 gene, which codes for schwannomin/merlin on chromosome 22. Typically, vestibular schwannomas present with progressive SNHL and tinnitus. Ten percent of patients present with sudden SNHL. Patients may also complain of imbalance, facial hypesthesia, and gradual onset of ipsilateral facial paralysis. Tumor expansion into the labyrinth resulting in spinning vertigo is rare.

Audiometric evaluation of hearing loss, including pure-tone audiometry and word discrimination, is necessary to evaluate patients with vestibular schwannomas. Auditory brainstem response testing may also be used for the electrophysiologic assessment of auditory function. MRI with gadolinium of the brain and brainstem remains the gold standard for diagnosis and can detect tumors as small as 1 mm.

Management

Management options for vestibular schwannomas include observation with serial imaging, stereotactic radiation, and microsurgical excision.[10,11] The optimal treatment varies according to tumor size, tumor location, hearing status, age of the patient, and medical comorbidities.

Because acoustic neuromas are usually slow growing, immediate intervention is not always necessary. For patients with very small, asymptomatic tumors, elderly patients, and patients with serious medical problems, a conservative approach with observation, including serial MRI studies, may be reasonable.

Intracranial stereotactic radiation therapy involves the administration of radiation to a precise location to limit tumor growth and minimize damage to any neighboring structures. Tumors typically expand immediately following radiation treatment, potentially compressing surrounding structures if the tumors are large. Thus, stereotactic radiation should only be used on tumors smaller than 2.5–3 cm in maximal diameter. The development of side effects is directly related to the radiation dose at the tumor periphery. These include hearing loss that can occur acutely or gradually, facial and trigeminal cranial neuropathies, hemifacial spasm, hydrocephalus, and chronic vestibular dysfunction.

Microsurgical resection of acoustic neuromas can be accomplished through multiple different operative approaches to the tumor, all of which have different advantages and disadvantages. These approaches may be combined for the treatment of very large tumors.

1. *Suboccipital (retrosigmoid)*: The craniotomy is performed behind the sigmoid sinus. The cerebellum typically needs to be retracted to allow visualization and removal of the tumor. This approach allows visualization of the cerebellopontine angle and the porus of the internal auditory canal. Following

drilling of the temporal bone, all but the most distal portion of the internal auditory canal can be visualized by this approach. Advantages of this approach include the potential for hearing preservation in appropriate patients and that it is a comfortable approach for most neurosurgeons. Disadvantages include a lack of visualization of the lateral portion of the internal auditory canal, the need for cerebellar retraction, and severe postoperative headaches.

2. *Translabyrinthine*: The neurotologist drills through the mastoid and bony labyrinth to the cerebellar plate, jugular bulb, cochlear aqueduct, tegmen mastoideum, into the internal auditory canal. This approach allows visualization of the cerebellopontine angle and the entire course of the facial nerve without retraction of the brain. Advantages of this approach include visualization of the complete course of the facial nerve with statistically better facial nerve function outcomes, the lack of need for cerebellar or temporal lobe retraction, and the familiarity of this approach to most neurotologists. The disadvantages of this approach are that hearing is not preserved by this approach and cerebrospinal fluid leak rates are higher than with other approaches.

3. *Retrolabyrinthine*: The neurotologist drills through the mastoid and outlines the bony labyrinth but does not violate it. Bone is removed from the tegmen mastoideum, sigmoid, and cerebellar plate, keeping the bony labyrinth intact. Advantages are potential hearing preservation and the lack of need for brain retraction. Disadvantages include lack of visualization of the most distal portion of the internal auditory canal and slightly decreased visualization of the cerebellopontine angle compared with the translabyrinthine approach.

4. *Middle fossa*: A craniotomy is made over the ipsilateral ear, the dura is elevated from the floor of the middle fossa, the temporal lobe is retracted extradurally, the internal auditory canal is drilled out, and the tumor is removed. This approach provides excellent results when used on small tumors (<10 mm) that mainly occupy the IAC with a minor

component of the cistern. Advantages of this approach include potential hearing preservation and access to the most lateral portion of the internal auditory canal. Disadvantages include the lack of familiarity of this approach to many neurosurgeons and the potential for facial nerve injury when the approach is performed by those unaccustomed to this procedure (http://thejns.org/doi/full/10.3171/2012.6.FOCUS12190).

DIAGNOSTIC WORKUP: "I CAN'T HEAR" (FLOWCHART 2.1)

History

"Is your hearing decreased or absent in one or both ears?"

"Was your hearing always absent, lost suddenly, or did your hearing change over days, weeks, months or years?"

"Do you have associated symptoms, such as tinnitus/ringing, imbalance, vertigo, ear drainage, or ear pain?"

"When did these associated symptoms start? Does it go away and then return?"

"Have you ever had problems with ear infections? Have you ever had ear surgery?"

"Do you have diabetes? Have you been treated with steroids on a long-term basis?"

"Have you noticed any popping or fullness in your ears?"

"Did you have a URI, head trauma, toxin exposure, changes in medications, surgery around the time you noticed a change in hearing?"

"Do you have headaches, visual disturbances, seizures, or memory loss?"

Physical Examination

1. *Assessment of the external ear*: Tenderness, inflammation.
2. *Otoscopic examination*: Look for signs of infection, foreign objects, inflamed ear canal, and colonies of bacteria or fungus. Assess the tympanic membrane for erythema,

Flowchart 2.1: Evaluation and management of hearing loss

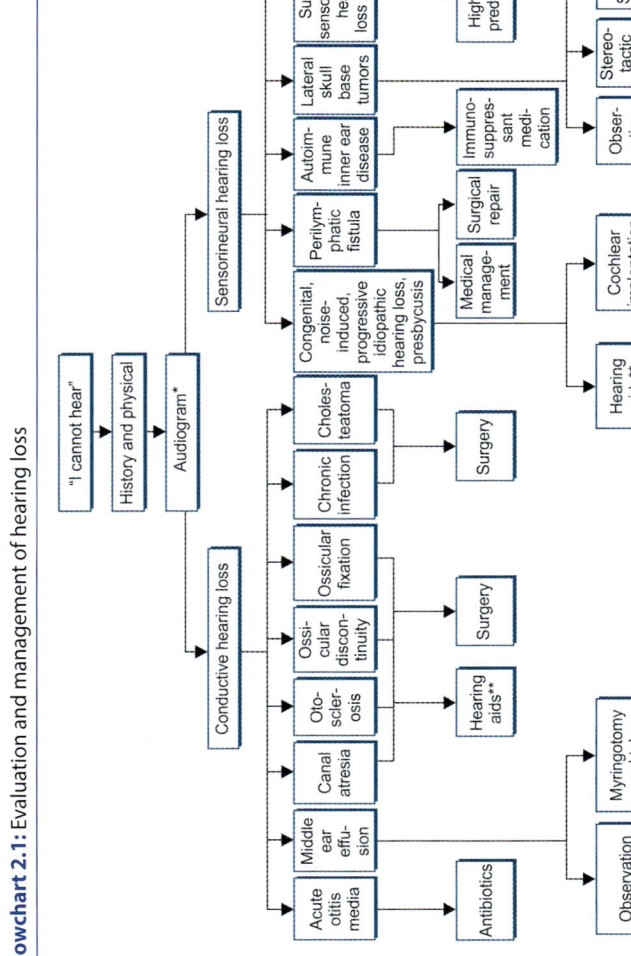

*For teaching purposes we have written a simplified decision tree solely based on audiogram findings. Imaging and treatment should be based on history and physical findings as well as audiogram.

** Includes bone anchored hearing aid options.

bulging, or perforation. Assess movement of the tympanic membrane using pneumo-otoscopy.
3. Cranial nerve assessment of CN II–XII.
4. Complete head and neck examination.
5. Clinical assessment of hearing loss using 512 and 1024 Hz tuning forks (Weber, Rinne) and responses to environmental and spoken sounds.

Audiology

An audiogram should be performed to determine whether there is a demonstrable decrease in auditory function compared with normative human hearing. Unless there is a perforation with purulent material within the external auditory canal, a tympanogram should also be performed to assess the status of the tympanic membrane and middle ear. Additional audiologic testing, including acoustic reflexes, otoacoustic emissions, and auditory brainstem response testing may be indicated in the evaluation of patients with hearing loss. Studies of vestibular dysfunction, including videonystagmogram, may also be indicated in the evaluation of patients presenting with hearing loss. Overviews of how to interpret audiograms can be found at http://www.aafp.org/afp/2013/0101/p41.html.

REFERENCES

1. Francis WH. Anatomy of the temporal bone, external ear and middle ear. In: Flint PW, Haughey BH, Lund VJ, et al. (Eds). Cummings Otolaryngology—Head & Neck Surgery, 5th edition. Philadelphia, PA: Mosby/Elsevier; 2010. pp. 1821-30.
2. Arts HA. Sensorineural hearing loss in adults. In: Flint PW, Haughey BH, Lund VJ, et al. (Eds). Cummings Otolaryngology—Head & Neck Surgery, 5th edition. Philadelphia, PA: Mosby/Elsevier; 2010. pp. 2116-30.
3. Hilderbrand MS, Husein M, Smith RJH. Genetic sensorineural hearing loss. In: Flint PW, Haughey BH, Lund VJ, et al. (Eds). Cummings Otolaryngology—Head & Neck Surgery, 5th Edition. Philadelphia, PA: Mosby/Elsevier; 2010. pp. 2086-99.

4. Kutz Jr JW, Isaacson B, Roland PS. Aging and the auditory and vestibular system. In: Rosen CA, Johnson JT (Eds). Bailey's Head and Neck Surgery—Otolaryngology, 5th edition. Philadelphia, PA: Wolters Kluwer Health/Lippincott Williams & Wilkins; 2014.

5. Rauch SD, Cohen MA, Ruckenstein MJ. Autoimmune inner ear disease. In: Flint PW, Haughey BH, Lund VJ, et al. (Eds). Cummings Otolaryngology—Head & Neck Surgery, 5th Edition. Philadelphia, PA: Mosby/Elsevier; 2010. pp. 2164-8.

6. Roland PS, Smith TL, Schwartz SR, et al. Clinical practice guidelines: cerumen impaction. Otolaryngol Head Neck Surg. 2008;139(3 Suppl 2):21.

7. Babu S, Lee KJ. Congenital hearing loss. In: Lee KJ (Ed). Essential Otolaryngology: Head and Neck Surgery, 10th edition. New York, NY: McGraw-Hill; 2012. pp. 117-43.

8. House JW, Cunningham CD. Otosclerosis. In: Flint PW, Haughey BH, Lund VJ, et al. (Eds). Cummings Otolaryngology—Head & Neck Surgery, 5th edition. Philadelphia, PA: Mosby/Elsevier; 2010. pp. 2028-35.

9. Stachler RJ, Chandrasekhar SS, Archer SM, et al. Clinical practice guideline: sudden hearing loss. Otolaryngol Head Neck Surg. 2012;146(3 Suppl):S1-35.

10. Brackmann DE, Arriaga MA. Neoplasms of the posterior fossa. In: Flint PW, Haughey BH, Lund VJ, et al. (Eds). Cummings Otolaryngology—Head & Neck Surgery, 5th edition. Philadelphia, PA: Mosby/Elsevier; 2010. pp. 2514-41.

11. Pickett BP, Crawley BK. Neoplasms of the ear and lateral skull base. In: Rosen CA, Johnson JT (Eds). Bailey's Head and Neck Surgery—Otolaryngology, 5th edition. Philadelphia, PA: Wolters Kluwer Health/Lippincott Williams & Wilkins; 2014.

SUGGESTED READING

1. Bewley AF, Ruckenstein MJ. Otologic manifestations of systemic disease: include autoimmune inner ear disease. In: Rosen CA, Johnson JT (Eds). Bailey's Head and Neck Surgery—Otolaryngology, 5th edition. Philadelphia, PA: Wolters Kluwer Health/Lippincott Williams & Wilkins; 2014. pp. 2519-29.

2. Choo DI, Greenwald Jr JH. Hereditary hearing impairment. In: Hughes GB, Pensak ML (Eds). Clinical Otology, 3rd edition. New York, NY: Thieme Publishers, Inc; 2007. pp. 289-99.

3. Monsell EM, Teixido MT, Slattery EL, et al. Nonhereditary hearing impairment. In: Hughes GB, Pensak ML (Eds). Clinical Otology, 3rd edition. New York, NY: Thieme Publishers, Inc; 2007. pp. 300-20.
4. Oliver E, Hashisaki GT. Sudden sensory hearing loss. In: Rosen CA, Johnson JT (Eds). Bailey's Head and Neck Surgery—Otolaryngology, 5th edition. Philadelphia, PA: Wolters Kluwer Health/Lippincott Williams & Wilkins; 2014. pp. 2589-96.

Chapter 3

Dizziness

Helen Xu, Yuan F Liu

Chief Complaint
"I feel dizzy, lightheaded, the room is spinning, unsteady, or off-balance".

DEFINITIONS

Vertigo: Illusion of oneself moving or one's environment moving without actual movement.

Central vertigo: Vertigo caused by disease of the central nervous system (CNS), including cranial nerve (CN) VIII.

Peripheral vertigo: Vertigo caused by disease of the peripheral vestibular system, within the membranous labyrinth.

ANATOMY AND PHYSIOLOGY OF VESTIBULAR SYSTEM

The vestibular system consists of five sensory organs within a bony labyrinth in the petrous portion of the temporal bone called the otic capsule. All vestibular end organs are lined by a membrane (membranous labyrinth) and contain endolymph. Perilymph flows between the bony and membranous labyrinths (Fig. 3.1).

1. Three semicircular canals
   a. Lateral (horizontal), superior (anterior), posterior canals
   b. Each semicircular canal is oriented at about 90° to the other two.

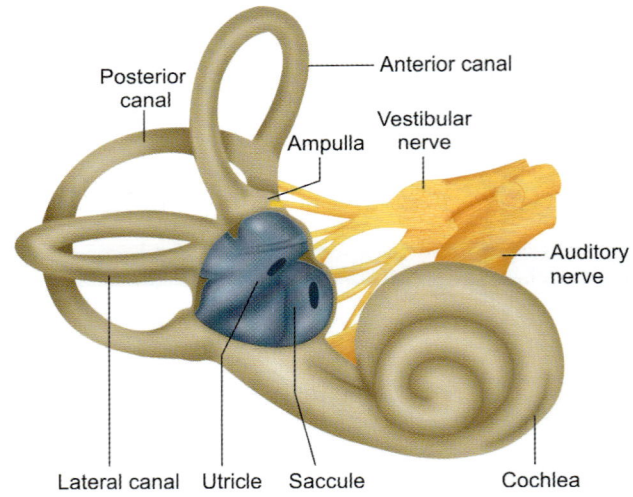

Fig. 3.1: The membranous labyrinth and vestibulocochlear nerve.

   c. Each detects angular (rotational) acceleration.
   d. Maximally sensitive to rotation in the plane of the canal.
   e. *Functional pairs*: Each canal has a corresponding canal on the contralateral side that lies roughly in the same plane (coplanar).
      i. Left horizontal to right horizontal
      ii. Left superior to right posterior
     iii. Left posterior to right superior
   f. Each canal has an ampulla, which contains the neuroepithelium with hair cells that detect motion.
   g. *Vestibular hair cells*: Modified columnar epithelial cells with elongated microvilli on apical surfaces called stereocilia. Each hair cell has a single long kinocilium. Stereocilia are embedded in a gelatinous mass called cupula. When the head rotates, endolymph and cupula lag behind due to inertia, thereby deflecting stereocilia in the direction opposite of head movement. Deflection of

stereocilia leads to depolarization or hyperpolarization of hair cells and initiates a change in the baseline rate of action potentials.

2. Two otolith organs
   a. Utricle (utriculus) and saccule (sacculus) are located in the vestibule: ovoid space within the bony labyrinth between the cochlea and the semicircular canals.
   b. Utricle is oriented in the horizontal plane and saccule in the vertical plane.
   c. Utricle and saccule detect linear acceleration. Saccule detects gravity in a standing position.
   d. Each contains a macula (analogous to ampulla).
   e. Each contains otolithic membranes (analogous to cupula), which contain embedded otoliths (otoconia). Otoliths are calcium carbonate deposits and have higher specific gravity than endolymph.
   f. Vestibular hair cells of the otolith organs work in a similar way to those of the semicircular canals.

3. Innervation
   a. The vestibulocochlear nerve (CN VIII) emerges from the brainstem at the cerebellopontine angle (CPA) and enters the internal auditory meatus (porus acusticus).
   b. Cranial nerve VIII branches into the cochlear, superior vestibular, and inferior vestibular divisions.
   c. Cell bodies of the vestibular divisions are located within the vestibular ganglion (Scarpa's ganglion), which sits within the internal auditory meatus. The vestibular ganglion is divided into superior and inferior ganglia. The superior ganglion gives rise to the superior vestibular nerve, which supplies the horizontal and superior semicircular canals, and the utricle. The inferior ganglion gives rise to the inferior vestibular nerve (IVN), which supplies the posterior semicircular canal and saccule.
   d. *Central vestibular pathway*: Cranial nerve VIII enters the brainstem at the pontomedullary junction and courses to the vestibular nuclei. Afferents to vestibular nuclei do

not cross midline. About 70% of afferents terminate in cerebellar vermis, which contributes to coordination of head and eye movement. Efferents from the vestibular nuclei project to the spinal cord (that stabilizes head and shoulders and maintains postural balance), contralateral vestibular nuclei, thalamus (visual processing and conscious perception of vertigo). Bilateral projections from vestibular nuclei to other parts of brainstem contribute to vestibulo-ocular reflex (VOR).

e. Afferent fibers have a resting potential (tonic activity) and detect excitation or inhibition by increasing or decreasing the firing rate.

f. The CNS can compensate for acute deficits in the peripheral vestibular system, but this central compensation process can take days to weeks.

g. A person can function near normal with only one intact labyrinth.

4. Vascular supply to the vestibular labyrinth

   a. Horizontal and superior semicircular canals, most of utricle, and some of saccule are supplied by the anterior vestibular artery, internal auditory (labyrinthine) artery, and anterior cerebellar, superior cerebellar, or basilar artery.

   b. Posterior semicircular canal, most of saccule, and some of utricle are supplied by the posterior vestibular artery, vestibulocochlear artery, common cochlear artery, internal auditory (labyrinthine) artery, and anterior cerebellar, superior cerebellar, or basilar artery.

5. Vestibular reflexes

   a. *Vestibulo-ocular reflex*: It has a role in retinal image stabilization. The VOR helps to maintain gaze by eliciting eye movements that are compensatory for head movement.

   b. *Vestibulocollic reflex (VCR)*: As the head moves, the VCR stabilizes the head through the activation of neck muscles.

COMMON CAUSES OF DIZZINESS

Benign Paroxysmal Positional Vertigo (BPPV)[1]

Most common peripheral vestibular disorder (20–40%)

1. *Epidemiology*: It occurs at all ages, with peak incidence at ages 40–60, with a female-to-male ratio being 2:1.
2. Presentation
    a. Rapid onset of vertigo after head movement (e.g. rolling in bed, looking up, and bending forward).
    b. Vertigo lasts for a few seconds, always <1 minute.
    c. It may recur over months and may cluster in time.
    d. It may follow head trauma, ear surgery, and vestibular neuritis.
    e. Half of BPPV cases are without identifiable causes.
3. Pathophysiology
    a. Dislodged otoconia deflect the cupula of a semicircular canal on movement.
    b. Posterior canal (~85%), horizontal canal (10–15%), superior canal (~2%).
    c. *Cupulolithiasis*: Otoconia are deposited and adhere to the cupula of a semicircular canal.
    d. *Canalithiasis*: Free-floating otoconia in a semicircular canal.
4. Workup
    a. *Dix–Hallpike maneuver*: It is the diagnostic gold standard and can be used to elicit posterior and superior semicircular canal diseases. Lower the patient quickly from sitting to supine with the head turned 45° to one side and end with the head extended 20° over the edge. Observe for nystagmus (up-beating and torsional toward dependent ear) with latency of a few seconds, duration <1 minute, crescendo–decrescendo intensity. Repeat with the head turned to the opposite side. The side that elicits nystagmus is the affected side. Nystagmus fatigues with repetition. Benign paroxysmal positional vertigo can be rarely bilateral in cases of head trauma.

b. *Supine roll test*: It can elicit horizontal semicircular canal disease. Perform the supine roll test when Dix–Hallpike is negative. The patient starts supine with the head resting on the table; then turn his/her head rapidly to the right. Monitor for nystagmus toward (geotropic) or away (apogeotropic) from the downward ear. Repeat with a head turn rapidly to the left. The affected ear is the side that elicits more intense nystagmus.

5. Management of BPPV
   a. Epley maneuver (canalith repositioning procedure)
      i. Start with Dix–Hallpike position of the head extended while supine; when nystagmus resolves, slowly roll 180° (90° at a time until nystagmus subsides) so that the affected ear is up, then sit upright.
      ii. Repeat until there is no more nystagmus.
      iii. It can unintentionally convert posterior to horizontal canal BPPV. After completing the Epley maneuver, the experienced physician will test for conversion of posterior BPPV to horizontal BPPV by performing the supine roll test.
   b. Horizontal canal BPPV usually spontaneously remits in a few days.
   c. Vestibular rehabilitation (physical therapy to help with habituation, adaptation, and compensation of balance disorder) and observation are options for initial treatment if the patient cannot tolerate the repositioning maneuvers.
   d. Reassess within 1 month.
   e. Surgery is an option if BPPV is disabling and not cured by repositioning maneuvers (posterior semicircular canal occlusion).

Vestibular Migraine

Vestibular migraine or migraine-associated vertigo is the most common cause for spontaneous episodic vertigo.

1. *Epidemiology*: All ages are affected, but migraine-associated vertigo usually starts in early adulthood. The female-to-male incidence ratio is 2:1.
2. Presentation
   a. Dizziness or vertigo lasting from 5 minutes to 72 hours.
   b. Symptoms may be triggered by head position change or visual stimulation (e.g. moving subjects in a busy mall), or may be spontaneous.
   c. It may or may not have a history of headaches.
   d. It may be associated with migrainous features: hypersensitivity to light, sound, or smell.
   e. A history of motion sickness is common.
   f. Frequently, there is a family history of migraine.
   g. It may be accompanied by bilateral sensorineural hearing loss or tinnitus.
   h. It may overlap with BPPV, Ménière disease.
3. Pathophysiology
   a. *Unclear etiology*: Neurovascular involvement
      i. *Neuronal dysfunction hypothesis*: Activation of the trigeminovascular system, cortical spreading depression, and neuronal sensitization, which can lead to triggering of pain receptors.
      ii. Pain may be due to vasodilation and stretching of pain fibers in vessel walls (less popular with new evidence).
   b. *Basilar migraine*: Migraine attributed to basilar artery ischemia.
4. Workup
   a. Diagnostic criteria[2]
      i. *Definitive*: Vestibular symptoms, current or history of migraine, and migrainous features.
      ii. *Probable*: Vestibular symptoms plus either the history of migraine or the migrainous features.
   b. Exclude other causes.

5.   Management
  a.   Lifestyle/diet modifications
    i.   Strict migraine diet for 6–8 weeks. If it helps, add back favorite foods one at a time.
  b.   *Prophylactic*: Tricyclic antidepressants, selective serotonin reuptake inhibitors, anticonvulsants, calcium channel blockers, β-blockers.[3,4]
    i.   Start with low dose, increase dose slowly, stay at the dose with good effect for 6 months, then wean off.

Ménière Disease (Idiopathic Endolymphatic Hydrops)[5]

The second most common cause of spontaneous episodic vertigo:

1.   *Epidemiology*: It occurs at all ages; peak age group 30–60. Ménière disease is more prevalent in Whites and slightly more prevalent in women.
2.   Presentation
  a.   Sudden onset of vertigo, recurring triad of vertigo, fluctuating sensorineural hearing loss, and tinnitus or aural fullness.
  b.   Atypical Ménière disease may have symptomatic overlap with vestibular migraine, and distinguishing between the two entities may be difficult.
  c.   Vertigo lasts from 20 minutes to 24 hours, usually 2–3 hours.
  d.   No symptoms versus disequilibrium between attacks.
  e.   Clusters of attacks with remission over years.
  f.   Sometimes bilateral.
  g.   About 10–20% familial (strongly associated with migraine).
3.   Pathophysiology
  a.   Ménière disease is caused by excess endolymphatic fluid (overproduction and/or underabsorption by endolymphatic sac). Etiology is unclear. There are

possible autoimmune, viral, ischemic, traumatic, and other infectious, congenital, or multifactorial causes.

4. Workup
   a. There is no definitive diagnostic test for Ménière disease.
   b. Refer to American Academy of Otolaryngology—Head and Neck Surgery guidelines for detailed diagnostic criteria.[5]
   c. "Definitive" Ménière disease per guideline: two or more episodes of vertigo of at least 20 minutes, audiometric-proven hearing loss, tinnitus or hearing loss, and other causes excluded.
   d. Magnetic resonance imaging (MRI) is recommended to exclude other causes of vertigo and hearing loss, such as vestibular schwannoma.
   e. *Audiometry*: Sensorineural hearing loss, typically at low frequencies.
   f. Vestibular testing
      i. *Caloric testing*: Depending on the timing of test, it varies from normal response to significant reduction or complete absence of response.
      ii. *Vestibular evoked myogenic potential*: Elevated thresholds (nonspecific) or absent response.
      iii. *Electrocochleography*: Summating potential (SP) to action potential (AP) ratio increases (threshold for diagnosis ranges from 0.35 to 0.5) in Ménière disease, but sensitivity and specificity are low.

5. Management
   a. Vertigo treatment
      i. Spontaneous improvement occurs in 60–80% of patients.
      ii. Salt restriction—a low-sodium diet is recommended.
      iii. Diuretics (not enough evidence to show efficacy).
      iv. *Symptomatic*: Vestibular suppressants (antihistamine, benzodiazepine, and anticholinergic), antiemetics, sedatives, and antidepressants.

v. Intratympanic injection of dexamethasone or gentamicin.
- *Dexamethasone (limited evidence on effectiveness)*: It possibly suppresses autoimmunity and can maintain residual hearing.[6]
- Gentamicin can result in a chemical labyrinthectomy. Gentamicin has high vestibulotoxicity, but it is also cochleotoxic and can cause severe hearing loss.[7]
- When titrated properly (e.g. gentamicin 40 mg/mL, one injection every 4 weeks, up to three injections as needed), gentamicin intratympanic injections can result in selective vestibulotoxicity with high successful control of vertigo (90%) without significant cochleotoxicity.[21]
- Gentamicin is also shown very effective (95%) in control of drop attacks.[21]

vi. Surgery (insufficient evidence for benefit)[8]
- Endolymphatic sac decompression (controversial efficacy).
- Vestibular neurectomy
  - Invasive and difficult neurosurgical procedure requiring a craniotomy.
  - Up to 85–95% vertigo control with 80–90% hearing maintenance.
  - It is less favored today because of the high efficacy of chemical ablation with gentamicin.
- Labyrinthectomy
  - It is most destructive and results in complete unilateral vestibular and hearing loss.
  - It may be offered to patients with no serviceable hearing and intractable vertigo.
  - It has higher vertigo control rate than vestibular neurectomy.
  - It is less favored today because of the high efficacy of chemical ablation with gentamicin.

Vestibular Neuritis[9,10]

1. Epidemiology
   a. Middle age.
2. Presentation
   a. Dramatic, sudden onset of vertigo, nausea, vomiting.
   b. Spontaneous, usually horizontal nystagmus suppressed with visual fixation.
   c. It may last hours to days with gradual improvement.
   d. Balance complaints related to head movement may last for months after resolution of the acute episode.
   e. Benign paroxysmal positional vertigo during recovery period is common.
   f. It can recur over years (unusual).
   g. There is no hearing loss or focal neurologic symptoms. There is sometimes a prior or concurrent upper respiratory infection (less than half).
3. Pathophysiology
   a. Vestibular nerve inflammation.
   b. The mechanism of dizziness is unclear: possibly viral, vascular, and immunologic causes.
   c. Herpes simplex virus 1 is responsible in some cases, but there is no identifiable cause in most cases.
   d. It affects the superior vestibular nerve more frequently, possibly due to the longer and narrower canal encasing the superior nerve (more susceptible to compression); however, vestibular neuritis involving the IVN can occur.
   e. Benign paroxysmal positional vertigo may occur infrequently following disease.
   f. Bilateral disease is possible.
4. Workup
   a. Physical examination
      i. Postural instability; the patient may be leaning toward the affected ear, but can walk without falling.
      ii. Slow phase of nystagmus beats toward the affected ear (dominant excitation from the unaffected side).

       iii. Nystagmus is intensified when looking away from the affected side and attenuated when looking toward the affected side (Alexander's law).

       iv. Head thrust test helps to determine which side is affected.

  b.   Vestibular testing

      i. *Caloric testing*: Reduced response on the affected side.

      ii. *Vestibular evoked myogenic potential*: Response attenuated or absent on the affected side.

  c.   Rule out central vertigo

      i. Magnetic resonance imaging scan with thin cuts to evaluate brainstem and cerebellum if there are risk factors for stroke, neurological abnormalities, or no improvement in 48 hours.

5. Management

  a. Corticosteroids (insufficient evidence for benefit).[11]

  b. Supportive

      i. Vestibular suppressants (antihistamine, benzodiazepine, and anticholinergic).

      ii. Antiemetics.

  c. Stop medications when possible to allow central vestibular compensation to take place.

  d. Vestibular rehabilitation (physical therapy to help with habituation, adaptation, and compensation of balance disorder) if the patient experiences residual symptoms.

Superior Semicircular Canal Dehiscence Syndrome[12]

1. Epidemiology

  a. Middle age.

2. Presentation

  a. Vertigo with loud sounds, pressure changes (e.g. tragal compression, nose-blowing, Valsalva, straining).

  b. Nystagmus (vertical and torsional) in the plane of the superior semicircular canal (SSC).

  c. Possible autophony (increased loudness of own voice), conductive hearing loss, pulsatile tinnitus, aural fullness.

    d. Spectrum from asymptomatic to auditory only to vestibular-only symptoms.

3. Pathophysiology
    a. A type of perilymphatic fistula between the SSC and epidural space.
    b. Absence of bone over the SSC, creating a "third window" that results in abnormal movement of endolymphatic fluid.
    c. It is possibly due to congenital or developmental abnormality.
    d. Conductive hearing loss may be due to dissipation of air-conducted acoustic energy from the third window.

4. Workup
    a. High-resolution computed tomography (CT) temporal bone without contrast.
    b. Physical examination
        i. *Tullio phenomenon*: Nystagmus elicited by sound.
        ii. *Hennebert's sign*: Nystagmus elicited by ear canal pressure.
    c. *Audiometry*: There may be a conductive hearing loss in the affected ear.
    d. Vestibular testing
        i. *Vestibular evoked myogenic potential*: Lower threshold or increased amplitude for response in the affected ear is a typical finding in superior semicircular canal dehiscence (SSCD) syndrome.

5. Management
    a. Treatment is based on the severity of symptoms. Observation alone is acceptable if symptoms are mild.
    b. Surgery
        i. Repair of dehiscence
            • Middle cranial fossa approach with or without obliteration of the SSC lumen is the standard surgical approach.
            • Transmastoid approach can be used if the anatomy of the middle cranial fossa allows access to the SSC.[13]

    ii. Transcanal reinforcement of round window ± oval window.[14]
- Dampens hypercompliance.
- Less invasive.

    iii. Tympanostomy tube placement may help with aural pressure symptoms.

Neoplasms

Neoplasms may cause compressive vestibular symptoms due to space-occupying lesions in the brainstem, cerebellum, CPA, or temporal bone.

Cerebellopontine Angle Tumors

The CPA is the most common location for posterior fossa neoplasms.

1. Epidemiology
   a. *Common primary CPA lesions*: Vestibular schwannoma (>90%), meningioma (~3%), facial nerve neuroma (1%), other CN neuromas, glomus tumors, arachnoid cyst, hemangioma.
2. *Presentation*: Presenting symptoms may include progressive sensorineural hearing loss, tinnitus, dysequilibrium (mild imbalance, vertigo uncommon because of slow progressive loss of vestibular function with compensation), facial hypesthesia, increased intracranial pressure (headache, nausea, and vomiting), ataxia.
3. Pathophysiology
   a. Compression of the following:
      i. Cranial nerves VIII, VII, and V.
      ii. Fourth ventricle leading to obstructive hydrocephalus.
      iii. Brainstem, possible cerebellar tonsillar herniation.
   b. Vestibular schwannoma
      i. Benign schwannoma of CN VIII.
      ii. It usually arises from the vestibular nerve, superior or inferior portion.
      iii. Slow-growing tumor, 1–2 mm per year.

      iv. It usually arises within the internal auditory canal, but can develop in the CPA.

      v. It is associated with neurofibromatosis type 2 (frequently bilateral schwannomas).

4. Workup
   a. Audiometry
      i. Asymmetric sensorineural hearing loss.
      ii. Impaired speech discrimination, worse than expected for the given extent of hearing loss.
   b. Auditory brainstem response testing
      i. Adjusted interaural latency for wave V > 0.2 milliseconds.
      ii. Auditory brainstem response is less used due to sensitivity of MRI.
   c. Magnetic resonance imaging with gadolinium.[15]
   d. Computed tomography with contrast: Computed tomography is not sensitive for detecting small tumors. This is used if MRI is contraindicated (e.g. pacemaker and cochlear implant).
5. Management[16]
   a. Surgical approach to vestibular schwannoma is based on the location and size of the tumor and hearing status.[17]
      i. Translabyrinthine
      ii. Retrosigmoid (suboccipital)
      iii. Middle fossa
   b. Stereotactic radiation.
   c. Serial imaging and observation.

Vascular Causes

Vertigo may occur with decreased blood flow through any of the three branches of the vertebral or basilar arteries: posterior inferior cerebellar artery (PICA), anterior inferior cerebellar artery, and superior cerebellar artery.

1. Permanent
   a. Arterial occlusion by atherosclerotic plaques.
   b. Hemorrhagic or ischemic infarction.

2. Transient
   a. Vascular spasm.
   b. Low perfusion pressure.
   c. Vascular steal syndromes
      i. *Subclavian steal*: Retrograde flow through the vertebral artery due to stenosis of the subclavian artery proximal to branching of the vertebral artery (decreased vascular resistance through distal subclavian branches leads to siphoning of blood from vertebral artery). Subclavian steal syndrome manifests as vertigo and other neurologic symptoms with arm exercise.

Vertebrobasilar Insufficiency

1. *Epidemiology*: It occurs in the elderly, often with known vascular risk factors.
2. *Presentation*: Abrupt onset of dizziness, lasting minutes. There may be vertigo, headache, nausea, vomiting, diplopia, ataxia, numbness, and weakness.
3. Pathophysiology
   a. Atherosclerosis in the vertebrobasilar system.
   b. Hypertension.
4. Workup
   a. Neurology consult.
   b. Computed tomography to rule out hemorrhagic event.
   c. Magnetic resonance angiography with contrast to identify vertebrobasilar artery stenosis.
5. Management
   a. Control diabetes, hypertension, and hyperlipidemia.
   b. Anticoagulation (aspirin or warfarin).
   c. Consider stenting or endarterectomy.

Lateral Medullary Syndrome (Wallenberg's Syndrome)

1. *Epidemiology*: It usually occurs in middle-aged patients.
2. Presentation
   a. Contralateral sensory deficits to trunk and extremities.

    b. Ipsilateral sensory and motor deficit to the face.

    c. Vertigo, ipsilateral facial pain (CN V), diplopia, dysphagia (CN X), dysphonia (CN X), ipsilateral Horner's syndrome (sympathetics).

3. Pathophysiology
   a. Infarction of the dorsolateral medulla.
   b. Occlusion of the vertebral artery, rarely the PICA.
4. Workup/Management
   a. Neurology consult.

Chiari Malformations

These are a group of developmental hindbrain and spinal cord abnormalities characterized by herniation of posterior cranial fossa content through the foramen magnum.

1. *Type 1*: Most common, least severe[18]
   a. Caudal displacement of cerebellar tonsils below foramen magnum. This is possibly a disorder of the para-axial mesoderm leading to small posterior fossa.
   b. Symptoms present around the age of 25–35 years.
   c. Headache is worse with Valsalva, neck pain, cerebellar symptoms, dysarthria, dysphagia, hand weakness, cape anesthesia.
   d. *Audiologic and vestibular symptoms*: Nystagmus, vertigo, dizziness, unsteadiness, hearing loss, tinnitus, aural fullness, and hyperacusis.
   e. About <10% hydrocephalus.
   f. About 30–70% syringomyelia.
2. *Type 2 (Arnold–Chiari Malformation)*: Less common, more severe
   a. Caudal displacement of lower brainstem (medulla, pons, fourth ventricle) through the foramen magnum.
   b. Always with myelomeningocele.
   c. Symptomatic in infancy or early childhood.
   d. Swallowing difficulty, stridor, apnea, weak cry, nystagmus, extremity weakness.
   e. Hydrocephalus and syringomyelia are common.

3. Chiari malformation types 3 and 4 are very rare and usually incompatible with life.
4. Workup
   a. Magnetic resonance imaging scan of brain.
   b. Computed tomography if the patient cannot undergo MRI.
5. Management
   a. Symptomatic medical treatment for type 1 if symptoms are mild and there is no syringomyelia.
   b. Surgery for decompression of the cervicomedullary junction.
   c. Ventricular–peritoneal shunt for hydrocephalus or drainage of syringomyelia.

DIAGNOSTIC WORKUP OF DIZZINESS
History

1. First, does the patient have true vertigo, dizziness, disequilibrium, lightheaded, or a combination of symptoms? True vertigo is the only specific symptom related to peripheral vestibular dysfunction.
2. Focus on vertigo—duration, spontaneous versus positional, associated ear symptoms, history of migraine headache or migrainous features—to rule out the four most common causes of vestibular dysfunction: BPPV, vestibular migraine, Ménière disease, and vestibular neuritis.

Common Questions

1. "Do you see or feel the room moving/spinning/tilting?" or "Do you feel yourself moving?"
2. "Do you have dizziness?"
3. "Are you off-balance?"
4. "Do you feel lightheaded or sometimes black out?"
   a. Presyncope
   b. Vasovagal reaction
   c. Cardiac etiology
   d. Orthostatic hypotension

5. "What triggered the vertigo?"
   a. *Spontaneous*: Ménière disease and vestibular migraine
   b. Loud sounds (Tullio phenomenon) or sudden pressure change (straining, Valsalva, cough) leading to vertigo may indicate SSCD or another type of perilymphatic fistula.
   c. Menstrual periods, foods, stress, lack of sleep, change in weather, or motion stimulation (e.g. ceiling fan and video games) may indicate migraine.
   d. Large salt load may suggest Ménière disease.
   e. *Head movement*: BPPV and vestibular migraine.
6. "Do the symptoms come and go or are they constant? How long do the symptoms last? How often do they occur?"
   a. *Vertigo lasting seconds*: BPPV.
   b. *Vertigo lasting minutes to hours*: Ménière disease, migraine (can last up to days).
   c. *Vertigo lasting days to weeks*: Vestibular neuritis (in most cases only one episode).
7. "Do you have other symptoms associated with the vertigo/dizziness?"
   a. Aural fullness or tinnitus preceding vertigo suggests Ménière disease.
   b. Sweating, dyspnea, and palpitations may indicate cardiac origin of presyncope.
   c. Aura, headache, photophobia, and phonophobia may occur in migraine.
   d. Focal neurologic signs may indicate vascular etiology or an intracranial mass.
   e. Anxiety, panic, agoraphobia, generalized imbalance for long periods of time may indicate a psychogenic cause.
8. "Do you have a family history of imbalance? Headache?"
   a. Familial migraine.
9. "What medications do you take?"
   a. Common drugs associated with vestibular dysfunction: aminoglycosides, cisplatin, alcohol, amiodarone, antihypertensives, diuretics, sedatives, methotrexate, and anticoagulants.

Physical Examination

1. Start with a complete otolaryngologic examination.
2. Neurologic examination.
3. Eye examination.
   a. Nystagmus (direction defined by quick phase)
      i. *Saccade*: Rapid change in gaze from one target to another.
      ii. *Frenzel lenses*: Multiple magnifying lenses that magnify the eye and prevent visual fixation; they can help to characterize nystagmus.
      iii. Dizziness of central origin is not suppressed with fixation and may change direction with gaze.
      iv. Dizziness of peripheral origin is always suppressed with visual fixation and never changes direction.
      v. In peripheral vertigo, such as vestibular neuritis, the horizontal component of the quick phase of nystagmus beats toward the intact side.
4. Head thrust test
   a. Rotate the head 10–15° very rapidly in one direction while having the patient fix his/her gaze on the examiner's nose.
   b. It tests semicircular canal function in the plane of thrust.
   c. Corrective saccade indicates hypofunction of the canal of the same side and is noted in patients with vestibular neuritis or after an acute attack of Ménière disease.
   d. Fistula test.
   e. *Tullio phenomenon*: Sound-induced vertigo.
   f. *Hennebert's sign*: Perception of movement in a stationary object after pressure is applied to the ear canal.
5. Postural tests (e.g. Romberg, tandem gait) have low sensitivity and specificity for locating the side of the lesion.
6. Dix–Hallpike maneuver; see BPPV above.

Ancillary Tools

1. Vestibular testing

a. *Electronystagmography or videonystagmography*: Fundamental array of tests involving recording of eye movement after visual or vestibular stimuli.[19]
   1. *Oculomotor*: Saccade, smooth pursuit, optokinetic nystagmus, gaze, fixation suppression testing.
   2. *Positional*: Analysis of eye movement with stationary head positions (gravity effects on nystagmus).
   3. *Caloric*: Irrigation of ear with different temperatures of water or air to induce cupula movement in the horizontal semicircular canal only, which helps to locate the side of the lesion based on the magnitude of induced nystagmus on each side. Irrigation temperatures are 7°C above and below body temperature. Since body temperature is 37°C, irrigation temperatures are 30°C and 44°C.
b. *Rotary chair (rotational testing)*: Evaluates pathway of horizontal VOR.
c. *Cervical vestibular evoked myogenic potential*: It evaluates stimulation of the sternocleidomastoid muscle with high-intensity acoustic stimuli to provide information on the saccule, IVN function and the vestibulocollic reflex.[20]
d. *Electrocochleography*: It measures cochlear function by an electrode placed in the ear canal as close to the cochlea as possible, which records electrical potentials (SP and AP) elicited by clicks. It can help to detect hydrops in Ménière disease.

2. *Audiometry*: It includes pure tone audiometry, speech audiometry, and tympanometry.

REFERENCES

1. Bhattacharyya N, Baugh RF, Orvidas L, et al. Clinical practice guideline: benign paroxysmal positional vertigo. Otolaryngol Head Neck Surg. 2008;139(5 Suppl 4):S47-81.
2. Lempert T, Olesen J, Furman J, et al. Vestibular migraine: diagnostic criteria. J Vestib Res. 2012;22(4):167-72.

3. Holland S, Silberstein SD, Freitag F, et al. Evidence-based guideline update: NSAIDs and other complementary treatments for episodic migraine prevention in adults: report of the Quality Standards Subcommittee of the American Academy of Neurology and the American Headache Society. Neurology. 2012;78(17):1346-53.

4. Silberstein SD, Holland S, Freitag F, et al. Evidence-based guideline update: pharmacologic treatment for episodic migraine prevention in adults: report of the Quality Standards Subcommittee of the American Academy of Neurology and the American Headache Society. Neurology. 2012;78(17):1337-345.

5. Committee on Hearing and Equilibrium guidelines for the diagnosis and evaluation of therapy in Ménière's disease. American Academy of Otolaryngology-Head and Neck Foundation, Inc. Otolaryngol Head Neck Surg. 1995;113(3):181-5.

6. Phillips JS, Westerberg B. Intratympanic steroids for Ménière's disease or syndrome. Cochrane Database Syst Rev. 2011;7:CD008514.

7. Pullens B, van Benthem PP. Intratympanic gentamicin for Ménière's disease or syndrome. Cochrane Database Syst Rev. 2011;3:CD008234.

8. Pullens B, Verschuur HP, van Benthem PP. Surgery for Ménière's disease. Cochrane Database Syst Rev. 2013;2:CD005395.

9. Baloh RW. Clinical practice. Vestibular neuritis. N Engl J Med. 2003;348(11):1027-32.

10. Strupp M, Brandt T. Vestibular neuritis. Semin Neurol. 2009;29(5):509-19.

11. Fishman JM, Burgess C, Waddell A. Corticosteroids for the treatment of idiopathic acute vestibular dysfunction (vestibular neuritis). Cochrane Database Syst Rev. 2011;5:CD008607.

12. Minor LB. Clinical manifestations of superior semicircular canal dehiscence. Laryngoscope. 2005;115(10):1717-27.

13. Zhao YC, Somers T, van Dinther J. Transmastoid repair of superior semicircular canal dehiscence. J Neurol Surg B: Skull Base. 2012;73(4):225-9.

14. Silverstein H, Kartush JM, Parnes LS, et al. Round window reinforcement for superior semicircular canal dehiscence: a retrospective multi-center case series. Am J Otolaryngol. 2014;35(3):286-93.

15. Lo W, Solti-Bohman L. Tumors of the temporal bone and the cerebellopontine angle. In: Som PM, Curtin HD (Eds). Head and Neck Imaging, Vol. 2, 3rd edition. Mosby-Year Book, St. Louis; 1996. p.1451.

16. Flickinger JC, Kondziolka D, Niranjan A, et al. Results of acoustic neuroma radiosurgery: an analysis of 5 years' experience using current methods. J Neurosurg. 2013;119(Suppl):1-6.

17. Ansari SF, Terry C, Cohen-Gadol AA. Surgery for vestibular schwannomas: a systematic review of complications by approach. Neurosurg Focus. 2012;33(3):E14.

18. Guerra Jiménez G, Mazón Gutiérrez A, Marco de Lucas E, et al. Audio-vestibular signs and symptoms in Chiari malformation type i. Case series and literature review. Acta Otorinolaringol Esp. 2015;66(1):28-35.

19. Bhansali SA, Honrubia V. Current status of electronystagmography testing. Otolaryngol Head Neck Surg. 1999;120(3):419-26.

20. Welgampola MS, Colebatch JG. Characteristics and clinical applications of vestibular-evoked myogenic potentials. Neurology. 2005;64(10):1682-8.

21. Viana LM, Bahmad F Jr, Rauch SD. Intratympanic gentamicin as a treatment for drop attacks in patients with Meniere's disease. Laryngoscope. 2014;124(9):2151-4.

Chapter 4

Tinnitus

Joseph Sciarrino, Michael Teixido

DEFINITIONS

ABR: Auditory brainstem responses, a neurophysiologic test that measures auditory evoked responses. The test is similar to electroencephalography but measures responses along the auditory pathway.

AVM: Arteriovenous malformation.

AVF: Arteriovenous fistula.

SNHL: Sensorineural hearing loss.

QOL: Quality of life.

Tinnitus: The perception of sound with no external source. Tinnitus is a symptom with multiple causes. Occasionally, it can be a symptom of serious disease.

Primary tinnitus: Idiopathic; it may or may not be associated with SNHL.

Secondary tinnitus: Associated with a specific cause other than SNHL, such as middle or inner ear dysfunction, auditory nerve pathology, vascular, intracranial hypertension, and myoclonus.

EPIDEMIOLOGY

- About 25% of people have experienced tinnitus. About 8% of people experience it frequently; approximately 20% of them will require intervention.

- The prevalence of tinnitus is higher in males, Whites, patients with body mass index ≥ 30 kg/m², patients with hypertension, diabetes mellitus, hyperlipidemia, anxiety, and history of loud noise exposure.
- Significant economic cost:
  - Estimated to be $2.75 billion annually in disability compensation for US veterans alone. Tinnitus is the most prevalent service-connected disability.
  - Tinnitus reduces employees' productivity.

PRESENTATION

There is great variability in the sound perceived (ringing, roaring, buzzing, clicking, and pulsations). Tinnitus may be unilateral or bilateral. There is variability in the effect on QOL. Patients may have insomnia, difficulty understanding speech, depression, and concentration difficulties. There is a 48–60% incidence of depression in tinnitus sufferers, with the severity related to the severity of tinnitus. The severity of tinnitus can fluctuate. Natural habituation may improve tolerance with time in some patients, while it worsens with time in others.

SUBJECTIVE VERSUS OBJECTIVE TINNITUS

The pathophysiology, evaluation, workup, and treatment differ significantly between primary and secondary tinnitus, and they will be presented separately.

PRIMARY TINNITUS

Pathophysiology

Primary tinnitus may result from central adaptation to hearing loss from injury in the cochlea. Peripheral injury releases inhibitory tone of frequency-specific afferents along tonotopic pathways. The frequency of tinnitus usually correlates with the frequency of hearing loss.

Workup

Targeted History and Physical

- Identify potentially treatable conditions (secondary tinnitus) or coexisting conditions such as depression and anxiety.
- Note the onset, duration, character, laterality, pulsations, effect on QOL, hearing loss [sudden, SNHL, conductive hearing loss (CHL), asymmetric, etc.], noise exposure, ototoxic medication use, vertigo/imbalance, depression/anxiety symptoms.
- Determine whether the patient has bothersome tinnitus affecting QOL, communication, sleep, and concentration.
- Tinnitus questionnaires/indices are helpful in quantifying QOL impact, and can guide treatment.
- Determine if tinnitus is persistent (>6 months)—less likely to resolve spontaneously. New-onset tinnitus may improve over time with habituation.
- Head and neck examination, otoscopy, focused neurologic examination, auscultation of head and neck.
- *Routine audiologic examination*: Indicated for all patients regardless of duration, laterality, or perceived hearing ability. Tinnitus may be a sign of hearing loss not appreciated by the patient. Identify hearing loss so that intervention can be started.
- A prompt, comprehensive audiologic examination is indicated for patients with tinnitus that is single sided, present ≤6 months, or associated with hearing impairment. If hearing loss is sudden, obtain an audiogram at the time of presentation or within 2 weeks.
- Unilateral tinnitus raises suspicion for a vascular pathology or schwannoma.

Imaging

This is useful only in unilateral or pulsatile tinnitus, asymmetric hearing loss, or in patients with focal neurologic abnormalities. Imaging is not useful in bilateral tinnitus with symmetric hearing.

Treatment

Patient Education

- Reassure the patient that tinnitus is a symptom and not itself a dangerous condition, and that the workup can identify or exclude a condition that would require treatment.
- Counsel the patient on hearing loss and hearing protection.
- *Management options*: Explain that there is no cure for primary tinnitus, but there are strategies to manage the symptoms.
- Hearing aid evaluation is indicated for patients with hearing loss and bothersome tinnitus. Hearing aids help with hearing loss and can make tinnitus more tolerable.

Cognitive Behavioral Therapy

- Identifies and restructures negative thoughts, relaxation techniques, and sleep hygiene.
- Performed by mental health professionals in weekly sessions for 8–24 weeks.
- Studies show improvement in questionnaire scores and QOL, not in subjective tinnitus loudness.

Sound Therapy (Masking)

- Alters the perception of tinnitus or the patient's reaction to tinnitus. Similarly, alters contrast between tinnitus and environment and promotes habituation.

Medications and Supplements

- Medications and supplements for primary tinnitus are of questionable benefit.
  - Antidepressants, anxiolytics, and anticonvulsants have been used, but have not been shown to be effective and may have side effects.
  - Anxiolytics may be helpful as a bridge in severely affected patients while cognitive behavioral therapy is arranged.

- No proven efficacy is found in high-quality studies for intratympanic injection of lidocaine. Steroid injection is helpful only in patients with hydrops and tinnitus.
- No proven efficacy is found in high-quality studies for ginkgo biloba, melatonin, zinc, or other dietary supplements.

Acupuncture

- Conflicting data regarding efficacy.

Repetitive Transcranial Magnetic Stimulation

- Conflicting data; no proof of long-term benefit.

SECONDARY TINNITUS

Pathophysiology

- Spontaneous, mechanical, or pulsatile.

Spontaneous

It may occur due to spontaneous otoacoustic emissions, which are present in 68% of normal-hearing infants and in 0% of people at the age of 70. Spontaneous tinnitus may be present in patients with CHL. This tinnitus may be reversible if CHL is corrected (e.g. serous otitis media and otosclerosis).

Mechanical

Myoclonus

- *Muscles involved in mechanical pulsatile tinnitus*: Tensor veli palatini, levator veli palatini, salpingopharyngeus, stapedius, tensor tympani (TT).
- This is the most common nonvascular cause of pulsatile tinnitus.
- Tinnitus sounds have irregular rhythm, may occur in bursts.
- Sounds may be objective.

- Usually, it occurs in the first 3 decades of life.
- Tensor tympani myoclonus is often associated with headache and may respond to headache treatment.

Patulous Eustachian Tube

- Autophony with recent weight loss, including weight loss after pregnancy or after cancer treatment. Tympanic membrane (TM) movements can be seen synchronous with respirations; may disappear when the patient is recumbent or when TM is mass loaded with paper or water.
- *Management*: Weight gain, tympanostomy tube placement, nasal drops to create edema of eustachian tube (ET), obstruction surgery in extreme cases, and mass loading of TM with cartilage tympanoplasty.

Pulsatile

- It accounts for about 4% of tinnitus patients; venous is much more common than arterial.
- Abnormal change in vascular contour from stenosis or compression leads to increased flow with turbulence.

Arterial

- Arteriovenous malformation, arteriovenous fistula, Paget's disease, aneurysm, atherosclerosis, fibromuscular dysplasia of the carotid artery, vascular loop, paraganglioma (Fig. 4.1).

Venous

- Benign intracranial hypertension (BIH), jugular bulb diverticula, lateral sinus stenosis, and superior canal dehiscence.

Benign intracranial hypertension:
- One of the most common causes of venous pulsatile tinnitus.
- May be associated with hearing loss, dizziness, and aural fullness.

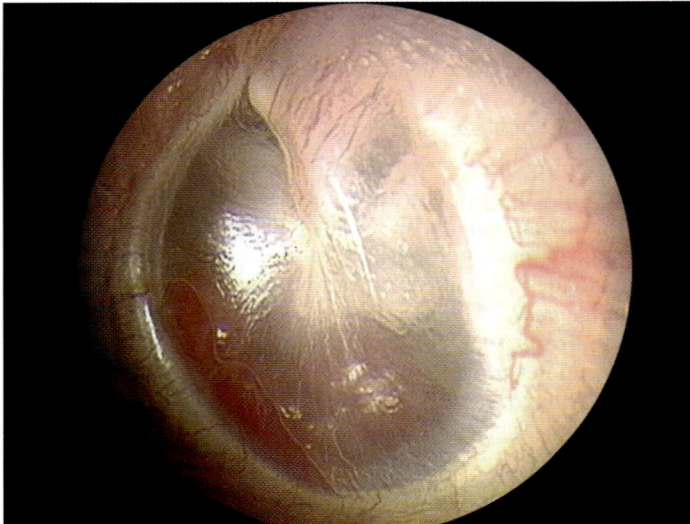

Fig. 4.1: Middle ear paraganglioma (glomus tympanicum) presents as a red pulsatile mass under the tympanic membrane.
Courtesy: Natasha Pollak, MD, USA.

- Occurs in obese women of childbearing age.
- Has increased intracranial pressure (ICP).

Superior semicircular canal dehiscence:

- Usually dehiscence at the superior petrosal sinus.

Sigmoid sinus diverticulum:

- Even small areas of exposed sinus can cause turbulent flow.

Stenosis of transverse sinus:

- Arachnoid granulations, thrombus.

Hyperdyamic flow:

- Anemia, pregnancy, thyrotoxicosis may cause a bruit in dominant jugular bulb (in 85% of patients, the right side is dominant).

Evaluation of Pulsatile Tinnitus

History:
- Note the onset, character, modifying factors (exercise, head/body position, and Valsalva), associated symptoms (hearing loss, aural fullness, and vertigo).
- *Age*: Benign intracranial hypertension occurs in women of childbearing age; AVMs become symptomatic in 5th to 6th decade of life, atherosclerosis in elderly, fibromuscular dysplasia in women between 20 and 60 years of age.
- *Factors associated with BIH*: Female gender, obesity, associated with hearing loss, aural fullness, headache, and visual disturbance.
- *Factors associated with atherosclerotic disease*: Hypertension, advanced age, diabetes, smoking, hyperlipidemia, and cerebrovascular disease.
- *Factors associated with glomus tumor (paraganglioma)*: Unilateral pulsatile tinnitus (often subjective), conductive hearing loss.
- *Factors associated with hyperdynamic flow*: Anemia, pregnancy, and thyrotoxicosis.

Examination:
- *Otoscopy*: Evaluate for middle ear pathology, jugular bulb, glomus tumor, respiratory TM movements with patulous ET or TM movements with TT myoclonus.
- *Auscultation*: Cranial, carotid, ear canal, orbits, and chest.
- Apply pressure over the internal jugular vein (IJV; head turn also obstructs the ipsilateral IJV) → decreased tinnitus ipsilaterally indicates a venous cause; there would be no change in tinnitus with an arterial cause. This is an important maneuver that drives the direction of workup.
- *Vital signs*: Blood pressure and pulse regularity.
- *Transnasal fiberoptic endoscopy*: Evaluate ET orifice, palatal myoclonus. Transoral examination of soft palate may reveal irregular contractions in palatal myoclonus.
- *Fundoscopic examination*: This may reveal papilledema.

- *Valsalva maneuver*: This reduces tinnitus associated with venous hum or patulous ET.
- *Weber/Ankle Weber*: Sound may lateralize to ear with superior canal.
- Dehiscence (any CHL may render internal sounds more audible).

Audiology:

Pure tone audiometry:
- Benign intracranial hypertension may manifest as a low-frequency hearing loss that reverses (normalizes) with IJV compression.
- In superior semicircular canal dehiscence (SCD) syndrome low-frequency CHL may be accompanied by supranormal bone thresholds.
- Any CHL may make any internal sound more evident, resulting in autophony.

Tympanometry:
- In patulous ET, tympanogram may show respiratory movements. Stapedius or TT myoclonus may be visible on tympanogram tracings.

ABR:
- Patients with BIH may show prolonged interpeak latencies in one third of cases (reverses with treatment).

Metabolic laboratory workup:
- *Complete blood count, thyroid function tests, and pregnancy test*: In patients with increased cardiac output, to rule out hyperthyroidism and anemia.
- *Lipid profile and fasting blood glucose*: If there is suspected atherosclerotic disease of the carotid system.
- Alkaline phosphatase is elevated in Paget's disease.

Ultrasound:
- Duplex carotid ultrasound including subclavian arteries; order before computed tomography angiography (CTA), if the patient has isolated carotid bruits.
- *Echocardiogram*: If there is suspected valvular disease.

Radiologic evaluation:

- The choice of radiologic studies is based on otoscopic findings and characteristics of the tinnitus: computed tomography (CT), CTA, magnetic resonance imaging (MRI)/magnetic resonance angiography (MRA)/magnetic resonance venography (MRV) (Flowchart 4.1)

Otoscopy normal and suspected venous pulsatile tinnitus:

- Computed tomography of the temporal bones.
- Identifies sigmoid sinus dehiscence/diverticula, SCD, thinning of temporal squamosa (associated with increased ICP/BIH), tegmen dehiscence (also associated with increased ICP/BIH).
- Magnetic resonance imaging /MR venogram.
- Identifies jugular bulb and dural venous sinus abnormalities, BIH signs (empty sella, small ventricles, and flattened posterior globe of eye).

Otoscopy normal and suspected arterial pulsatile tinnitus:

- Computed tomographic angiogram, which includes upper neck, may identify cervical vascular pathology (carotid body tumor), tortuous carotid vessels, AVF/AVM, carotid artery dissection or aneurysm, cervical or intracranial atherosclerotic disease of carotid, fibromuscular dysplasia, and aneurysm.

Otoscopy abnormal:

- Computed tomographic angiogram of the temporal bones first, which identifies ectopic carotid artery, jugular bulb abnormalities, glomus tumor, and associated carotid body tumor.
- Carotid angiography is ordered only if there is a strong suspicion of AVF/AVM (loud retroauricular bruits) or for prospective surgical candidates.

Other testing:

- Lumbar puncture with the measurement of opening pressure for patients with BIH.

Flowchart 4.1: Workup of pulsatile tinnitus.

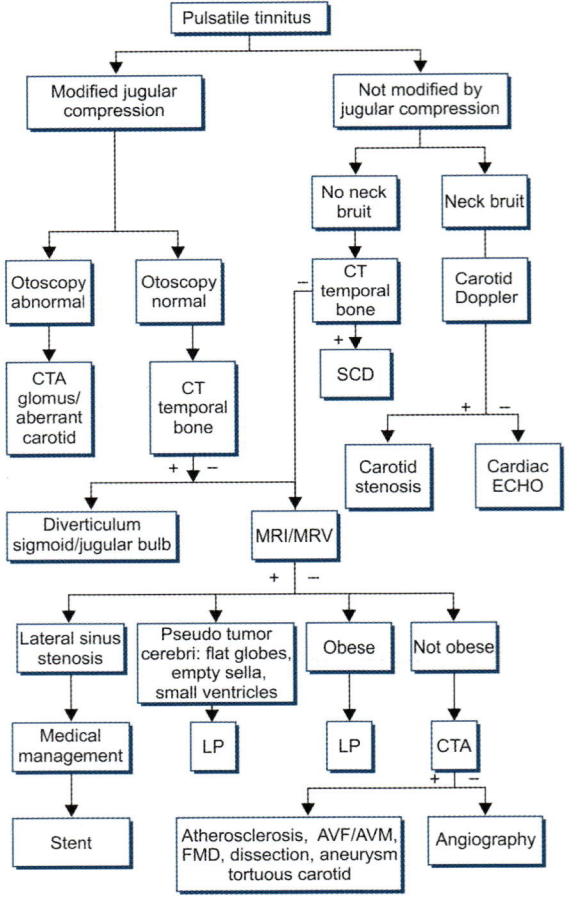

(CT: Computed tomography; CTA: Computed tomography angiography; SCD: Semicircular canal dehiscence; MRI: Magnetic resonance imaging; MRV: Magnetic resonance venography; ECHO: Echocardiogram; LP: Lumbar puncture; AVF: Arteriovenous fistula; AVM: Arteriovenous malformation; FMD: Fibromuscular dysplasia of the carotid).

Management of Pulsatile Tinnitus

- Management is directed at the underlying cause.

BIH

- Educate the patient on association with obesity.
- *Weight reduction*: It will reduce or eliminate pulsatile tinnitus in most patients.
- *Acetazolamide*: Causes decrease in cerebrospinal fluid production. It may reduce intensity, but rarely eliminates tinnitus.
- Ventriculoperitoneal shunt, if tinnitus is disabling, or if there is a progressive effect on vision or persistent headaches.
- Weight-reduction surgery.
- Need follow-up with ophthalmologists and neurologists.

Atherosclerotic Carotid Artery Disease

- Consider surgical intervention if pulsatile tinnitus is bothersome.
- Carotid endarterectomy and angioplasty with stenting are the possible options.

Glomus Tympanicum

- *Surgical excision via tympanotomy*: Larger tumors may require a mastoidectomy with an extended facial recess approach or a transcanal hypotympanotomy.

Glomus Jugulare

- Surgery versus stereotactic radiation versus combined treatment.

Carotid Artery Dissection

- Anticoagulants may be effective in preventing emboli.

High/Dehiscent Jugular Bulb

- Surgical repair with bone dust, perichondrium, or cartilage graft in severely symptomatic cases.

Middle Ear Myoclonus

- Pulsatile tinnitus due to TT or stapedius myoclonus responds to migraine prophylaxis, if headache is present. Surgical section of the TT and/or stapedius may be offered.

Palatal Myoclonus

- Botox injections of the tensor veli palatini muscle are helpful in some cases.

Dural AVF

- Coiling/embolization.

Ligation of Ipsilateral IJV

- Poor results for venous pulsatile tinnitus.

Superior Semicircular Canal Dehiscence at Superior Petrosal Sinus

- Middle fossa or transmastoid surgical repair if symptoms warrant (dehiscence is often not visible from the standard middle fossa approach).

Lateral Sinus Stenosis

- Venous stenting in severely affected individuals.

SUGGESTED READING

1. Baomin L, Yongbing S, Xiangyu C. Angioplasty and stenting for intractable pulsatile tinnitus caused by dural venous sinus stenosis: a case series report. Otol Neurotol. 2014;35(2):366-70.
2. Eisenman DJ. Sinus wall reconstruction for sigmoid sinus diverticulum and dehiscence: a standardized surgical procedure for a range of radiographic findings. Otol Neurotol. 2011;32(7): 1116-9.
3. Pollak N, Azadarmaki R, Ahmad S. Endoscopic treatment of middle ear myoclonus with stapedius and tensor tympani section:

a new minimally-invasive approach. Br J Med Med Res. 2014; 4(17): 3398-405.

4. Sismanis A. Pulsatile tinnitus: contemporary assessment and management. Curr Opin Otolaryngol Head Neck Surg. 2011;19:348-57.

5. Teixido MT, Seymour P, Kung B, et al. Transmastoid middle fossa craniotomy repair of superior semicircular canal dehiscence using a soft tissue graft. Otol Neurotol. 2011;32(5):877-81.

6. Tunkel D, Bauer CA, Sun GH, et al. Clinical practice guideline: tinnitus. Otolaryngol Head Neck Surg. 2014;151(2 Suppl):S1-40. Available from www.entnet.org/content/clinical-practice-guideline-tinnitus. Accessed October 2014.

Chapter 5

Trauma to the Ear

Natasha Pollak

> **Chief Complaint**
> *"I had an accident and injured my ear or head. Ear is bleeding or draining".*

DEFINITIONS

Alexander's law: Describes horizontal nystagmus that occurs after an acute peripheral vestibular injury. The fast phase of the nystagmus is directed toward the healthy ear. Nystagmus worsens when looking toward the healthy ear and is attenuated when gaze is directed toward the affected ear.

Anterior tympanostomy: Approach to the tympanic membrane (TM) and middle ear cleft via the external auditory canal. This is in contrast to a posterior tympanostomy, which approaches the middle ear cleft via the mastoid and facial recess.

ATLS: Advanced trauma life support.

Battle sign: Postauricular ecchymosis, sometimes seen in patients with temporal bone fractures.

Cauliflower ear: Pinna deformity resulting from an untreated auricular hematoma.

EcochG (electrocochleography): Neurophysiologic test performed by audiologists, often used to support the diagnosis of Ménière's disease.

ENoG (electroneurography): A neurophysiologic test that examines the integrity and conductivity of a peripheral nerve. It is often used for serial testing of the facial nerve after acute onset of unilateral facial paralysis.

Hemotympanum: Blood behind the eardrum, in the middle ear space.

Myringoplasty: Surgical repair of the tympanic membrane.

SP/AP: The summating potential (SP) and action potential (AP) are measured during the EcochG test. If the ratio of the SP and AP is > 0.5, then EcochG supports the presence of endolymphatic hydrops or Ménière's disease in the tested ear.

Tympanoplasty: Surgical repair of the tympanic membrane and/or exploration and repair of the structures of the middle ear.

VEMP (vestibular-evoked myogenic potential) test: An electrophysiologic test of the otolith organs, specifically the saccule innervated by the inferior vestibular nerve. It also tests the integrity of the vestibulo-collic reflex.

EXTERNAL EAR TRAUMA (TRAUMA TO THE PINNA)
Pinna Laceration

Anatomy and Physiology

Although the principles for pinna laceration repair are essentially the same as for any other laceration, the complex three-dimensional anatomy of the pinna often makes repairs challenging. Even minor distortions of the normal pinna contour can be perceived as disfiguring.

Treatment

Treatment of a pinna laceration begins with administration of adequate local anesthesia or a regional nerve block of the auriculotemporal nerve and/or great auricular nerve. Preparations such as lidocaine with dilute epinephrine are acceptable. The wound is examined and thoroughly cleansed of debris. Lacerations are repaired primarily if possible. Deeper or full-thickness wounds require a layered repair. Cartilage lacerations are repaired by approximating the perichondrium with 5-0 or 6-0 absorbable suture. Any exposed cartilage should be covered with skin. If skin cannot be repaired primarily, a local skin advancement or rotation flap should be designed. The goal of repair is to close the wound and achieve an esthetically acceptable outcome. The repair is covered with bacitracin ointment. A compression dressing may be needed to prevent formation of a hematoma. Prophylactic antibiotics may be used if cartilage was lacerated. Sutures are removed 5–7 days after repair. The patient may need a tetanus vaccination booster.

Complications

Possible complications after pinna laceration repair include chondritis, hematoma, keloid formation, and wound infection.

Pinna Avulsion

Anatomy and Physiology

A pinna avulsion is defined as loss of a portion of the pinna or the entire pinna, without any skin bridges or other soft tissue attachments to the head. A simple reattachment of the avulsed pinna as a compound graft usually results in graft necrosis and complete loss of the pinna. Multiple approaches to management of pinna avulsions have been described in the literature, with microvascular repair techniques showing consistently better results over the others. The blood supply to the pinna comes from branches of the external carotid artery. The posterior auricular artery—a direct branch of the external carotid—supplies the posterior surface of the pinna and the helix. The terminal branch of the external carotid is the superficial temporal artery (STA). The STA gives off several auricular branches, which supply most of the anterior surface of the pinna. The superior auricular branch gives off the helical artery, which enters the pinna at the helical root.

Treatment

Microvascular repair: If the helical artery can be identified and is of adequate caliber, a microvascular repair and reattachment of the pinna can be attempted.[1] As there is no venous anastomosis, therapeutic bleeding or leeches can be used to relieve venous congestion.

Pocket techniques: The classic Mladick pocket technique, described in 1971, involves de-epithelializing the avulsed pinna using microdermabrasion, then reattaching the pinna cartilage to its stump. A postauricular pocket is developed and the pinna cartilage placed in that pocket. After a few months, a second procedure is needed to elevate the pinna and recreate the postauricular groove with a partial-thickness skin graft.[2] The classic Mladick pocket technique is now rarely used and has been supplanted by several modified pocket procedures. One such modification involves removing only the postauricular skin, then making several fenestrations in the cartilage to allow contact of the anterior skin with the vascular bed. The pinna is reattached to its stump. The skin edges along the helix are sutured to the postauricular vascular bed. A second-stage procedure is needed at a few months later to recreate the postauricular sulcus.[3] With this technique, dermolysis and cartilage shrinkage can be seen.

Pinna Hematoma

Anatomy and Physiology

Auricular hematoma is often seen in wrestlers and in practitioners of martial arts or other contact sports. The hematoma presents as a fluctuant swelling on the pinna with a dark discoloration. A pinna hematoma occurs when shearing forces separate the perichondrium from the auricular cartilage. As the cartilage receives its blood supply from the perichondrium, it is important to drain the hematoma in a timely manner to prevent cartilage necrosis and subsequent pinna deformity, called a "cauliflower ear."

Treatment

Auricular hematomas can be drained via a large-bore needle or a small incision. Recurrence of hematoma is common. For that reason, a bolster is placed to press the perichondrium against the cartilage. An example of an appropriate bolster may be a dental roll or cotton ball wrapped in petrolatum gauze, placed on both sides of the pinna, and secured with a through-and-through prolene or nylon suture. Prophylactic antibiotics may be used for 5–7 days until the bolster is removed.

Ear Canal Trauma

Ear Canal Abrasions

These occur most often when the patient self-instruments the ear in an attempt to remove cerumen or relieve pruritus. Most ear canal abrasions do not require any treatment and are managed expectantly. Sometimes, debridement may be necessary under office otomicroscopy. Stenting may be helpful if there is a partial avulsion of the ear canal skin.

Ear Canal Bony Fractures

These are often seen in temporal bone fractures. An ear canal bony fracture raises suspicion for a more extensive temporal bone fracture. History usually reveals a recent head trauma. Examination shows bloody otorrhea and a deeper ear canal laceration with possible exposed bone. Computed tomography (CT) of the temporal bones without contrast is indicated. Most ear canal bony fractures are managed conservatively, but can sometimes result in ear canal stenosis.

MIDDLE EAR TRAUMA

Tympanic Membrane Perforation

Diagnosis

A tympanic membrane (TM) perforation can occur after ear probing, after explosive trauma, barotrauma, an open-handed slap, or iatrogenically during attempts to remove cerumen or an ear foreign body. Symptoms may include bloody otorrhea, pain, hearing loss, and tinnitus. A traumatic TM perforation is usually diagnosed by otoscopy and confirmed with tympanometry. A full audiogram is usually performed as well.

Treatment

Ototopic medications are not routinely used, but should be considered in a "dirty injury" where contaminants may have entered the middle ear space through the perforation, or if the ear becomes infected. TM perforations are managed conservatively, and even larger perforations usually heal spontaneously. Dry ear precautions are recommended. Surgery is indicated if the perforation has not healed after 2 months. A myringoplasty or tympanoplasty can be performed via anterior tympanostomy.

Ossicular Trauma

Diagnosis

Ossicular dislocation may occur in conjunction with TM perforations. Penetrating trauma can cause ossicle displacement, dislocation, or fracture, resulting in discontinuity of the ossicular chain and associated conductive hearing loss.

Treatment

These ossicular injuries do not heal spontaneously and need to be surgically repaired. A tympanoplasty is performed, either via a transcanal or postauricular approach, with the goal of repairing the TM perforation and re-establishing ossicular continuity using native ossicles or a partial or total ossicular reconstruction prosthesis (PORP or TORP).

INNER EAR TRAUMA

Perilymph Fistula

Diagnosis

A perilymph fistula (PLF) can result from a penetrating ear injury, other concussive head injury, or barotrauma. The patient might experience sensorineural hearing loss and dizziness in addition to the symptoms encountered with a traumatic TM perforation. The round window or oval window niche may be disrupted, resulting in a small leak of perilymph from the inner ear into the middle ear. As the total volume of perilymph is only ~0.07 mL, the fluid leak can rarely be seen even intraoperatively with the use or otomicoscopy while the anesthesiologist performs a Valsalva maneuver. The presence of a PLF is inferred in a patient with ear or head trauma who also has acute sensorineural hearing loss in the affected ear and dizziness that worsens with coughing, sneezing, or blowing the nose. The presence of a PLF can be supported by performing a fistula test, which involves applying positive pressure to the external auditory canal while observing for development of nystagmus. Several other otologic conditions may results in a positive fistula test, such as superior semicircular canal dehiscence (SSCD) syndrome and Ménière's disease; in those cases, however, the patient would not have a history of recent head trauma. An audiogram is also performed in a patient with a suspected PLF and may show unilateral sensorineural hearing loss in the affected ear. EcochG may show an elevated SP/AP ratio in both PLF and Ménière's disease. VEMP may show elevated thresholds in both PLF and SSCD. Computed tomography (CT) and magnetic resonance imaging (MRI) have no role in the diagnosis of a PLF, except to rule out other conditions. MRI may rule out a vestibular schwannoma. CT of the temporal bones may rule out SSCD or a congenital malformation of the otic capsule in children. Diagnosis of a PLF is difficult and indications for surgical repair are controversial.

Treatment

Treatment of a PLF involves avoidance of strenuous activity, elevation of the head of the bed, and stool softeners. The patient is followed with serial audiograms. Most PLFs resolve spontaneously; however, if symptoms persist or hearing worsens, surgery can be considered. An exploratory tympanotomy is performed, the round (and oval) window niche is denuded of native mucosa, and then sealed with a fascia plug. PLF recurrence is seen in a significant minority of patients, even after surgery.

TEMPORAL BONE FRACTURE

General Considerations

For all trauma patients (except minor trauma), first initiate the primary survey of the ATLS protocol:

1. *Airway*: Establish a secure airway while protecting the cervical spine.
2. *Breathing*: Ensure patient is breathing; provide assisted ventilation and intubation if necessary.
3. *Circulation*: Ensure patient is hemodynamically stable; control any hemorrhage.
4. *Disability and neurologic assessment*: Perform a neurologic survey, including the 12 cranial nerves.
5. *Exposure and environmental control*: Remove garments; warm the patient.

Diagnosis

Patients with temporal bone fractures have a recent history of head trauma. They may have unilateral hearing loss, dizziness, or nausea. Examination may show a Battle sign, serous or bloody otorrhea, hemotympanum, or even facial nerve paralysis. The status of the facial nerve should be documented in all patients with temporal bone fractures. Tuning fork tests may indicate conductive or sensorineural hearing loss.

Radiology

Patients with head trauma usually have a CT head scan performed after initial resuscitation. A temporal bone fracture may be apparent. Dedicated high-resolution CT imaging of the temporal bones is useful and is indicated in cases of suspected otic capsule fracture, facial nerve palsy, or cerebrospinal fluid (CSF) otorrhea. CT imaging may show a longitudinal or transverse temporal bone fracture (Fig. 5.1). True longitudinal fractures are infrequent. Instead, most often an oblique fracture is seen, approximately

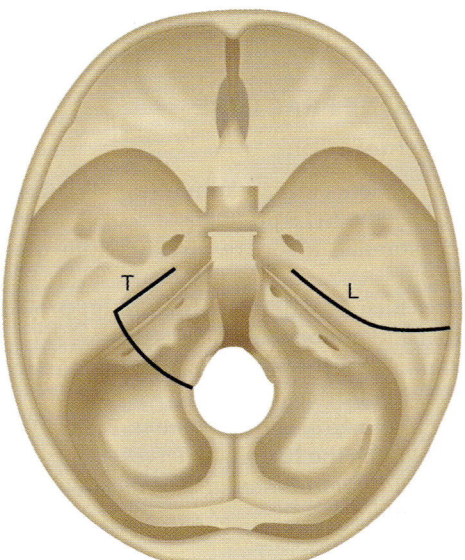

Fig. 5.1: A transverse temporal bone fracture (T) occurs after a blow to the occipital region. It originates at the foramen magnum, crosses the petrous ridge, involves the facial canal and otic capsule, and ends near the foramen lacerum. A longitudinal temporal bone fracture (L) occurs after a blow to the temporoparietal region. It originates at the squamous portion of the temporal bone, runs parallel to the petrous ridge avoiding the otic capsule, and ends at the foramen lacerum.

paralleling the petrous ridge. These fractures occur from a blow to the temporoparietal region and usually do not involve the dense bone of the labyrinth. Conductive hearing loss and ossicular disruption are common, but sensorineural hearing loss is rare. Facial nerve injury is uncommon in longitudinal/oblique fractures and is usually delayed onset and temporary. Transverse temporal bone fractures are less frequent and occur from a blow to the occipital region. These fractures carry a higher morbidity. Facial nerve paralysis occurs in approximately half of transverse fractures and is immediate and permanent. The otic capsule is frequently fractured, resulting in sensorineural deafness and loss of peripheral vestibular function, which results in horizontal nystagmus following Alexander's law.

Treatment

Temporal bone fractures usually do not require surgical reduction, and the vast majority are treated expectantly. Specific treatment approaches are needed for some complications that can occur as a result of a temporal bone fracture.

Complications

Hemotympanum

A blood collection can often be seen under an intact TM after a temporal bone fracture. This can cause temporary hearing loss. Hemotympanum usually resolves within a few weeks after injury and does not require any specific treatment.

Hearing Loss

A temporal bone fracture can result in both conductive and sensorineural hearing loss. A bedside tuning fork examination may help distinguish between the two types of hearing loss. The Weber test is performed by placing the base of the tuning fork on the patient's forehead in the midline. A patient with normal hearing will not localize the sound to either ear, but rather report that the sound is heard in the midline. A patient with a conductive hearing loss will localize the sound to the affected ear, while a patient with a sensorineural hearing loss will localize the sound to the contralateral, unaffected ear. Conductive hearing loss can occur due to hemotympanum or ossicular disruption, while sensorineural hearing loss can occur due to disruption of the otic capsule, which more commonly happens in transverse temporal bone fractures. Otic capsule disruption usually results in a deaf ear and cannot be recovered. All patients with temporal bone fractures should have a baseline audiogram about a month after the injury, to assess the status of their hearing and counsel them on hearing rehabilitation options as appropriate.

Cerebrospinal Fluid (CSF) Leak

A CSF leak occurs in fewer than 20% of temporal bone fractures. Patients may have CSF otorrhea that leaves a classic "halo sign" on their pillow. While testing of otorrhea fluid for beta-2 transferrin may be helpful, it is often difficult to collect the necessary fluid volumes required to complete these tests. Most CSF otorrhea after temporal bone fractures can be treated conservatively with bed rest, head-of-bed elevation, and other CSF leak precautions, including placement of a lumbar drain. If CSF otorrhea persists after conservative treatment, a thorough radiologic investigation with high-resolution CT of the temporal bones may be helpful in identifying the site of the leak. MRI, CT cisternography, and radionuclide cisternography may help localize the site of the leak. The choice of surgical approach depends upon the site of the leak.

Facial Nerve Injury

Delayed-onset facial nerve palsy after a temporal bone fracture is almost always temporary and is treated with a course of steroids and counseling on corneal protection as needed. Management of facial nerve paralysis that occurs immediately after the injury is more complex and is the subject of some debate.

Surgical decompression may be needed. A high-resolution CT of the temporal bones is obtained to examine the course of the facial nerve in detail. If the site of injury can be identified, then surgical decompression can be limited to the affected segment. In longitudinal fractures, bony spicules may impinge upon the facial nerve, or the nerve may be edematous from crush injury or have an intraneural hematoma. Less frequently, the facial nerve may be transected. In transverse fractures, the facial nerve is nearly always transected. The nerve may require decompression or reanastomosis. Anastomosis is performed by approximating the epineurium with several 7-0 or smaller sutures. A cable graft may be required if primary anastomosis is not possible. A cable graft can be harvested from the great auricular or sural nerve. If the site of facial nerve injury cannot be identified radiologically, the patient may be followed using a protocol similar to that used for Bell's palsy. The role of ENoG in the management algorithm for traumatic facial nerve paralysis is not well defined. Paralleling the protocol for Bell's palsy, ENoG can be performed every 3 days. If ENoG shows < 95% degeneration within 14 days, prognosis for full recovery of facial function is good. Otherwise, surgical exploration of the entire course of the facial nerve may be indicated, which requires a translabyrinthine or middle fossa approach, depending on the status of the patient's hearing.

BAROTRAUMA

Physics

Barotrauma to the ear occurs mostly in divers, but also sometimes with air travel. Air-filled spaces in the body are affected by sudden pressure changes according to Boyle's law. Boyle's law states that, given a constant temperature, the volume of a gas varies inversely with the pressure. For each 10 m (33 ft) of seawater through which a diver descends, pressure increases by 1 atm. In relative terms, therefore, the greatest pressure changes occur in shallow waters. More frequent ear-pressure equalization maneuvers are needed near the water surface. Divers are trained to perform several different maneuvers to allow them to equalize their middle ear pressure through the eustachian tube.

Middle Ear Barotrauma

Diagnosis

Symptoms of middle ear barotrauma include a sensation of ear fullness, otalgia, or hearing loss. Findings on otoscopy may include a tympanic membrane (TM) retraction, erythema, or localized hemorrhage within the drum. Hemotympanum or TM perforation may be seen. Tuning fork testing and audiometry may show conductive hearing loss.

Treatment

Treatment is conservative, mostly with oral and topical decongestants. Antibiotic ear drops may be used if there is suspicion of a bacterial superinfection. TM perforations in the setting of barotrauma usually heal spontaneously, but some may require surgical repair. A perforated TM precludes diving.

Inner Ear Barotrauma (Perilymph Fistula)

Diagnosis

The diver may experience sudden onset of dizziness, hearing loss, tinnitus, and nausea, usually on descent. An otoscopic examination may reveal concomitant signs of middle ear barotrauma or no visible abnormalities at all. The presence of sensorineural hearing loss and dizziness indicates inner ear involvement. The mechanism of injury is thought to be a PLF of the round or oval window.

Treatment

Treatment involves bed rest with the head of the bed elevated, steroids, and avoidance of any coughing or straining. If hearing loss and vertigo persist after a few days, surgical exploration may be indicated to repair the presumed PLF.

Inner Ear Decompression Sickness

Diagnosis

Inner ear decompression sickness (IEDS) can occur as part of a known syndrome of decompression sickness ("the bends"). In a classic scenario, a professional diver using a helium-containing breathing mixture exceeds the recommended depth or diving time and, upon ascending or shortly after surfacing, develops sudden dizziness, hearing loss, tinnitus, and nausea. The mechanism of injury is thought to be formation of gas bubbles in the fluids of the inner ear, as the dissolved gasses come out of solution at lower pressures. More commonly, IEDS occurs in divers with a cardiac right-to-left shunt such as a patent foramen ovale (PFO). PFO is present in about a quarter of the population. Otoscopic examination is usually normal, and tuning fork testing may show a unilateral sensorineural hearing loss.

Treatment

Treatment involves prompt recompression in a hyperbaric chamber, breathing 100% oxygen.

REFERENCES

1. Pennington DG, Lai MF, Pelly AD. Successful replantation of a completely avulsed ear by microvascular anastomosis. Plast Reconstr Surg. 1980;65(6):820-3.
2. Mladick RA, Horton CE, Adamson JE, et al. The pocket principle: a new technique for the reattachment of a severed ear part. Plast Reconstr Surg. 1971;48(3):219-23.
3. Baudet J, Tramond P, Goumain A. A new technique for the reimplantation of a completely severed auricle. Ann Chir Plast. 1972;17:67-72.

Chapter 6

Microbiology and Antimicrobial Therapy of the Ear

Purva Gumaste, Rafik Samuel

> ***Chief Complaint***
> *"My ear hurts", "My ear drains".*

DEFINITION

PICC: Peripherally inserted central catheter.

OTITIS EXTERNA (SWIMMER'S EAR)

Otitis externa (OE) is defined as a diffuse inflammation of the external ear canal, which may also involve the pinna or the tympanic membrane (TM).

Types of OE:
1. Acute OE
2. Fungal OE (otomycosis)
3. Chronic OE
4. Malignant OE (skull base osteomyelitis)

ACUTE OTITIS EXTERNA

Etiology

Aerobic bacteria such as *Pseudomonas aeruginosa* (38%), *Staphylococcus epidermidis* (9%), *Staphylococcus aureus* (8%)

and, less commonly, *Haemophilus influenza* and *Escherichia coli*. Anaerobic pathogens are present in 4–25% of general population, most commonly *Bacteroides* and *Peptostreptococci* spp.[1-3]

Treatment

- *Mild external otitis*: Gentle cleansing to remove debris along with use of a topical preparation with an acidifying agent such as acetic acid with hydrocortisone.
- *Moderate and severe external otitis*: Use a topical medication that contains an antibiotic, an antiseptic, and a glucocorticoid.
- Commonly used topical glucocorticoids such as hydrocortisone, dexamethasone, and prednisolone decrease inflammation, resulting in relief of pruritus and pain.
- Topical antibiotics are highly effective and should cover most common pathogens such as *Pseudomonas* and *S. aureus*. Fluoroquinolones such as ciprofloxacin and ofloxacin are frequently used. Polymyxin B and neomycin combinations are available that cover both organisms.
- Ensure adequate pain control with oral nonsteroidal anti-inflammatory agents. Systemic antibiotics are reserved for extensive deep tissue infection and immunosuppressed patients.
- *Duration of treatment*: 7–10 days. Failure of symptoms to improve in 2 weeks warrants re-evaluation.

FUNGAL OTITIS EXTERNA

Fungal OE (otomycosis) accounts for 10% of cases of OE in the United States.

Etiology

- *Aspergillus* species: *A. niger, A. flavus, A. fumigatus*
- *Candida* species: *C. albicans, C. parapsilosis*
- Rarely *Phycomycetes, Rhizopus, Penicillium*.

Predisposing Conditions

Diabetes mellitus, immunocompromised state, prior history of OE, prolonged use of antibiotics and corticosteroid drops, moist ear canals, and chronic ear probing.

Treatment

Meticulous cleaning and topical antifungal therapy: All debris and visible fungal elements should be removed under direct supervision. Clotrimazole is the commonly used antifungal agent. Administer clotrimazole 1% solution twice daily for 2 weeks and then reassess the ear canal. Systemic oral antifungals may be used in refractory cases, and intravenous antifungals are reserved for invasive otomycosis.

CHRONIC OTITIS EXTERNA

Thickening of the external auditory canal skin secondary to a persistent low-grade infection and inflammation. It affects 3–5% of general population, involving both ears in at least half of them.[4]

Etiology

- *Infectious*: Caused by irritation from chronic drainage secondary to chronic suppurative otitis media or wet mastoid cavity. Rarely due to tuberculosis, syphilis, yaws, and leprosy.
- *Autoimmune*: Sarcoidosis, granulomatosis with polyangiitis. (Wegener granulomatosis), Sjögren disease, psoriasis, and cutaneous Crohn's disease.
- *Allergic/dermatological*: Dermatophytid reaction, contact allergen (nickel, neomycin), contact dermatitis.

Treatment

The goal is to restore the external auditory canal skin to a healthy state and to promote normal cerumen production. Medium- and high-potency topical steroid preparations such as betamethasone 0.1% and triamcinolone 0.1% have been shown to provide some improvement. Tacrolimus 0.1% ointment has shown efficacy in atopic dermatitis and noninfectious chronic OE. Bacteriophage therapy has shown some improvement in symptoms of patients with chronic otitis externa due to antibiotic-resistant *P. aeruginosa*. Bacteriophages are viruses that specifically infect and kill the bacteria causing the infection.

NECROTIZING (MALIGNANT) OTITIS EXTERNA

Malignant OE is an invasive infection of the external auditory canal, spreading and resulting in osteomyelitis of the temporal bone and skull base. The infection typically begins at the bony–cartilaginous junction of the external auditory canal and spreads, possibly through the Santorini fissures into the mastoid bone and along the base of the skull.

Etiology

P. aeruginosa is almost always the causative agent. Rarely, other organisms have been reported.[5]

Risk Factors

Diabetes mellitus, advanced age, and immunocompromised state. Increasing incidence is seen in AIDS patients. Many reports suggest an association between aural irrigation and onset of necrotizing OE.

Treatment

Systemic antipseudomonal antibiotics are the mainstay of therapy. For adults, ciprofloxacin (400 mg every 8 hours or 750 mg every 12 hours) remains the drug of choice. Levofloxacin has antipseudomonal activity also, but clinical experience has not been reported. In case of ciprofloxacin resistance, antipseudomonal beta-lactam drugs such as piperacillin, ceftazidime, or cefepime can be used based on susceptibility.

These must be administered intravenously, usually through a PICC line. Prolonged treatment for 6–8 weeks is recommended.

CHRONIC OTITIS MEDIA

Chronic otitis media (COM) is defined as an ear with a TM perforation in the setting of recurrent or chronic ear infections.

COM is classified as:

- *Chronic serous otitis media*: Characterized by continuous serous drainage.
- *Chronic suppurative otitis media (CSOM)*: Diagnosed when there is persistent purulent drainage through a perforated TM or tympanostomy tube. Usually follows an episode of AOM.
- *Cholesteatoma*: A keratinized, desquamated epithelial collection in the middle ear or mastoid that may occur as a primary lesion or may be secondary to TM perforation or surgery.

Microbiology

P. aeruginosa and *S. aureus* are the most commonly isolated aerobic bacteria. Enteric gram-negative rods such as *Proteus, Klebsiella*, and *E. coli* are common in areas with poor hygienic conditions. Several studies reported anaerobic isolates ranging from 8% to 59%.

Biofilms have also been associated in the pathogenesis of CSOM. A biofilm is a community of bacteria, embedded in a matrix they created, that adheres to a foreign body or a mucosal surface. The role of biofilms in patients with cholesteatoma is better defined. In several small studies, biofilms were detected in 14–92% of patients with CSOM.[6,7]

Treatment

Aural Toilet

The goal is to stop otorrhea. Lukewarm irrigation solutions such as 1:1 dilutions of distilled white vinegar, saline, or povidone iodine with water can be used. Aural irrigation is typically performed two to three times daily until discharge disappears.

Antibiotics

Topical antibiotics are the first-line treatment for uncomplicated otorrhea as they can achieve increased concentration in the middle ear cavity. Topical ciprofloxacin and ofloxacin are the ototopical agents used in case of TM perforation. Topical corticosteroid combination drops with an antibiotic can be used if granulation tissue is present.

Treatment failure can occur in case of a resistant organism, presence of a cholesteatoma, or poor adherence to the prescribed medical regimen. Treatment is considered to have failed if otorrhea persists despite 3 weeks of medical therapy. Cultures directly from the middle ear should be obtained in such cases. Systemic antibiotics may have decreased efficacy secondary to inflammation and scarring in CSOM as well as with limited blood supply to the middle ear mucosa.

ACUTE OTITIS MEDIA

Acute otitis media (AOM) is defined by moderate to severe bulging of the TM or new onset of otorrhea not due to acute OE, accompanied by acute signs of illness and signs or symptoms of middle ear inflammation.

Etiology

Bacterial and/or viral respiratory tract pathogens can be isolated from most middle ear aspirates from children with AOM. The most common bacteria are *Streptococcus pneumoniae*, *H. influenza*, and *Moraxella catarrhalis*. Rarely, *Streptococcus pyogenes*, *S. aureus*, enteric gram-negative bacteria and *Mycoplasma pneumoniae* have been reported. Viruses including respiratory syncytial virus, picornaviruses (e.g. rhinovirus, enterovirus), coronaviruses, influenza viruses, adenoviruses, and human metapneumovirus can cause AOM.

Treatment

Observation

Used in unilateral AOM in children 6 months to 23 months or AOM ≥2 years without severe signs and symptoms. When observation is used, ensure follow-up and instructions to the caregiver to begin antibiotic if the child worsens or fails to improve in 48–72 hours of onset of symptoms.

Antibiotic Therapy

Used in AOM (unilateral or bilateral) in children ≥ 6 months of age with severe signs and symptoms. Physicians should not prescribe prophylactic antibiotics to reduce the frequency of AOM.

Amoxicillin 90 mg/kg/d divided in two doses (maximum 3 g/d) if there is a low suspicion of resistance.

If there is a high suspicion for resistance, such as prior use of beta-lactam antibiotic in the previous 30 days or concomitant purulent conjunctivitis (conjunctivitis–otitis media syndrome mainly caused by *H. influenzae*), the recommendation is to use amoxicillin–clavulanate.

Pain Control

Oral ibuprofen or acetaminophen for pain control in children with AOM. Topical benzocaine preparations are an alternative for children ≥2 years, but should not be used in children with a perforated TM.

Duration of Treatment

Children <2 years, children with AOM and TM perforation, and children with a history of recurrent AOM should be treated for 10 days.

Children ≥2 years without TM perforation or a history of recurrent AOM should be treated for 5–7 days (Tables 6.1 and 6.2).

Other Measures

In order to reduce the incidence of AOM, the physician may recommend avoidance of tobacco smoke, exclusive breastfeeding for the first 6 months of life, and annual influenza vaccine per published guidelines.

Table 6.1: Recommendations for initial management of uncomplicated AOM.

Age	Unilateral AOM* without otorrhea	Bilateral AOM* without otorrhea	Unilateral or bilateral AOM* with severe symptoms†	Otorrhea with AOM*
6 months to 2 years	Antibiotic therapy or additional observation	Antibiotic therapy	Antibiotic therapy	Antibiotic therapy
≥2 years	Antibiotic therapy or additional observation‡	Antibiotic therapy or additional observation	Antibiotic therapy	Antibiotic therapy

(AOM: Acute otitis media).

*Applies only to children with well-documented AOM with high certainty of diagnosis.

†A toxic-appearing child, persistent otalgia more than 48 hours, temperature ≥39°C (102.2°F) in the past 48 hours, or if there is uncertain access to follow-up after the visit.

‡This plan of initial management provides an opportunity for shared decision-making with the child's family for those categories appropriate for additional observation. If observation is offered, a mechanism must be in place to ensure follow-up and begin antibiotics if the child worsens or fails to improve within 48–72 hours of AOM onset.

Source: From Lieberthal AS, Carroll AE, Chonmaitree T, et al. The diagnosis and management of acute otitis media. Pediatrics. 2013;131(3):e964-99.

Table 6.2: Recommended antibiotics for (initial or delayed) treatment of acute otitis media and for patients who have failed initial antibiotic treatment.

Initial immediate or delayed antibiotic treatment		Antibiotic treatment after 48–72 hours of failure of initial antibiotic treatment	
Recommended first-line treatment	*Alternative treatment (if penicillin allergy)*	*Recommended first-line treatment*	*Alternative treatment*
Amoxicillin (80–90 mg/kg/d in two divided doses)	Cefdinir‡ (14 mg/kg/d in one or two doses)	Amoxicillin-clavulanate* (90 mg/kg/d of amoxicillin, with 6.4 mg/kg/d of clavulanate in two divided doses)	Ceftriaxone, 3 days Clindamycin (30–40 mg/kg/d in three divided doses), with or without third-generation cephalosporin
Or	Cefuroxime‡ (30 mg/kg/d in two divided doses)	Or	Failure of second antibiotic

Contd ...

Contd ...

Initial immediate or delayed antibiotic treatment		Antibiotic treatment after 48–72 hours of failure of initial antibiotic treatment	
Recommended first-line treatment	Alternative treatment (if penicillin allergy)	Recommended first-line treatment	Alternative treatment
Amoxicillin-clavulanate* [90 mg/kg/d of amoxicillin, with 6.4 mg/kg/d of clavulanate (amoxicillin to clavulanate ratio, 14:1) in two divided doses]	Cefpodoxime‡ (10 mg/ kg/d in two divided doses) Ceftriaxone‡ (50 mg IM or IV per day for 1 or 3 days)	Ceftriaxone (50 mg IM or IV for 3 days)	Clindamycin (30–40 mg/ kg/d in three divided doses) plus third-generation cephalosporin Tympanocentesis† Consult specialist†

(IM: Intramuscular; IV: Intravenous).

*May be considered in patients who have received amoxicillin in the previous 30 days or who have the otitis–conjunctivitis syndrome.

†Perform tympanocentesis/drainage if skilled in the procedure, or seek a consultation from an otolaryngologist for tympanocentesis/drainage. If the tympanocentesis reveals multidrug-resistant bacteria, seek an infectious disease specialist consultation.

‡Cefdinir, cefuroxime, cefpodoxime, and ceftriaxone are highly unlikely to be associated with cross-reactivity with penicillin allergy on the basis of their distinct chemical structures.

Source: From Lieberthal AS, Carroll AE, Chonmaitree T, et al. The diagnosis and management of acute otitis media. Pediatrics. 2013;131(3):e964-99.

REFERENCES

1. Roland PS, Stroman DW. Microbiology of acute otitis externa. Laryngoscope. 2002;112(7 Pt 1):1166-77.
2. Brook I, Frazier EH, Thompson DH. Aerobic and anaerobic microbiology of external otitis. Clin Infect Dis. 1992;15(6):955-8.
3. Clark WB, Brook I, Bianki D, et al. Microbiology of otitis externa. Otolaryngol Head Neck Surg. 1997;116(1):23-5.
4. Kesser BW. Assessment and management of chronic otitis externa. Curr Opin Otolaryngol Head Neck Surg. 2011;19(5):341-7.
5. Gordon G, Giddings NA. Invasive otitis externa due to Aspergillus species: case report and review. Clin Infect Dis. 1994;19(5):866-70.
6. Gu X, Keyoumu Y, Long L, et al. Detection of bacterial biofilms in different types of chronic otitis media. Eur Arch Otorhinolaryngology. 2014;271(11):2877-83.
7. Saunders J, Murray M, Alleman A. Biofilms in chronic suppurative otitis media and cholesteatoma: scanning electron microscopy findings. Am J Otolaryngol. 2011;32(1):32-7.

Section

2

The Face

Section Editor: *Oren Friedman*

Chapter 7

Wounds and Healing

Sarah A Gitomer, Anthony E Brissett

> ***Chief Complaint***
> *"My wound will not heal".*

DEFINITIONS

Acute wound: A wound that is in the early stages of healing, often within the first 24 hours to 1–2 weeks of the injury, and appears to be following a normal course.

Delayed wound: A wound that is slower to heal but continues to show progress along the wound-healing continuum.

Nonhealing wound: A simple wound that is >3 weeks to 1 month old and has failed to complete the early phases of wound healing.

Hypertrophic scar: Excessive scarring and fibrous tissue overgrowth that remains within the confinement of the original wound.

Keloid: Fibrous tissue overgrowth and excessive scarring that spread beyond the boundaries of the original wound.

Scar contracture: Continued contractile healing in an adequately healed and epithelialized wound (Figs. 7.1A to C).

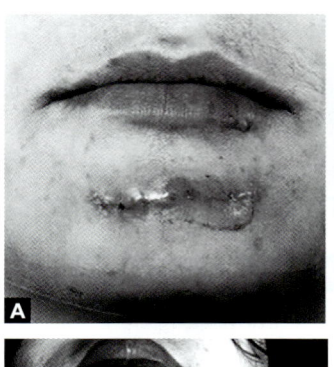

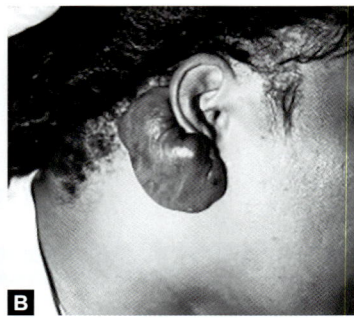

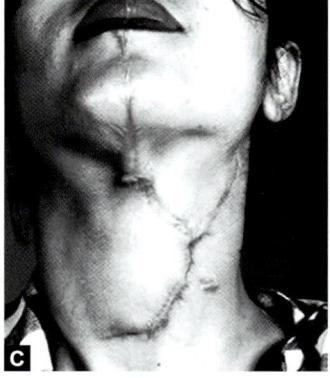

Figs. 7.1A to C: (A) A hypertrophic scar of the chin after traumatic injury. (B) A keloid of the ear lobule after ear piercing. (C) A scar contracture after neck dissection.
Source: Brissett AE, Sherris DA. Scar contractures, hypertrophic scars, and keloids. Facial Plastic Surg. 2001;17(4): 263-72.

PHYSIOLOGY OF WOUND HEALING
Stages of Healing (Figs. 7.2A to D)

1. *Hemostasis*: Wound healing begins with injury followed by a vascular response to the traumatic event. In order to obtain hemostasis, the coagulation cascade and kinin cascade are triggered, and damaged tissues secrete hormones to induce arteriolar vasoconstriction. Platelets adhere to the damaged tissues and are activated forming a clot. The initial injury also activates the complement cascade as part of the innate immune response. After this step, local cytokines

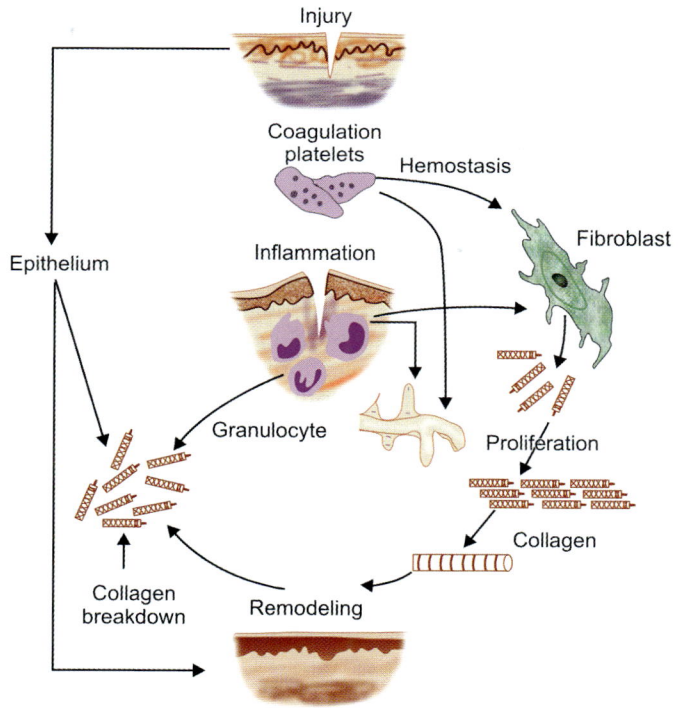

Figs. 7.2A to D: The normal wound-healing cascade. (A) *Hemostasis*: The coagulation cascade, platelets, and kinin cascade are initiated to form an initial barrier to further infection. (B) *Inflammation*: Surrounding vessels dilate and polymorphonuclear cells enter the injury to debride necrotic tissue and bacteria. (C) *Proliferation*: Fibroblasts migrate to the wound to initiate ground substance formation, collagen synthesis, and granulation tissue formation. Neoangiogenesis occurs. (D) *Remodeling*: Maturation of the scar begins with fibroblasts and macrophages secreting collagenase to break down and cross-link collagen to improve wound strength.

and hormones induce increased vascular permeability and arteriole vasodilation to begin the next stage.

2. *Inflammation*: The immune response continues in this step, and polymorphonuclear neutrophils (PMNs) migrate to the site of injury to remove bacteria and devitalized tissue.

3. *Proliferation*: The defining factor of the proliferation phase is fibroblast proliferation and the formation of granulation tissue. After PMNs arrive, monocytes reach the injured tissue and convert it into macrophages. Growth factors promote fibroplasia and formation of granulation tissue. Fibroblasts migrate from healthy surrounding tissue into the wound and form ground substance, fibronectin, collagen, elastin, and integrins. Vascular endothelial growth factor (VEGF) promotes angiogenesis. Epithelialization begins, and the basement membrane is formed.

4. *Remodeling*: Once the granulation tissue is formed, the maturation phase of wound healing begins. Macrophages and fibroblasts release collagenase to break down excess collagen. To organize the structure of the scar and to increase the strength, collagen cross-linking begins, and there is regression of the new vascular structures.

Review

Growth factors involved in wound healing are as follows:

- PDGF (platelet-derived growth factor)—attracts neutrophils and macrophages
- TGF (transforming growth factors)—stimulates epithelial cells and fibroblast proliferation
- EGF (epidermal growth factor)—activates fibroblasts and epithelial cells, angiogenic
- TNF (tumor necrosis factor)—stimulates fibroblast proliferation
- FGF (fibroblast growth factors)—angiogenic, stimulates fibroblast proliferation
- Interferon—inhibits fibroblast proliferation

PATHOGENESIS OF ABNORMAL WOUND HEALING

- *Keloids and hypertrophic scars*: Although the exact etiology of hypertrophic scars and keloids is unknown, both begin with trauma to the affected area. Excessive mechanical tension and strain are thought to contribute to the formation of overdeveloped scars, but this might not always be the case. Foreign body reaction (e.g. to an earring) may also contribute. Overexpression of growth factors PDGF and TGF-B has been proposed as contributors to production of excessive extracellular matrix and stimulation of fibroblasts to produce excess collagen within a healing wound.
- *Nonhealing wounds*: Any number of factors that disrupt the normal healing process can convert an acute wound into a nonhealing wound. Poor vascularity of the wound site, which leads to hypoxia, can prevent migration of inflammatory cells to the wound. Illnesses that impair the immune system, such as hyperglycemia, excess glucocorticoid use, or liver failure, also interfere with every stage of wound healing. Another important cause of a chronic "nonhealing wound" is malignancy. For instance, Marjolin's ulcer is a type of squamous cell carcinoma that arises in a nonhealing wound.

BARRIERS TO WOUND HEALING

- Wound characteristics:
  - Tension
  - Infection, including biofilms
  - Retained foreign body
  - Malignancy
  - Ischemia
  - Desiccation
- Patient characteristics:
  - Smoking
  - Diabetes
  - Poor nutrition
  - Radiation

- Vascular insufficiency
- Immunocompromise autoimmune disorders (such as vasculitis)
- Coagulation disorders
- Liver or renal failure
- Excess glucocorticoids

DIAGNOSTIC WORKUP

When faced with a nonhealing wound, it is the surgeon's responsibility to rule out generalized patient factors, such as vascular disease or nutritional deficiencies that may contribute to poor wound healing, including smoking. In addition, it is necessary to evaluate for other causes of nonhealing wounds such as malignancy, acute or chronic infection, biofilms, or foreign bodies. The diagnostic workup can be directed toward answering these questions.

History

- "How did this happen?"
- "Do you have a history of previous wounds that took longer than expected time to heal?"
- "Do you have a history of keloids or hypertrophic scars?"
- "Have you had recent fevers, increased redness, or foul-smelling drainage from the wound?"
- It is important to conduct a thorough patient history, to evaluate for past medical history that may predict poor wound healing such as diabetes or vascular disease, and to evaluate for social history, including current smoking.

Physical Examination

- First conduct a thorough head and neck physical examination, and evaluate vital signs for systemic disease.
- Then evaluate the new wound, taking into consideration its size, the presence of foreign bodies or contamination, and its location, as this will have implications for closure technique.

- If the wound is old, examine for signs of poor wound healing such as increased odor or purulence, more than a week of inflammation, dehiscence, or necrotic tissue.

Ancillary Tools

- Preoperatively, or in patients with poor wound healing, laboratory work can help screen for systemic or wound-specific causes of delayed healing.
- Laboratory work: Prealbumin, HgbA1C, complete blood count (CBC), basic metabolic panel (BMP), wound cultures

Closure Techniques

- *Primary closure*: The wound edges are reapproximated at the time of presentation. This can be done using suture, fibrin glue, tissue sealants (2-octyl cyanoacrylate), staples, or tapes.
- *Secondary intent*: The wound is left open and allowed to heal with contraction and epithelialization forces. This requires dressings that help debride the wound, prevent infection, and maintain moisture at the site of granulation.

Adjuvant Therapies to Improve Healing

- *Hyperbaric oxygen*: Hyperbaric oxygen exposes patients to higher than atmospheric pressure, which increases the partial pressure of oxygen in the air. At the level of the wound, this induces vasoconstriction and improves partial pressure of oxygen in the blood, which, in turn, stimulates angiogenesis and fibroblast production. Nowadays, this therapy is commonly used to treat osteoradionecrosis, poorly healing, or nonhealing wounds.
- *Wound Vacuum-assisted closure (VAC)*: A polyurethane foam dressing that is covered with occlusive tape is put under negative pressure using a vacuum. This dressing removes interstitial edema, which is thought to promote blood flow and granulation. It removes proinflammatory mediators, proteolytic enzymes, and excess fluid from the wound bed,

which helps decrease bacterial load and edema and increases granulation.

- *Growth factors*: A more recent adjuvant in wound therapy used in conjunction with traditional wound care. The first growth factor used in chronic wounds was rhPDGF (becaplermin), which is used to induce fibroblast proliferation and collagen production in order to promote granulation tissue formation. In the head and neck, rhPDGF has been used in previously irradiated tissue, to close pharyngocutaneous fistulas, and combined with bone matrix to promote bone replacement, with modest results. Phase I and II clinical trials of rhTGFβ3 (avotermin)—which inhibits collagen and extracellular matrix deposition—have shown promising results with preinjury and postinjury injections improving the appearance of scars. Another growth factor that is being studied is δ-like ligand 4 (DLL4), which inhibits angiogenesis by blocking VEGF. The DLL4-inhibitors have been shown to improve the rate of healing in animal studies. It is important to recognize that there is a theoretical risk of malignant transformation of wounds treated with growth factors, and growth factors should not be used in patients with malignancy.
- *Bioengineered skin*: It is useful for patients who are not candidates for autologous skin grafts. Many products have been approved for use in burns and diabetic foot ulcers; however, their use is increasing in off-label indications to help heal large wounds of the head and neck.

Scar Care

There are many adjuncts to wound healing that are promoted to help improve the appearance of a scar. Some are based on evidence, and some treatments are based on popular opinion without evidence of their efficacy.

- *Vitamin E*: Vitamin E is an important cofactor in the synthesis of collagen. It has been used extensively to help improve the appearance of scars, but there are limited data supporting its efficacy. In the dermatology literature, it has been shown to cause a high frequency of contact dermatitis reactions and not to improve the cosmetic appearance of scars when used alone while wounds are healing. There are, however, some data to support its use in hypertrophic scars when used in combination with silicone sheeting.

- *Onion extract*: Allium cepa, the main ingredient in popular scar creams such as Mederma, is frequently used by patients. It is thought to improve scars because of its anti-inflammatory properties and down-regulatory effects on collagen. However, multiple randomized controlled trials in humans have failed to show improved appearance of scars when compared to petroleum ointment alone. It is also proposed that the consistent massaging that is used to apply these creams may be the variable responsible for scar improvement when using creams and lotions.

- *Silicone sheets*: Silicone sheeting or silicone gels combined with occlusive dressings have been shown in multiple randomized controlled trials to help improve the cosmetic appearance of scars and decrease the formation of hypertrophic scars and keloids. Silicone gel can be used in new scars or previously formed scars and has been shown to improve the color, depth, elasticity, size, and induration of scars.

- *Imiquimod cream*: This is a topical immune response modifier that stimulates proinflammatory cytokines, in particular interferon α. Interferon α stimulates collagen breakdown, and therefore this medication is used to help prevent formation of keloids and hypertrophic scars. Randomized controlled trials have shown benefit in preventing keloid formation in animal models, but no human trial has shown its efficacy in prevention of hypertrophic scar formation.

SUGGESTED READING

1. Brissett AE, Hom DB. The effects of tissue sealants, platelet gels, and growth factors on wound healing. Curr Opin Otolaryngol Head Neck Surg. 2003;11(4):245-50.

2. Brissett AE, Sherris DA. Scar contractures, hypertrophic scars, and keloids. Facial Plast Surg. 2001;17(4):263-72.

3. Chen MA, Davidson TM. Scar management: prevention and treatment strategies. Curr Opin Otolaryngol Head Neck Surg. 2005;13(4):242-7.

4. Hershcovitch MD, Hom DB. Update in wound healing in facial plastic surgery. Arch Facial Plast Surg. 2012;14(6):387-93.

5. Hom DB, Sun GH, Elluru RG. A contemporary review of wound healing in otolaryngology: current state and future promise. Laryngoscope. 2009;119(11):2099-110.

6. Mac Cornick S, de Noronha SAAC, Chominski V, et al. Clinical use of growth factors in the improvement of skin wound healing. Open J Clin. Diagn. 2014;4(04):227.

Chapter 8

Facial Palsy

Carly J Stewart, Andrew A Winkler

> ***Chief Complaint***
> *"My face droops".*

DEFINITIONS

Paralysis: Inability to perform voluntary movement in one particular area of the body or globally

Paresis: Incomplete paralysis

Palsy: Paralysis, often accompanied by involuntary muscle movements and twitching

Diplegia: Paralysis affecting symmetrical parts of the body (e.g. both sides of the face).

ANATOMY AND PHYSIOLOGY OF FACIAL MOVEMENT

Facial Movement Pathway

1. *Central pathways*: Facial movement starts in the cerebral cortex at the lateral precentral gyrus of the frontal lobe and travels through the corticobulbar tract through the internal capsule to the pons.
2. *Facial nerve nucleus*: It is located in the pons.

3. Facial nerve (Fig. 8.1)
   a. *Meatal segment*: Pons to internal auditory canal
      i. The facial nerve travels through the cerebellopontine angle, a common location for tumors.
   b. *Labyrinthine segment*: Fundus of internal auditory canal to the geniculate ganglion, which is the location of the facial nerve afferent fiber cell bodies. The geniculate ganglion is located at the first bend (called a "genu") of the facial nerve near the distal end of the labyrinthine segment.
      i. This is the narrowest segment of the facial nerve, making it vulnerable to compression injury.

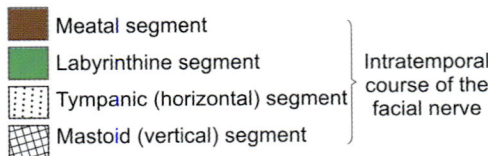

Meatal segment
Labyrinthine segment   ⎫
Tympanic (horizontal) segment ⎬ Intratemporal course of the facial nerve
Mastoid (vertical) segment   ⎭

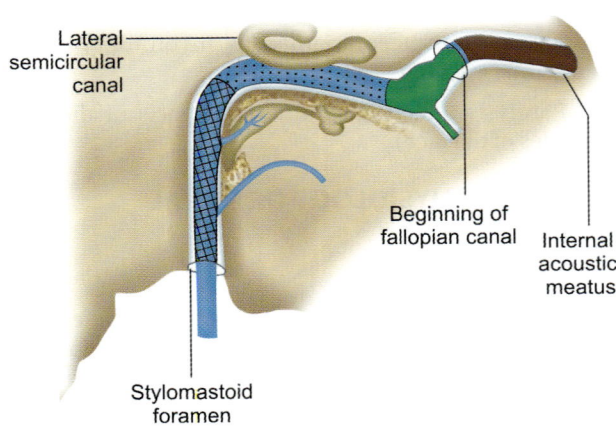

Lateral semicircular canal

Beginning of fallopian canal   Internal acoustic meatus

Stylomastoid foramen

Fig. 8.1: Facial nerve anatomy.

ii. The nervus intermedius, which carries afferent fibers for taste to the anterior two-thirds of the tongue, joins the facial nerve at the geniculate ganglion.

iii. The facial nerve runs in the anterior, superior quadrant of the internal auditory canal.

c. *Tympanic segment*: Geniculate ganglion to the horizontal semicircular canal at the pyramidal eminence, which is the location of the second genu of the facial nerve.

d. *Mastoid segment*: Pyramidal process to the stylomastoid foramen.

e. *Extratemporal segment*: Distal to stylomastoid foramen; the facial nerve splits into superior and inferior divisions at the pes anserinus (goose's foot) and then further divides into five branches: temporal (aka frontal), zygomatic, buccal, marginal mandibular, and cervical.

4. *Neuromuscular junction*: Acetylcholine is released into the synaptic cleft, which binds to neurotransmitter-gated ion channels.

5. *Muscle*: Binding of acetylcholine to the ion channels causes depolarization of muscle fibers and contraction.

SEDDON'S CLASSIFICATION OF PERIPHERAL NERVE INJURY

1. *Class I*: Neuropraxia—temporary conduction block and demyelination at site of injury.
2. *Class II*: Axonotmesis—axonal loss but connective tissue layers are preserved.
3. *Class III*: Neurotmesis—nerve is divided.

SUNDERLAND'S CLASSIFICATION OF PERIPHERAL NERVE INJURY

- *Class I*: Same as neuropraxia above
- *Class II*: Same as axonotmesis above
- *Class III*: Damage to endoneurial tubes
- *Class IV*: Damage to perineurium
- *Class V*: Damage to epineurium

CAUSES OF FACIAL PALSY

Congenital

1. *Birth trauma*: Forceps delivery, molding.
2. *Mobius syndrome*: Congenital facial diplegia with abducens palsy; 1:50,000 newborns.

Trauma

1. Cortical or brainstem injuries.
2. *Intratemporal injury*: About 7–10% of temporal bone fractures cause facial nerve paresis.[1]
3. *Extratemporal injury*: Both blunt and penetrating trauma.

Treatment

- *Conservative measures*: Observation and oral corticosteroids.
- Surgical procedures including primary reanastomosis, cable grafting, and supportive/symptom-relief surgery (see surgical procedures below).

Vascular

Cerebrovascular accidents of the motor cortex or brainstem.

Infectious

1. *Bell's palsy* (*Treatment*): Strong recommendation for oral steroids and consider combination oral antiviral therapy if within 72 hours of symptom onset if the patient is >15 years old.[2]
2. Ramsay Hunt syndrome (herpes zoster oticus)
3. Malignant otitis externa
4. Otitis media/mastoiditis
5. Cholesteatoma
6. Encephalitis and meningitis
7. Lyme disease
8. *Miscellaneous*: Varicella zoster, poliomyelitis, mumps, mononucleosis, human immunodeficiency virus, influenza, coxsackie, syphilis, tuberculosis, botulism, parotitis

Neoplastic

Tumors of the cerebellopontine angle (CPA), middle ear, temporal bone, and parotid gland can result in facial nerve paralysis. Proximal tumors may also cause hearing loss, tinnitus, vertigo, and imbalance, while facial nerve paralysis due to tumors of the parotid gland is limited to affected branches. The vast majority of CPA tumors are benign, the most common of which is the vestibular schwannoma, making up 80.7% of CPA tumors.[3] The most common benign parotid tumor is pleomorphic adenoma, and the most common malignant tumor is mucoepidermoid carcinoma.

Iatrogenic

The facial nerve can be injured during resection of tumors in the cerebellopontine angle and during middle ear, mastoid, parotid, and neck surgery. Not uncommonly, the facial nerve is naturally dehiscent in the tympanic segment, a potential site of injury. Of note, local anesthesia can cause a temporary paralysis.

Toxic

Toxins such as thalidomide, tetanus toxin, diphtheria, carbon monoxide, and lead may cause facial nerve paralysis, which tends to be bilateral. Botulinum toxin is the most common cause of facial nerve paralysis, which is typically undertaken for aesthetic indications.

Systemic

1. Multiple sclerosis
2. Guillain–Barré
3. Myasthenia gravis
4. Amyotrophic lateral sclerosis
5. *Melkersson–Rosenthal syndrome*: Orofacial swelling, recurrent facial nerve paralysis, and plicated tongue
6. Other neuromuscular and autoimmune disorders (Charcot–Marie-Tooth syndrome, myotonic dystrophy, etc.).

DIAGNOSTIC WORKUP: "MY FACE DROOPS"

History

"Is your face moving some or not at all?"

"Are any other areas of your body affected?"

"Are both sides of your face affected?"

"Did you have any trauma, surgery, upper respiratory infection, or toxin exposure around the time this started?"

"Did the difficulty moving your face come on suddenly or gradually over days, weeks, or months?"

"Do you have pain?"

"Do you have associated symptoms such as headache, hearing loss, tinnitus, seizures, vertigo, or imbalance?"

Physical Examination

- Complete cranial nerve examination including detailed facial nerve examination (degree of facial nerve paralysis, branches of facial nerve involved, presence of fasciculations, other CN involvement)
  - House-Brackmann grading system for facial nerve paresis (Table 8.1)[2]—originally developed in 1983 to standardize facial nerve injury grading after neurotologic surgery.
- Otoscopy (middle ear masses, effusions, signs of infection, or cholesteatoma)
- Parotid examination (signs of trauma, masses)
- Skin examination (rashes, scars to indicate previous trauma or surgery)

Imaging

- Magnetic resonance imaging for suspected cerebrovascular accident, intracranial tumor, or parotid mass
- Computed tomography to investigate middle ear pathology, basilar skull fractures, or parotid mass.

Table 8.1: House-Brackmann classification.		
Grade		*Description*
1	Normal	Normal function in all areas.
2	Mild dysfunction	Weakness noticed on close inspection only. Face has good symmetry at rest. Able to close eyes completely with minimal effort. No synkinesis, contracture, or spasm.
3	Moderate dysfunction	Weakness obvious but not disfiguring. Face has good symmetry at rest. No functional impairment. Able to close eyes completely with maximal effort. Mild synkinesis, contracture, or spasm. Can move corners of mouth with maximal effort but with obvious asymmetry.
4	Moderately severe dysfunction	Weakness and asymmetry can be disfiguring. Face has good symmetry at rest. No forehead movement visible. Cannot close eyes completely with maximal effort. Synkinesis, contracture, and spasm can impair function.
5	Severe dysfunction	Motion is only barely perceptible. Asymmetry present at rest. No visible forehead movement. Only slight motion of eyelid with maximal effort. Slight movement present at the corner of mouth. Synkinesis, contracture, and spasm are usually absent
6	Total paralysis	No perceptible facial movement. Loss of tone present. No synkinesis, contracture, or spasm.

Treatment

Medical

Conservative management includes anything from treating the underlying medical condition causing facial palsy to administering corticosteroids for a traumatic intratemporal facial nerve injury. Medical treatments are listed above under the specific condition.

Surgical

Nerve repair in traumatic injuries

1. Decompression for intratemporal injuries
   - Consider for patients with complete paralysis and >95% degeneration on electroneuronography testing performed after 72 hours from injury.[4]
2. *Reanastomosis*: End-to-end neurorrhaphy
3. *Cable grafting*: Great auricular or sural nerves are most common graft sources.
   - Cross-face cable grafting is performed if the ipsilateral proximal facial nerve segment is not available for grafting. The nerve graft travels from segmental branches of the contralateral facial nerve to the ipsilateral distal facial nerve branches.
   - About 9–12 months before, muscle movement begins to occur.
4. *Jump anastomosis grafting*: End-to-side anastomosis of cranial nerve XII proximally to the facial nerve distally.

Note: Generally with all of these anastomosis and grafting techniques, the best House-Brackmann score that can be achieved is nerve III.

Upper one-third of the face:

1. *Brow ptosis*: Browlift botulinum toxin to the opposite side for symmetry
2. *Upper eyelid closure*: Tarsorrhaphy, lid loading (gold or platinum weight placement)
3. *Paralytic ectropion*: Tarsal strip canthoplasty

Lower two-thirds of the face:

1. *Static slings*: Acellular dermis, expanded polytetrafluoro-ethylene (GoreTex), tensor fascia lata, suture suspension, rhytidectomy
2. Dynamic slings[5]
   - *Muscle transposition flaps*: Temporalis or masseter. These flaps are considered when the distal facial nerve is not viable for grafting because the neuromuscular unit is absent or fibrosed (>2-year-old injury).

- *Free tissue transfer*: Gracilis, pectoralis minor, latissimus dorsi. Consider free tissue transfer when there is a concomitant soft tissue defect. The proximal facial nerve segment is grafted to the free tissue flap. Movement is possible beginning at 7–8 months.

ACKNOWLEDGMENT

The authors would like to thank the Department of Otolaryngology, University of Colorado, Denver in Aurora, Colorado, USA.

REFERENCES

1. Nash JJ, Friedland DR, Boorsma KJ, et al. Management and outcomes of facial paralysis from intratemporal blunt trauma: a systematic review. Laryngoscope. 2010;120:1397-404.
2. Baugh RF, Basura GJ, Ishii LE, et al. Clinical practice guidelines: Bell's palsy. Otolaryngol Head Neck Surg. 2013;149:S1-27.
3. Moffat DA, Ballagh RH. Rare tumours of the cerebellopontine angle. Clin Oncol. 1995;7:28-41.
4. Chang CYJ, Cass SP. Clinical forum: management of facial nerve injury due to temporal bone trauma. Am J Otol. 1999;20:96-114.
5. Tatea JR, Tollefsonb TT. Advances in facial reanimation. Curr Opin Otolaryngol Head Neck Surg. 2006;14:242-8.

Chapter 9

Nasal Deformities

Jarrod Keeler, Charles Woodard, Sam P Most

> ***Chief Complaint***
> *"I do not like the appearance of my nose". "I cannot breathe through one side of my nose".*

ANATOMY OF THE EXTERNAL NOSE

In general, the nose can be considered to be a triangular pyramid with each nasal sidewall making up one side and the ala and the tip forming the other side.

External Nasal Landmarks[1-3]

- Nasal tip—the most anterior projection of the nose at the caudal end.
- Nasal dorsum—the anterior surface along the length of the nose.
- Nasal sidewall—the lateral surface along the length of the nose.
- Ala—the soft tissue laterally at the base of the nose forming a pyramid with the nasal tip.
- Columella—the central and most caudal portion of the nasal base, soft tissue made up by the medial crural footplates of the lower lateral cartilages.
- Radix—the root of the nose.

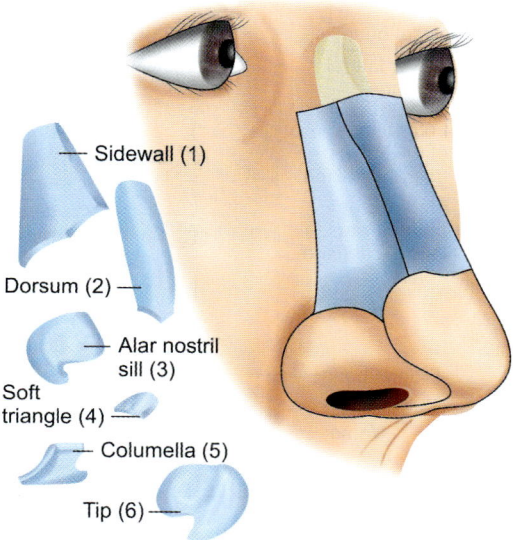

Fig. 9.1: Nasal subunits.

- Nasion—the depression at the root of the nose representing the start of the nose, where the nasal bones meet the frontal bone.
- Rhinion—the junction of bony/cartilaginous nasal dorsum.
- Tip-defining point—the most anterior part of the nasal tip made up by the intermediate crura of the lower lateral cartilages.
- Nasal subunits—any defect of >50% of one subunit should have the entire subunit removed and repaired (Fig. 9.1).

Internal Nasal Landmarks[1,3] (Fig. 9.2)

- Anterior septal angle—most caudal and dorsal portion of the cartilaginous septum.

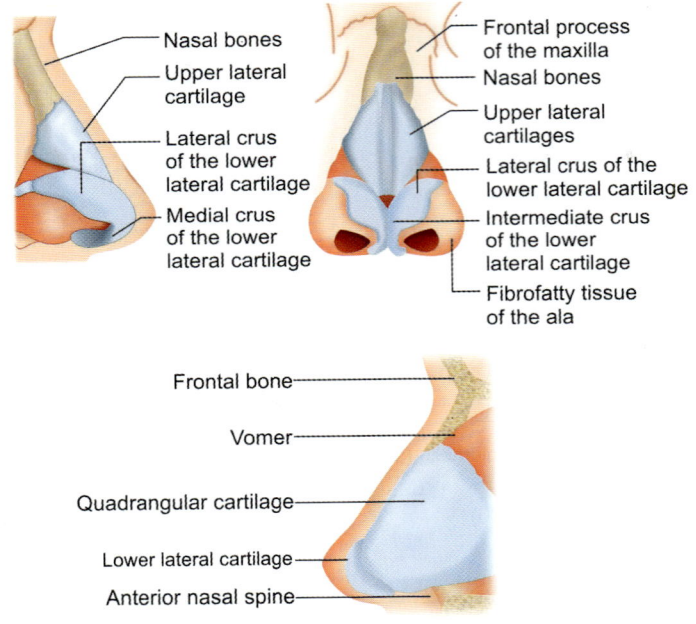

Nasal bones
Upper lateral cartilage
Lateral crus of the lower lateral cartilage
Medial crus of the lower lateral cartilage

Frontal process of the maxilla
Nasal bones
Upper lateral cartilages
Lateral crus of the lower lateral cartilage
Intermediate crus of the lower lateral cartilage
Fibrofatty tissue of the ala

Frontal bone
Vomer
Quadrangular cartilage
Lower lateral cartilage
Anterior nasal spine

Fig. 9.2: Internal nasal landmarks.

- Internal nasal valve—region of greatest resistance to nasal airflow made up by the septum, lower lateral cartilage, upper lateral cartilage, inferior turbinate, and piriform aperture.
- External nasal valve—region caudal to the internal valve consisting of the ala laterally and septum and columella medially.
- Scroll region—junction of the upper and lower lateral cartilages.

Bony[1,3]

- Nasal bones—paired bony framework of the nasal pyramid joining laterally with the frontal process of the maxilla bilaterally.

- Nasal turbinates—three sets of paired bone and soft tissue that travel the length of the nose and serve to heat and moisturize incoming air.
- Piriform aperture—the inferior-most border of the nose formed by the paired maxillary bones.

Cartilage[1,3]

- Anterior septum—midline cartilaginous structure made up by the quadrangular cartilage.
- Upper lateral cartilages—paired structures with the rough form of an obtuse triangle pointed laterally; they join in the midline with the anterior septum, cranially with the nasal bones, and caudally with the lower lateral cartilages.
- Lower lateral cartilages—paired structures with the rough form of an L with three confluent portions (lateral, intermediate, and medial crura); cranially they interdigitate with the upper lateral cartilages (lateral crus), caudally they come together to form the dome (intermediate crus), and medially they join to form the columella (medial crus).

Soft Tissue[1,3]

- Fibrofatty tissue—form bilateral ala and soft tissue triangles.
- Interdomal ligament—binding ligament between the intermediate crus of the lower lateral cartilages, securing them together.
- Membranous septum—ligamentous structure binding the medial crus of the lower lateral cartilages.
- Nasal vestibule—entrance to the nasal cavity continuing to the inferior turbinate; contains the nasal hairs called vibrissae.

DORSAL DEFORMITIES[1-5]

- Nasal bone fracture—one of the most common nasal deformities and the most common facial bone fracture.
- Twisted nose deformity—complex deformity of the bony pyramid and the upper and the lower cartilaginous vault, and

the septum; may be traumatic or congenital, and often affects nasal function as well as aesthetics.

- Saddle nose deformity—depression of the nasal dorsum due to loss of septal support at the rhinion, creating a "saddle" within the nasal dorsum.
- Dorsal hump—common nasal deformity in esthetic rhinoplasty. A dorsal hump is reduced with the aid of osteotomies or rasps.
- Open roof deformity—iatrogenic deformity caused by over-resection of the nasal dorsum without appropriate osteotomies to reform the nasal pyramid.
- Inverted V deformity—over-resection of a dorsal hump with inadequate support of the upper lateral cartilages can result in an inferomedial collapse of the upper lateral cartilages.
- Pollybeak deformity—undesirable supratip fullness; typically a postsurgical complication.

TIP DEFORMITIES[1-5]

- Over/under rotation—normal tip rotation at the nasolabial angle should be 95°–105° in women and 90°–95° in men.
- Over/under projection—projection is ideally 60% of nasal length, although this varies somewhat by culture and gender.
- Bulbous/boxy tip—tip shape is affected by the intermediate portions of the lower lateral and the soft tissue envelope, and can result in either a bulbous or a boxy tip depending on the soft tissue envelope.
- Twisted tip—most frequently due to nasal trauma with scar contracture, although it can be iatrogenic. This entity represents many different changes to the anterior septum, lower lateral cartilages, and ala.
- Bifid tip—splaying of the medial crura of the lower lateral cartilages.
- Bossae—a rebending of the lower lateral cartilage at the tip due to posterior retraction acting on weakened lower lateral cartilages.

NASAL ALA/COLUMELLAR DEFORMITIES[1-5]

- Retracted/hanging columella or ala—normal columellar show should be 2–4 mm. Changes to this can be due to either retracted or hanging columella or ala.
- Alar notching—notch in the ala, usually due to previous surgery or trauma.

DIAGNOSTIC WORKUP[2-6]

- "When did this start? When does this occur? Is there anything that makes it better or worse?"
- "Any history of recurrent sinus infections or allergies? What is your previous medical history? Are you using any nasal medications, either over the counter or prescription?"
  - The history of chronic sinusitis, allergies, or other nasal disease all affects how we will treat the problem. Comorbidities can confound surgical correction. Use of nasal decongestants can be a common cause of nasal obstruction and must be halted months before treatment. Blood thinners, vitamin E supplementation, fish oil, and many herbal supplements increase bleeding risk and should be stopped, if it is safe to do so.
- "Do you have any history of facial injuries? Have you had any previous surgical procedures especially those of the nose and the face? Any history of keloids in your past or in your family?"
  - A history of these should help the surgeon to pause and assess how the previous injuries/procedures could affect the result or material available to work with for grafts. Skin healing should always be in mind.
- "Do you smoke, drink alcohol, or use illegal drugs? Any history of use of inhaled nasal stimulants (i.e., cocaine)?"
  - Most rhinoplasty surgeons will not operate on someone who uses tobacco products or has any recent history of use of inhaled nasal stimulants.
- "What are your goals?"

- This is possibly the most important question as it will lead your surgery. Order the concerns from the greatest to the least, if possible. This question can also help uncover any underlying psychiatric issues the patient may have.

- *Physical examination*: Full head and neck examination should be performed. A highly focused nasal examination should include the evaluation from the outside, including skin color, texture, thickness, and type. The ala and columella should be evaluated in pairs. The nose should be evaluated for projection, rotation, tip support, and defects. Watch the patient breathe through his or her nose both silently and with deep inspiration. Cotton applicators can be used to support the inner cartilage to simulate graft material. Finally, the internal nose should be evaluated thoroughly. Nasal masses can cause obstruction as well. The remainder of the face should be fully evaluated for position, symmetry, and defects as other distant structures can cause appearance changes of the nose.

- Photographs should be taken from the frontal view, bilateral side views, and base view at a minimum. Other views include 45° angle view and top–down view. These should be brought to the operating room.

SURGICAL MANAGEMENT[2-6]

External rhinoplasty is the most frequent treatment modality.

Prior to surgery, the patient should have an informed consent discussion, with any grafts that need to be taken specifically. The patient should be taken to the Operating Room and intubated. The nose should be anesthetized with either 1% lidocaine with epinephrine or 4% cocaine. The entire face should be prepped sterilely. Incision should start with a broken line incision at the thinnest portion of the columella using an inverted V, gull wing, or similar incision. Marginal incisions should be made sharply along the leading edge of the lower lateral cartilage. The soft tissue envelope should then be sharp and bluntly dissected in a sub-Superficial Musculo-Aponeurotic System plane along the lower lateral cartilages. Maintain meticulous hemostasis. The anterior septal angle should be identified and the nose degloved. This can be combined with a septoplasty through one of the standard hemitransfixion or transfixion incision. The upper lateral cartilages can be freed from the septum and any resected septum can be removed. Specific procedures to alleviate nasal deformities mentioned above are beyond the scope of this chapter.

The soft tissue envelope is redraped over the nose and the columellar incision is closed with 6-0 nonabsorbable suture. The marginal incisions may be closed or left to heal by second intention. The nose is then taped based on the surgeon's preference and a nasal splint/cast is placed. Sutures should be removed within a week. The patient should avoid physical activity for 3–4 weeks and any contact sports for 6 weeks to 3 months.

REFERENCES

1. Bailey B. Head and Neck Surgery—Otolaryngology. 3rd edition. Philadelphia, PA: Lippincott Williams & Wilkins; 2006.
2. Higgins TS, Hwang PH, Kingdom TT. Systematic review of topical vasoconstrictors in endoscopic sinus surgery. Laryngoscope. 2011;121(2):422-32.
3. Papel, I (Ed). In: Facial Plastic and Reconstructive Surgery. New York; Theime Medical; 2009.
4. Park SS. Fundamental principles in aesthetic rhinoplasty. Clin Exp Otorhinolaryngol. 2011;4(2):55-66.
5. Powell N, Humphrey B. Proportions of the Aesthetic Face. New York: Thieme-Stratton; 1984.
6. Rohrich RJ, Ahmad J. Rhinoplasty. Plast Reconstr Surg. 2011;128:49-73e.

SUGGESTED READING

1. Fang F, Clapham PJ, Chung KC. A systematic review of interethnic variability in facial dimensions. Plast Reconstr Surg. 2011;127: 874.

2. Farkas LG, Hreczko TA, Kolar JC, et al. Vertical and horizontal proportions of the face in young adult North American Caucasians: revision of the neoclassical canons. Plast Reconstr Surg. 1985;75:328-38.
3. Hoss RA, Ramsey JL, Griffin AM, et al. The role of facial attractiveness and facial masculinity/femininity in sex classification of faces. Perception. 2005;34(12):1459-74.

Chapter 10

Deformities of the External Ear

Paul Sabini

Chief Complaint
"The child has an abnormal ear" or "Part of the ear is missing".

DEFINITIONS

Deformity: A condition in which a part of the body does not have the normal or expected shape.

Anotia: Complete absence of the auricle.

Microtia: Literally, "small ear"; an auricular deformity ranging from a small, slightly misshapen external ear to a major deficit of internal and external structures.

Deformities of the external ear range from a preauricular pit to complete absence of the external ear. For the reconstructive surgeon, it is helpful to determine whether or not the deformity requires reshaping the existing structure or rebuilding some or the entire auricular framework. This chapter focuses on the congenital deformity commonly referred to as microtia. Patients with anotia will benefit from the same techniques. The treatment most often involves rebuilding the framework, although many of these patients will also benefit from reshaping the contralateral ear. Reconstructive techniques used for patients who have had cancer or sustained trauma are helpful particularly for revision cases.

EMBRYOLOGY AND ANATOMY OF THE EXTERNAL EAR

The ear is derived from the mesenchyme of the first and second pharyngeal arches. Tissue from the same area forms the mandible as well as portions of the middle ear. Six buds of tissue (auricular hillocks of His) work in concert to build the external ear. This process begins around the 4th week of gestation and continues until the 12th week when the auricle reaches its home (Figs. 10.1A and B).[1] While this is happening, the facial nerve, derived from the second arch, must find its way through and around the developing ear.[2]

The position of the auricle with respect to other structures of the face has some variability, but in general the superior helical rim rests at the level of the lateral aspect of the eyebrow in a horizontal plane. A lateral view of the ear reveals that the long axis of the ear tilts ~15°–20° forward compared to the nasal dorsum (Fig. 10.2). When everything is properly synchronized,

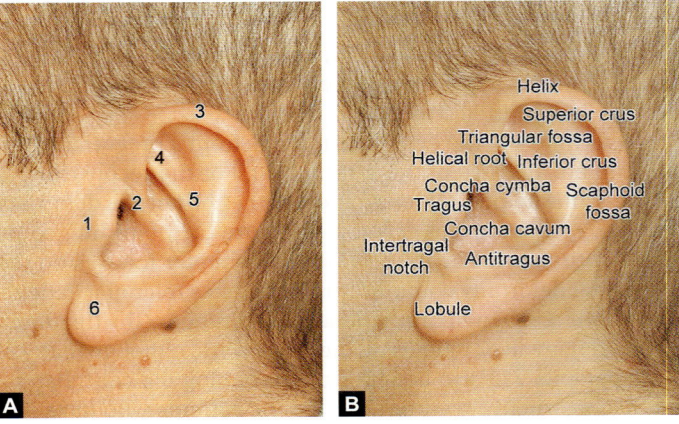

Figs. 10.1A and B: (A) The corresponding parts of the ear formed by the six hillocks of His. (B) The components of a normal ear.

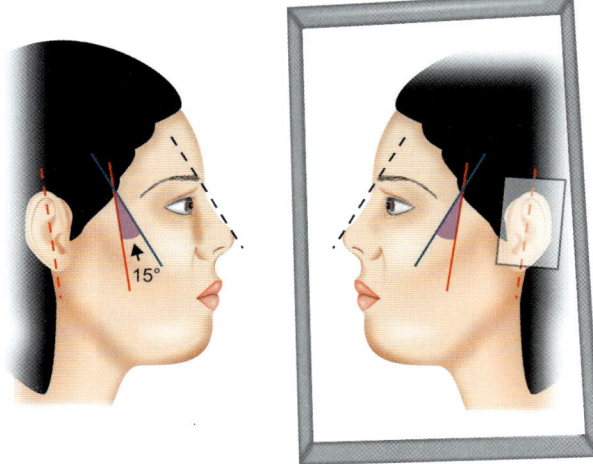

Fig. 10.2: The axis of orientation of a normal ear relative to the face.

the end result is a normal ear and mandible, with a properly positioned and functioning facial nerve (Fig. 10.3).

Disruption of these events occurs in at least 0.03% of live births, resulting in an incidence of microtia of 1 in 10,000–20,000 people. At least half of these patients have associated anomalies of the first and second branchial arch derivatives.[3] Therefore, most patients with microtia have other issues for the surgeon to consider before planning reconstruction of the external ear. This ranges from a mild mandibular hypoplasia to oculo auricular vertebral dysplasia. Obvious concerns such as hemifacial microsomia are evident from the physical examination; anomalous positioning of the facial nerve or cervical spine anomalies may not be apparent, yet are critically important to the surgeon and anesthesiologist (Fig. 10.4).

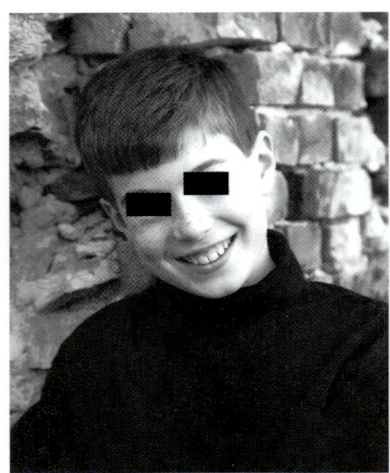

Fig. 10.3: Normal anatomy and function.

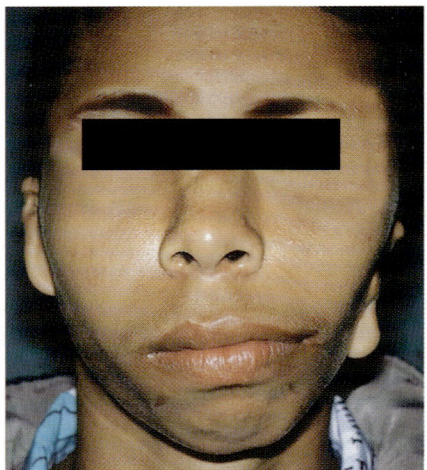

Fig. 10.4: A patient with bilateral microtia and left mandibular hypoplasia.

TREATMENT OF THE EXTERNAL AURICULAR DEFORMITY

The shape of the external ear may aid in audition, but the loss of the auricle in trauma and cancer patients does not seem to appreciably alter hearing. The overwhelming impact of the absence of the external ear is psychological. Very often, the impact extends beyond the individual patient to include the family.

Reshaping

Lop ear deformities or prominent ears are among the more common ear issues leading to consultation with a facial plastic surgeon. The placement of Mustarde sutures with or without conchal setback sutures is a well-established and reliable approach for this concern. The operation decreases projection and either creates or sharpens the superior crus of the antihelix (Fig. 10.5). The human ear is near its adult size by the age of 5 years, so it is possible to perform the procedure at that point

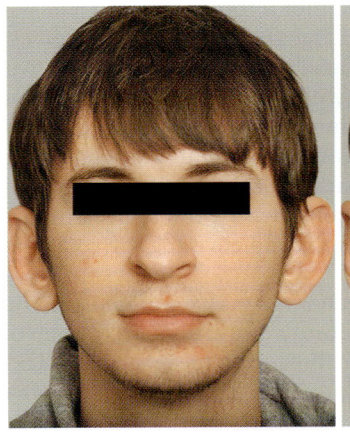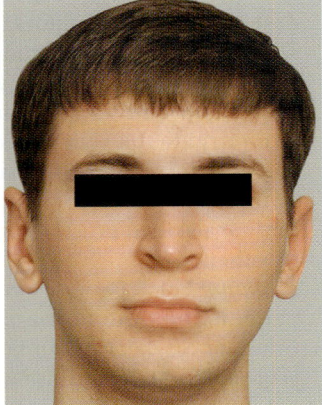

Fig. 10.5: Before and after otoplasty.

without appreciably altering the natural course of the ear's growth. Nevertheless, most 5-year-olds are not ideal candidates for any elective surgery. Waiting until the deformity is a concern for the patient, as opposed to his or her parents, ensures that the patient is motivated.

Patients with unilateral microtia can benefit from these same techniques on the nonreconstructed ear when it remains relatively overprojected in comparison to the new ear.

Rebuilding

For the reconstructive surgeon, the ear is a complex three-layered structure. The anterior and posterior skin layers cover a soft, pliable, cartilaginous framework and the adipose tissue of the earlobe. It should be stated upfront that no current technique can match the pliability of the normal framework, but imperceptibly matching the contour is now a realistic goal.

Options for Rebuilding the Ear

1. *Prosthetics*: A well-made prosthetic can be attached to the side of the scalp with either a topical adhesive or with osseointegrated implants (Fig. 10.6). The latter involves a slight risk related to infection of the posts, but it is a relatively straightforward procedure with low morbidity. The former requires a daily application of an adhesive, which can often irritate the skin or, worse, can fail in a public setting. Nevertheless, for many patients this can be an excellent option. The issue for patients who want a prosthetic is finding a skilled prosthodontist and covering the cost of the prosthetic.

2. *Implants*: For >20 years, some surgeons have offered microtia patients the option of a porous polyethylene framework (Medpor, Stryker Craniomaxillofacial, Chicago, Illinois, USA) (Fig. 10.7). Medpor implants have a clear advantage over autologous costal cartilage; there is less donor site morbidity. The donor site is the temporal scalp and not the thoracic

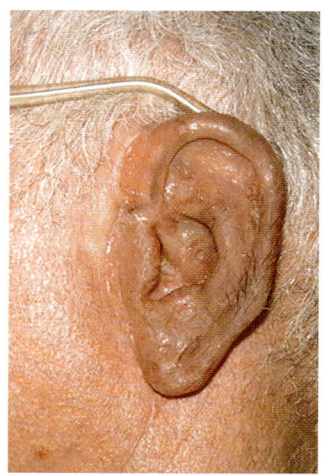

Fig. 10.6: An osseointegrated implant with its attached prosthesis.

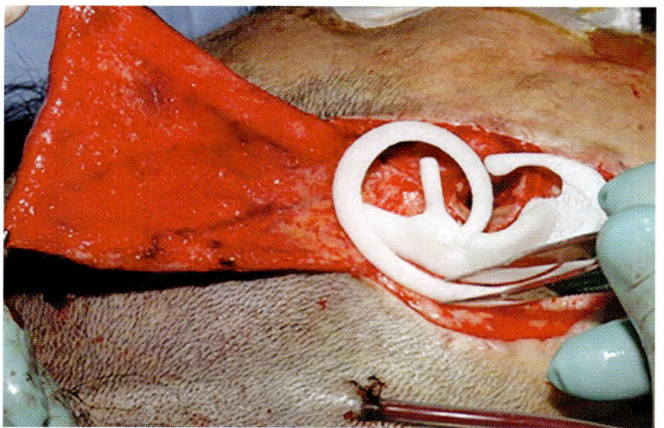

Fig. 10.7: Placement of a temporoparietal fascial flap over a Medpor framework.

cavity. In any patient who has a viable temporoparietal fascial flap (TPFF), the implant should be discussed. Even in the absence of a TPFF, a free flap surgeon can utilize the radial forearm flap to provide soft-tissue coverage for the implant. Reconstruction of the ear with Medpor, a TPFF, and skin grafts is typically a one-stage procedure. Implant exposure and loss is the disadvantage of Medpor. A simple adjacent pimple or folliculitis can undo the entire reconstruction (Fig. 10.8). Autologous tissue can handle exposure from this as well as from minor trauma, but Medpor cannot.

At this point in time, there are a few centers with experienced surgeons who offer the procedure. Medpor cannot and should not be discounted; however, patients and surgeons would be better served to wait for these centers to publish long-term data (15- to 20-year follow-up) for scrutiny. These reports are not yet available. Until that time, surgeons can rely on the track record of a patient's own tissue.

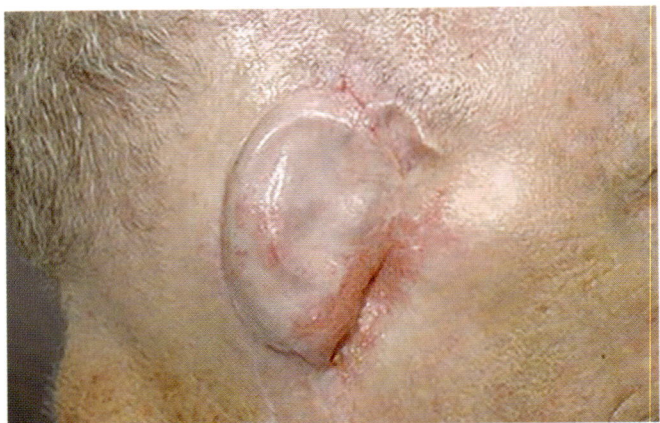

Fig. 10.8: Breakdown of the anterior edge of the soft tissue overlying Medpor 2 years after placement.

3. *Autologous tissue*: It can be used to create the three layers of a normal ear. The costal cartilaginous framework is usually covered by the pre-existing scalp soft tissue on its anterior surface and a skin graft on its posterior surface. Tanzer first described the operation and used six stages to achieve the goal.[3] Brent reduced the technique to four stages, and Nagata then refined the overall framework and pocket in order to achieve a two-stage reconstruction.[4,5] More recently, Firmin has offered nuances on Nagata's approach while Kasrai and Fisher have described a single-stage adaptation of Nagata's technique.[5–7]

Nagata's approach is well-described and diagrammed in his paper published in 1993.[5] A few key points can be emphasized. The operation includes an ipsilateral costal cartilage harvest (Fig. 10.9) of ribs 6 through 9. A subperiosteal dissection decreases the risk of pneumothorax and, in Nagata's opinion, it may allow for some regrowth of cartilage at the donor site. A significant difference between this procedure and Brent's technique is the amount of cartilage harvested (Figs. 10.10A

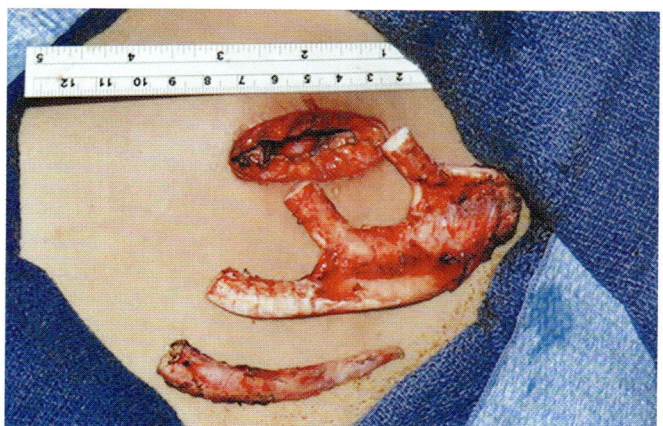

Fig. 10.9: Cartilage harvest for the framework.

and B). The framework has tiers to it, and it includes the tragus. It consumes more cartilage in its creation. Although the procedure can be performed in patients as young as the age of 5, waiting until the age of 8 allows further development of the costal cartilage. This increased volume of the framework stresses the pocket to a greater extent, but the preservation of a soft-tissue pedicle in the location of the concha cavum is a critical step that cannot be overemphasized. This pedicle helps one avoid flap necrosis and the subsequent loss of some or the entire framework (Figs. 10.11A and B). The technique includes transposition of the lobule with the placement of the framework. A block of cartilage is also harvested for the second stage in order to provide projection. This can be banked in the subcutaneous tissue of the chest. At the second stage, the cartilaginous block provides projection from the mastoid surface and is covered with a TPFF and a full-thickness graft (Figs. 10.12A to C).

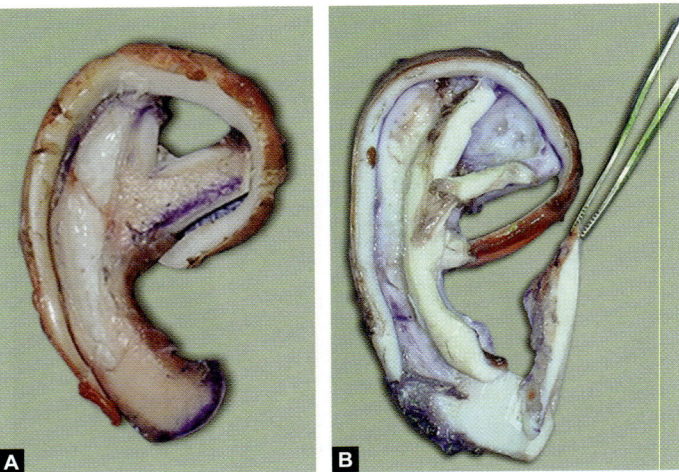

Figs. 10.10A and B: (A) A carved framework after the method described by Brent. (B) A carved framework after the method described by Nagata.

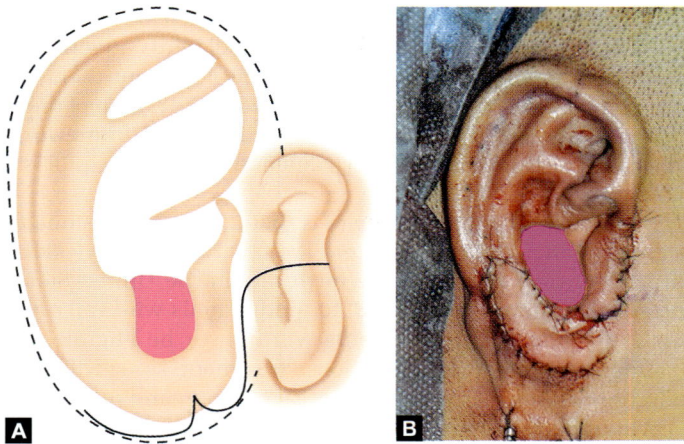

Figs. 10.11A and B: (A) The dark "w"-shaped line corresponds to the posterior incision for the pocket described by Nagata. The shaded pink area is undissected and provides additional blood supply to the pocket. (B) A framework in position after the first stage as described by Nagata. The shaded area is not dissected and ultimately sits in the conchal bowl. The lobule has been transposed.

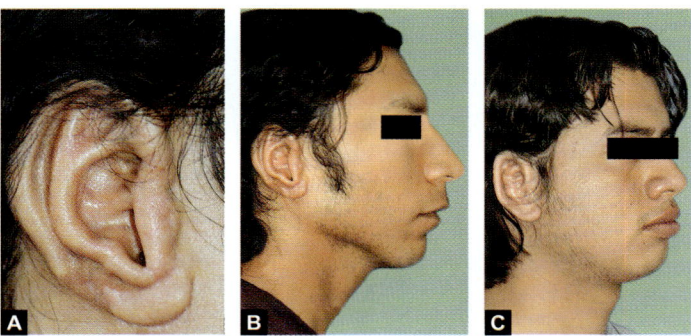

Figs. 10.12A to C: Microtia repair utilizing the two stage approach. (A) A close up view of the detail made possible by Nagata's technique. (B) The same patient as seen in lateral view (C) An additional patient with a two stage reconstruction.

Nagata has developed his own needles, which are essentially small Keith needles with the stainless steel wires attached to them. It is possible to perform this surgery without them (or something like them), but it is more difficult. The design of these sutures allows for very precise construction of the framework. Other than a scalpel, another instrument that is very helpful is a sharp gouge (Fig. 10.13).

A paradox of microtia surgery is that it takes a long time to become proficient, and yet there are few cases for any given surgeon to treat per year. The birth rate in the United States translates to between 200 and 400 individuals with microtia. Not every one of these patients will opt, or be eligible, for treatment. Among those who choose treatment, some will elect to have prosthetics, some will choose Medpor, and others will have autologous costal cartilage grafts. Some of these patients may travel overseas, so the number of surgeons trained in the technique quickly outstrips the number of patients in need. This, in turn, limits each surgeon's ability to maintain proficiency. One

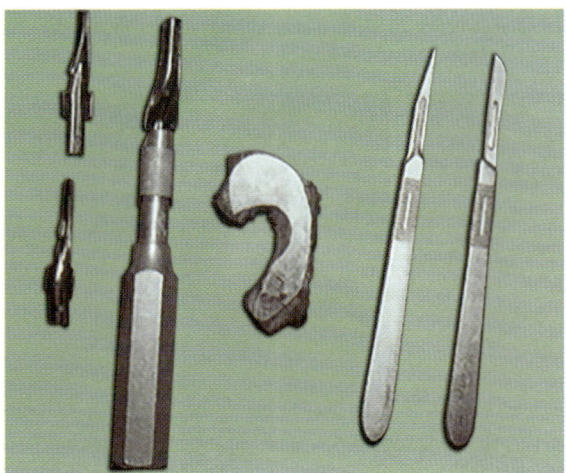

Fig. 10.13: Instruments for carving.

surgeon's ability to learn and master the procedure may vary from another, but no one can dispute the notion that repetition builds proficiency while also creating a track record from which to learn and develop modifications.

This raises the following question: why learn to perform a rarely performed procedure? The techniques used for microtia have applications for far more common maladies affecting the external ear, namely, skin cancer and trauma. While a given surgeon may never have multiple opportunities to carve the perfect framework, he or she is likely to encounter patients who will benefit from these ideas (Figs. 10.14A to E).

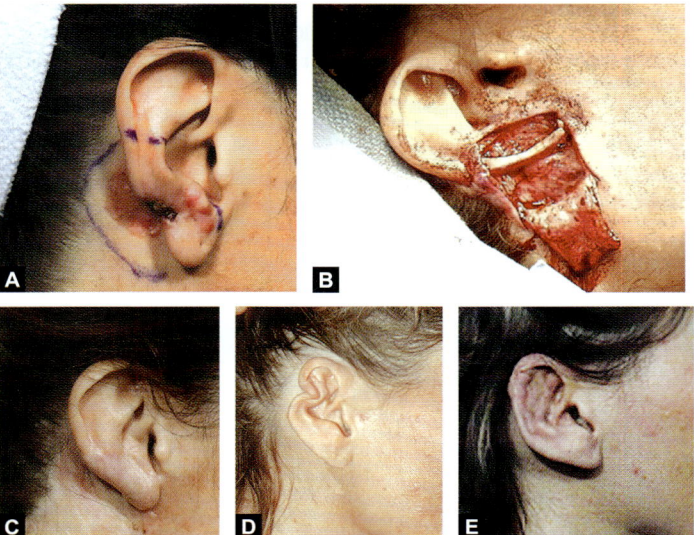

Figs. 10.14A to E: Reconstructive cases utilizing the concepts of microtia surgery. (A) Skin cancer eroding the lower half of the auricle. (B) Following excision, a rib graft is placed under a postauricular flap. (C) After elevation of the rib graft and creation of a lobule. (D) An ear piercing gone awry. (E) After a single-stage reconstruction with a septal cartilage graft.

REFERENCES

1. Murakami CS, Quatela VC. Reconstruction surgery of the ear. In: Cummings CW, Richardson MA (Eds). Otolaryngology Head and Neck Surgery. St. Louis: Mosby; 1998;439-41.
2. Gasser RF, May M. Embryonic development. In: May M, Schaitkin BM (Eds). The Facial Nerve. New York: Thieme; 2000;1-15.
3. Tanzer RC. Total Reconstruction of the external ear. Plast Reconstr Surg Transplant Bull. 1959;23 (1):1-15.
4. Brent B. Ear reconstruction with an expansile framework of autogenous rib cartilage. Plast Reconstr Surg. 1974;53(6):619-28.
5. Nagata S. A new method of total reconstruction of the auricle for microtia. Plast Reconstr Surg. 1993;92(2):187-201.
6. Firmin F, Marchac A. A novel algorithm for autologous ear reconstruction. Semin Plast Surg. 2001;25(4):257-64.
7. Kasrai L, Snyder-Warwick AK, Fisher DM. Single-stage autologous ear reconstruction for microtia. Plast Reconstr Surg. 2014;133(3):652-62.

Chapter 11

Facial Aesthetics

Benjamin Marcus

> ***Chief Complaint***
> *"I look older than my age".*

DEFINITIONS

Dermatochalasis: Excess upper lid skin.

Blepharochalasis: Intermittent and recurrent swelling of the upper lids.

Brow ptosis: Vertical descent of the brow, often leading to lateral hooding.

Liposis: Excessive facial fat, especially in the submental region.

Elastosis: Descent and loss of elasticity of the facial skin.

Rhytidosis: Wrinkling of the skin.

ANATOMY AND PHYSIOLOGY OF THE AGING FACE

Facial features that change with aging *are as follows*:

- *Facial skin*: As we age the facial skin loses elasticity. In addition, photoaging causes rhytids and pigment irregularities. Aging skin also frequently has excess capillaries.
- *Facial volume:* As we age we often lose facial fat. This leads to hollowing in a number of specific regions:
    - Lower lids (tear troughs)

- Cheeks (malar fat pads)
- Temples
- *Elastosis:* Aging results in loss of skin elasticity. Significant aesthetic impact occurs at the following:
  - Jowls
  - Nasolabial folds
  - Neck
- *The upper third*: Upper lid aging is often a combination of dermatochalasis of the upper lid combined with brow ptosis. The upper lid can also undergo pseudoherniation of fat, especially at the medial upper lid.
- Lower lid aging is a combination of rhytidosis, pseudoherniation of fat and volume loss.
- An area of special consideration for facial aging is the midface. The malar fat pad can undergo significant descent. This area often requires specific evaluation to determine its role in facial rejuvenation.

THE AGING FACE: CAUSES

Physiologic

- *Aging*: Loss of elasticity combined with volume loss and age-related changes in the skin are a normal part of the aging process. This can be accelerated through a variety of pathologies.
- *Treatment*: A variety of therapies are available, including laser resurfacing, face lifting, and volume replacement. Resurfacing should be considered to improve skin texture. Face lifting is inclusive of lower facelift and neck lifting, and upper and lower lid blepharoplasty. Brow lifting can also be considered. Volume enhancement can be achieved with commercial fillers or the use of autologous fat transfer.

Extrinsic

Chronic exposure to the sun is a key element of early aging for skin. Repeated photodamage leads to the formulation of solar lentigines, telangiectasias, and loss of skin elasticity.

Treatment: Photodamage is often best treated with resurfacing. This can be done with lasers, chemical peels, and even dermabrasion.

Endocrine

Early-onset menopause and loss of the estrogen response can lead to premature aging of the skin.

Treatment: A variety of therapies are available, including laser resurfacing, face lifting, and volume replacement. A more controversial therapy is hormone replacement. This type of treatment should be advised when all the risks and benefits have been thoroughly discussed with the patient and her primary physician.

Iatrogenic

Patients who undergo bariatric surgery may experience significant weight loss. This often leads to significant volume shifts within the face and subsequent significant elastosis.

Treatment: In the setting of massive weight loss, patients do best with surgery that removes excess skin. Precise volume replacement can also be helpful to fill in specific hollows.

Toxic

Smoking causes premature fine lines that typically appear on places where the skin is very thin, such as the sides of the eyes (smile lines) and above the upper lip. These typical smoking lines may appear 10–15 years before they appear among nonsmokers. The reason for the premature wrinkles among smokers is a decrease in vitamin C level in their blood. Vitamin C is a key component in the production of collagen fibers, which are responsible for the elasticity and appearance of youthful and healthy skin; lack of vitamin C affects the proper production of collagen.

Treatment: Rhytidosis is often best treated with resurfacing. This can be done with lasers, chemical peels, and even dermabrasion.

DIAGNOSTIC WORK UP— "I LOOK OLDER THAN MY AGE."

History

"What bothers you the most about your appearance?"

"Have the changes that concern you happened slowly over time, or have things changed rapidly?"

"What is your history of sun exposure? Are you currently using protection for your skin?"

"Are you an active smoker? Have you ever smoked?"

"Are you looking for noninvasive treatments, or are you willing to consider surgery?"

Physical Examination

- The skin should be evaluated for:
    - Fine lines
    - Excess pigmentation (solar lentigines)
    - Telangiectasias
- The upper third of the face should be evaluated for:
    - Brow ptosis
    - Upper lid dermatochalasis
    - Lower lid skeletonization; volume loss and rhytidosis
- The middle third should be evaluated for:
    - Midface descent
    - Prominence of the nasolabial fold
- The lower third of the face should be evaluated for:
    - Jowling
    - Submental elastosis, liposis, and platysmal banding.

Ancillary Tools

- *Traditional photography*: A mainstay of facial aesthetics; this is essential for documentation and standardized evaluation of outcomes.
- *Three-dimensional image capture*: A newer form of imaging; this ancillary tool allows practitioners to simulate a variety of rejuvenation procedures.

Chapter 12

Facial Trauma: Soft Tissue Trauma and Bony Fractures

Samuel Hahn

FACIAL SKELETAL ANATOMY

The facial bones are arranged in a complex and intricate three-dimensional (3D) manner. They function to sustain masticatory forces, provide support for the soft tissue envelope of the face, and protect vital organs housed within the head. Traumatic injury to the face can result in both aesthetic and functional deficits.

The facial skeletons are supported through a system of horizontal and vertical buttresses (Fig. 12.1).

- Horizontal buttresses:
  - Frontal bar
  - Infraorbital rim and nasal bone
  - Maxillary alveolus and hard palate
- Vertical buttresses:
  - Mandibular ramus
  - Pterygomaxillary buttress
  - Zygomaticomaxillary (ZM) buttress
  - Nasomaxillary buttress.

PRINCIPLES OF EVALUATION AND MANAGEMENT OF FACIAL TRAUMA

Initial evaluation of the head and neck trauma patient should begin with resuscitation of the patient. Once the patient has

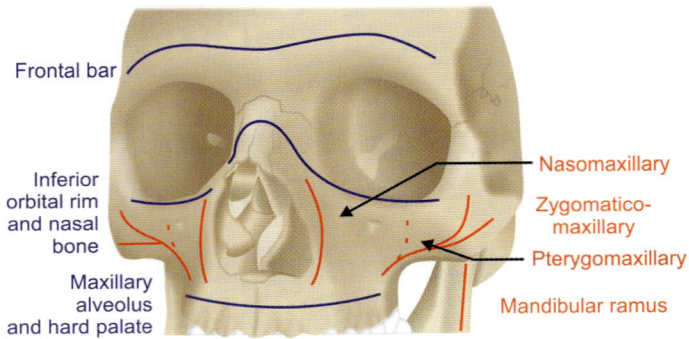

Fig. 12.1: Facial buttresses provide support for the facial skeleton. Horizontal buttresses (blue): 1, frontal bar; 2, inferior orbital rim and nasal bone; 3, maxillary alveolus and hard palate. Vertical buttresses (red): 1, mandibular ramus; 2 (dotted line), pterygomaxillary buttress; 3, zygomaticomaxillary buttress; 4, nasomaxillary buttress.

been stabilized, understanding the mechanism of injury, tissue damage, and impact of the injury on facial form and function is important in determining the treatment algorithm for facial trauma.

Mechanism of Injury

Assess the angle and velocity of impact as well as whether the injury was blunt or penetrating. The energy imparted during the traumatic event will determine the degree of soft tissue and skeletal injury as well as injury to vital organs within the head and neck region.[1]

Soft Tissue Management

The initial management of soft tissue trauma includes cleaning and thoroughly irrigating open wounds to remove any foreign material, debridement of devitalized tissue, and local wound care. Administer antibiotics and check tetanus immunization status.

Definitively manage open wounds within 24 hours of injury. Clean wounds with minimal tissue loss can be closed primarily, while contaminated wounds or wounds with significant tissue loss should be managed with delayed closure or wound healing by secondary intention. Additional reconstructive surgery may be required to correct the defect.[2]

Imaging

Evaluation of the facial skeleton following trauma is now largely performed by computed tomography (CT) scans. The CT scan allows for fast, high-resolution imaging of bony facial structures in multiple dimensions. Three-dimensional images can be constructed from the CT images to further assist with spatial positioning of the fractures. Panoramic radiography plays an important role in diagnosis and treatment of mandibular fractures, especially with evaluation of the alveolar-ridge and tooth root fractures.[3]

Surgical Planning

The reconstructive goals of surgery involve restoring facial form (e.g. facial symmetry, height, and width) and function (e.g. mastication and vision).

EVALUATION AND MANAGEMENT OF FACIAL FRACTURES

Facial fractures can be divided by subsites:
1. Upper third—frontal sinus and skull base
2. Middle third—midface
3. Lower third—mandible

Facial Fractures of the Upper Third

The frontal bone forms the upper third of the face and houses the frontal sinus and anterior cranial vault. Fractures involving the upper third of the face are at higher risk for intracranial involvement and may require concomitant management with neurosurgery. Surgical access to the upper third can be obtained via the use of existing facial lacerations, a coronal incision, a brow incision (gull wing incision), or endoscopic approaches.

Frontal Sinus Fracture

Frontal sinus fractures can be classified as anterior and/or posterior table fractures. Assessment of the nasofrontal recess is important to avoid postinjury complications.

Anterior Table Fractures

- Minimally displaced fractures (<2 mm) can be managed conservatively.
- Displaced fractures without severe comminution should be reduced and internally fixated.
- Severely comminuted fractures require obliteration of the frontal sinus.

Posterior Table Fractures

- High risk of intracranial injury and cerebrospinal fluid (CSF) leak; consider neurosurgical consultation.
- Minimal displaced fractures (<2 mm) without CSF leak can be managed conservatively; if CSF leak is present and persistent, they will require obliteration or cranialization of the frontal sinus.
- Displaced fractures without severe comminution should be treated with obliteration; if CSF leak is present and persistent, they will require cranialization.
- Severely comminuted fractures require cranialization of the frontal sinus.

Nasofrontal Recess Injury

- Minimal displaced fractures with patent nasofrontal recess can be managed conservatively.

- Mildly displaced fractures may be treated with stents or widening ostium.
- Significantly displaced fractures require obliteration of the frontal sinus to prevent postinjury complications, e.g. traumatic mucocele.

Facial Fractures of the Middle Third

Fractures of the middle third of the face include nasal, orbital, naso-orbitoethmoid, ZM complex (ZMC), and Le Fort type maxillary fractures.

Nasal Fractures

- Most common facial fractures.
- Evaluate for epistaxis, septal hematoma, and nasal obstruction.
- Closed reduction within the first 3 hours or 3–10 days following fracture, after edema has subsided.
- Open reduction with internal fixation (septorhinoplasty) in instances of failed closed reduction or delayed treatment.

Orbital Fractures

- Obtain ophthalmologic evaluation to evaluate for serious ocular injury.
- Surgical access to the orbit is obtained via lower eyelid transconjunctival, subciliary, or subtarsal approaches.
- *Surgical indications*: Enophthalmos, hypophthalmos (> 2 mm), entrapment, diplopia, defects with >50% of orbital floor (high risk for delayed enophthalmos).
- *Contraindications to surgery*: Hyphema, retinal tear, globe rupture, and only seeing eye.
- Orbital floor reconstruction can be performed with bone graft, titanium mesh, or porous polyethylene sheets.

Nasoorbitoethmoid Fracture

- Fracture involving the nasal bone, nasal process of frontal bone and maxilla, lacrimal bone, and medial orbit.

- Presenting signs can include rounding of the medial canthus/ traumatic telecanthus [medial canthal ligament (MCL) involvement], CSF rhinorrhea (cribriform plate injury), and epiphora (injury to lacrimal system).
- Surgical access is obtained via coronal, transconjunctival, or transcutaneous lower eyelid, and midfacial degloving approaches.
- Technically very challenging to repair; it requires accurate resuspension of MCL, dacryocystorhinostomy for repair of lacrimal system (it can be staged).

Zygomaticomaxillary Complex Fracture

- Four sutures are involved in ZMC fracture: (1) zygomaticofrontal (ZF) suture, (2) ZM suture, (3) zygomaticotemporal suture, and (4) zygomatic sphenoid suture.
- *Surgical indications:* Facial asymmetry, trismus, and orbital complication (diplopia and enophthalmos).
- Surgical access is obtained via multiple incisions to visualize the fracture segments.
  - *Orbital region:* Lateral brow or upper eyelid approach (ZF suture), transconjunctival or subciliary approach (inferior orbital rim and orbital floor).
  - *Zygoma:* Coronal approach (ZF and zygomatic arch), Gilles or Keen approach (isolated arch fracture).
  - *Maxillary:* Sublabial approach (ZM suture and inferior orbital rim).
- *Open reduction and internal fixation:* Minimum of two-point fixation required for stabilization of ZMC fracture.

Le Fort Type Maxillary Fractures

- Classification of maxillary fractures based on patterns of fractures along lines of minimal resistance (Fig. 12.2).[4]
  - *Le Fort classification:*

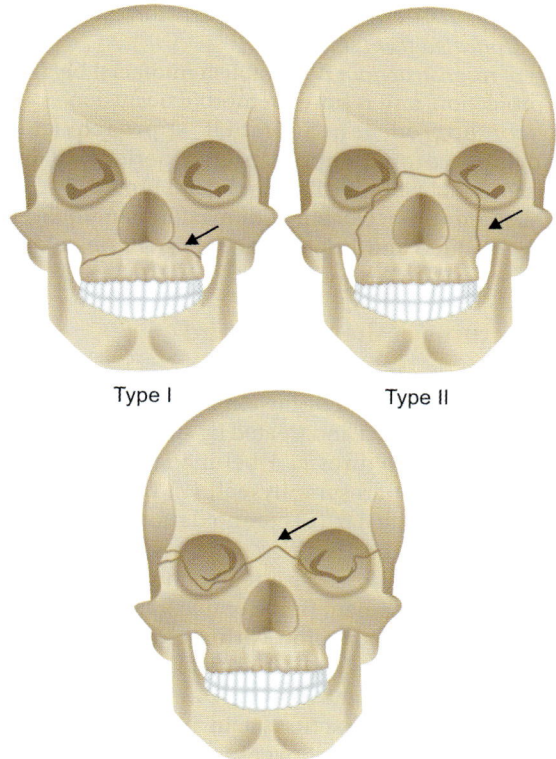

Type I

Type II

Type III

Fig. 12.2: Le Fort classification of maxillary fractures. Type I: Transverse maxillary fracture; Type II: Pyramidal midface fracture; Type III: Craniofacial separation.

- *Type I—transverse maxillary fracture, upper alveolus (above tooth roots) separated from craniofacial skeleton.*
- *Type II—pyramidal midface fracture.*

> - *Type III—craniofacial separation, facial skeleton separated from skull base.*

- *Goals of reconstruction*: Re-establish midfacial height, width, and projection, and restore premorbid occlusion.
- *Surgical approaches*: Sublabial approach (midfacial degloving), coronal approach, and periorbital incisions (transconjunctival, subciliary, or lateral brow).
- Establish normo-occlusion with maxillomandibular fixation (MMF), reduce and internally fixate fractures along facial buttresses.

Facial Fractures of the Lower Third

Fractures of the lower third of the face involve the mandible. Re-establishing premorbid occlusion is critical. The mandibular fracture can be classified and treated by site.

- The mandible fractures can be divided into seven types: (1) symphyseal/parasymphyseal, (2) body, (3) angle, (4) ramus, (5) subcondylar, (6) coronoid (nonoperative), and (7) condylar.
- Strong masticatory forces exerted on the mandible can result in fracture displacement (unfavorable fracture).
- Maxillomandibular fixation with arch bars, intermaxillary screws, or interdental wires is used to re-establish occlusion and restore facial height.
- Some mandibular fractures can be treated with closed reduction (MMF) for 2–6 weeks, depending on the site of fracture.[5]
- Open reduction and internal fixation are indicated in displaced and comminuted fractures, edentulous, multiple/bilateral fractures, patients with seizure disorders, noncompliant patients (alcoholism), and pregnant patients.
- Surgical approaches to the mandible include the intraoral incision (with care taken to preserve the mental neurovascular bundle) and/or external approach (submandibular, retromandibular, or preauricular incisions).

EVALUATION OF A FACIAL TRAUMA PATIENT

History

- "How and when did you get hurt? What was the mechanism of injury (e.g. assault, motor vehicle accident, and gunshot wound)?"
- "Do you have double or blurry vision?"
- "Do your teeth feel like they come together normally?"
- "Do you have normal sensation over your forehead, face, and chin?"
- "Do you have normal movement of your face?"
- "Do you have nose bleeds, nasal obstruction, or difficulty breathing?"
- "Do you have hearing loss or vertigo?"

Physical Examination

- *Resuscitation*: Check ABCs (airway, breathing, and circulation)—establish airway (it may require intubation or emergent tracheostomy, or cricothyroidotomy).
- *Eye examination*: Assess for pupillary defect, conjunctival hemorrhage, eye movement (check for entrapment, forced duction testing), proptosis, enophthalmos, telecanthus, orbital rim step off, and tearing.
- *Ear examination*: Assess for hemotympanum, CSF leak, tympanic membrane perforation, Battle's sign (mastoid ecchymosis), and auricular hematoma.
- *Nasal examination*: Assess for external nasal deviation or deformity and septal hematoma.
- *Oral examination*: Assess for loose or missing teeth, malocclusion, open bite, trismus, mucosal lacerations, loose maxilla and midface (Le Fort I, II, or III fractures).
- *Facial examination*: Assess for facial numbness [cranial nerve (CN) V1–V3 distribution), facial weakness (CN 7), facial asymmetry, and open wounds.

Radiologic Examination

- *Computed tomography*: Most commonly used form of radiologic examination performed for facial trauma to obtain axial and coronal images, possible 3D reconstruction.
- *Panoramic radiography (e.g. Panorex)*: Frequently used for mandibular fracture; it shows condyle-to-condyle view.
- *Facial plain films*: Largely replaced by CT, anterior–posterior axial (Towne) view, posterior–anterior view, and bilateral oblique.
- *Computed tomography angiography*: It is indicated when there is concern for vascular injury.

Consultations to Consider

- *Neurosurgery*: Intracranial involvement of facial trauma, fractures involving posterior table of frontal sinus or skull base, and CSF leak.
- *Ophthalmology*: Orbital fractures, retrobulbar hematoma, globe injury, retinal injury, and ophthalmoplegia.

REFERENCES

1. Nahum AM. The biomechanics of facial bone fracture. Laryngoscope. 1975;85(1):140-56.
2. Futran ND. Maxillofacial trauma reconstruction. Facial Plast Surg Clin North Am. 2009;17(2):239-51.
3. Wilson IF, Lokeh A, Benjamin CI, et al. Prospective comparison of panoramic tomography and helical computed tomography in the diagnosis and operative management of mandibular fractures. Plast Reconstr Surg. 2001;107(6):1369-75.
4. Tessier P. The classic reprint. Experimental study of fractures of the upper jaw. I and II. Rene Le Fort MD. Plast Reconstr Surg. 1972;50(5):497-506.
5. Fayazi S, Bayat M, Bayat-Movahed S, et al. Long term outcome assessment of closed treatment of mandibular fractures. J Craniofac Surg. 2013;24(3):735-9.

SUGGESTED READING

1. Fox AJ, Kellman RM. Mandibular angle fractures: two-miniplate fixation and complications. Arch Facial Plast Surg. 2003;5:464-9.
2. Gonty AA, Marciani RD, Adornato DC. Management of frontal sinus fractures: a review of 33 cases. J Oral Maxillofac Surg. 1999;57:372-9.
3. Kellman R. Maxillofacial trauma. In: Flint PW (Ed). Cummings Otolaryngology Head and Neck Surgery, 5th edition, Vol 1. Philadelphia: Mosby Elsevier; 2010. pp. 318-41.
4. Manson PN, Hoopes JE, Su CT. Structural pillars of the facial skeleton: an approach to the management of Le Fort fractures. Plast Reconstr Surg. 1980;66(1):54-61.
5. Nguyen M, Koshy JC, Hollier LH Jr. Pearls of naso-orbital-ethmoid trauma management. Semin Plast Surg. 2010;24(4):383-8.
6. Ondik MP, Lipinski L, Dezfoli S, et al. The treatment of nasal fractures. Arch Facial Plast Surg. 2009;11(5):296-302.
7. Raveh J, Laedrach K, Vuillemin T, et al. Management of combined frontonasoorbital/skull base fractures and telecanthus in 355 cases. Arch Otolaryngol Head Neck Surg. 1992;118:605-14.
8. Sorel B. Open versus closed reduction of mandible fractures. Oral Maxillofac Surg Clin North Am. 1998;10:541-65.
9. Worsaae N, Thorn JJ. Surgical versus nonsurgical treatment of unilateral dislocated low subcondylar fractures: a clinical study of 52 cases. J Oral Maxillofac Surg. 1994;52:353-60.

Sleep Medicine

Section Editor: *Fredric Jaffe*

Chapter 13

Sleep Disordered Breathing

Fredric Jaffe, Maria Elena Vega

> ***Chief Complaint***
> *"I am sleepy during the day".*

DEFINITION

- Sleep disordered breathing refers to upper airway partial or total obstruction and the partial or complete cessation of airflow.
    - There can be respiratory effort (obstructive) or no respiratory effort (central) associated with this airway obstruction.
    - These events while the individual is sleeping are a normal phenomenon.
    - If the number of events rises during the sleep period above a certain threshold (> 5 events per hour), they are considered pathologic.
- Obstructive events consist of two types of airflow limitation that exists on a continuum from snoring to frank apneas:
    - A hypopnea is defined as noncomplete cessation of airflow with either an associated arousal from sleep or a significant desaturation from baseline.
    - An apnea is near-complete cessation (>90%) of airflow with no need for associated criteria. Snoring to frank apneas is a continuum of upper airway patency (Flowchart 13.1).

SLEEP DISORDERED BREATHING SEVERITY

- The apnea hypopnea index (AHI) is measured by the total number of apneas plus the total hypopneas divided by the number of hours of sleep (Table 13.1).
- Apnea hypopnea indices in the mild range need clinical symptoms to be present to diagnose a patient with sleep apnea syndrome.
  - Those with an AHI of >15 do not need to have symptoms to be classified as having sleep apnea syndrome.

Flowchart 13.1: The spectrum of sleep disordered breathing.

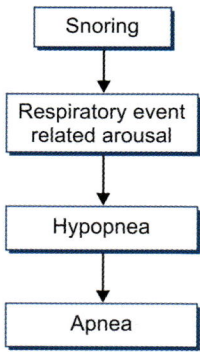

Table 13.1: Severity definition in sleep disordered breathing.	
Severity	*AHI*
Normal	<5
Mild	5–15
Moderate	16–30
Severe	>30

(AHI: Apnea hypopnea index).

History

- Dates back to *Pickwick Papers* published in 1836 by Charles Dickens, who described a character named "Joe the Fat Boy" who was obese, sleepy, and red in the face (Fig. 13.1).
- Later this syndrome was labeled as the Pickwickian syndrome in 1956 by Dr Burwell in patients with the same characteristics as Joe.

Prevalence

- There has been a relative increase of up to 55% in some segments of the American population.
  - Two large epidemiologic studies in the United States defined the prevalence of obstructive sleep apnea (OSA) and OSA syndrome.
    - In one study, 12,000 women and 4,000 men ranging in age from 20 to 100 years old were interviewed.

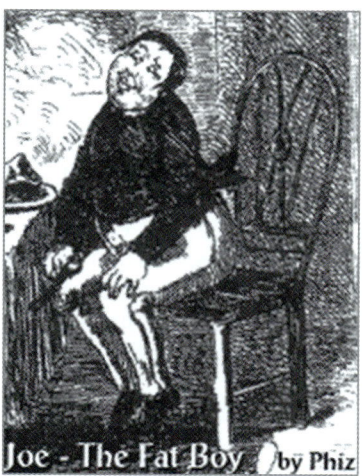

Fig. 13.1: "Joe the Fat Boy" from Charles Dickens' *Pickwick Papers*.

In another study 1,000 women and over 700 men performed one night of sleep laboratory evaluation.

1. Sleep apnea was defined as an AHI >10 events per hour and daytime symptoms including daytime sleepiness.
   a. The prevalence was 3.9% for men and 1.2% for women.
   b. The prevalence of sleep apnea for postmenopausal women who were not taking hormone replacement therapy was 2.7% versus 0.6% in premenopausal women.

- The Wisconsin Sleep Cohort Study (WSCS)
  - This was a longitudinal epidemiology study designed to investigate the natural history of sleep disordered breathing.
    - Overnight polysomnography (PSG), repeated at 4-year intervals, on a random sample of the general population.
    2. The estimated prevalence in the WSCS was high for both men and women, with a prevalence of 9% for women and 24% for men for mild OSA, and 4% for women and 9% for men for an AHI >15 events per hour.

- Some of the first data on the incidence of sleep disordered breathing came from the Cleveland Family Study.
  - The 5-year incidence was estimated to be 7.5% for moderate-to-severe OSA (AHI of ≥15) and 16% for mild OSA (AHI of at least 10 events per hour).
    - This study also suggested that with aging, male gender and body mass index (BMI) lose importance as risk factors for OSA.
    3. By age 50 the incidence rates between men and women are similar.
  - In an epidemiologic study in 2013, Peppard found that the prevalence in those with moderate-to-severe (AHI >15 events/hour) sleep disordered breathing in the

population had increased to 10% in men 30- to 49-years-old and in women to 3%.

4. In those 50- to 70-years-old the incidence was 17% in men and 9% in women.

Evaluation of the Patient

Sleep History

- Sleep habits including bedtime and wakeup time.
  - Bed partner can be helpful in obtaining the sleep history.
  - Common symptoms
    - Excessive daytime sleepiness (see below)
    - Loud snoring (>80 decibels)
    - Witnessed apneas
    - Choking and gasping
  - Daytime sleepiness
    - Epworth sleepiness scale
      a. This is an eight-question self-reported test that measures the patient's subjective sleepiness in several situations (Table 13.2).
         i. A score of >10 indicates excessive daytime sleepiness.
         ii. A score of <6 is considered no daytime sleepiness.
- Risk factors for sleep apnea
  - Obesity
  - Advancing age
  - Airway anatomic phenotypes
    - The strongest of those risk factors are obesity and age >65 years:
    - Obesity is the strongest risk factor (Fig. 13.2).
      1. Obesity is the main epidemiologic risk factor increasing the risk of OSA 2- to 10-fold.
      2. Obesity rates in 2014 published by the Centers for Disease Control:
         a. In the United States one in three persons in that population is considered obese with a BMI of over 30 kg/m^2.

Table 13.2: Epworth sleepiness scale.

How likely are you to doze or fall asleep in the following situations?
Answer considering how you have felt over the past week or so.

0 = Would never doze
1 = Slight chance of dozing
2 = Moderate chance of dozing
3 = High chance of dozing

1. Sitting and reading
2. Watching TV
3. Sitting inactive in a public place (e. g., theater or meeting)
4. As a passenger in a car for an hour without a break
5. Lying down to rest in the afternoon when able
6. Sitting and taking to someone
7. Sitting quietly after a lunch without alcohol
8. In a car while stopped for a few minutes in traffic

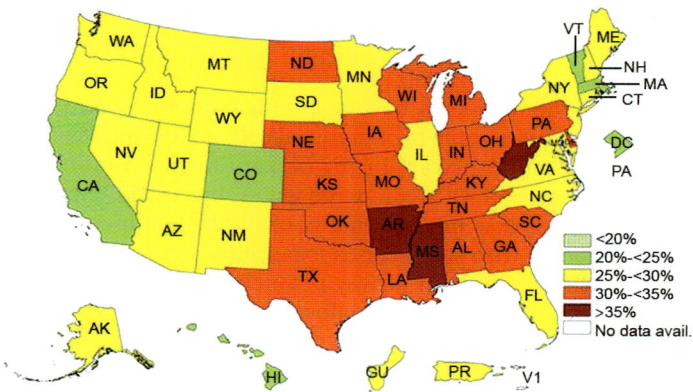

Fig. 13.2: Prevalence of self-reported obesity among US adults by state and territory.
Source: Centers for Disease Control and Prevention, 2014 Behavioral Risk Factor Surveillance System.

- – A less strong factor that helps raise the suspicion of sleep apnea is a positive family history. This can increase the risk of OSA by as much as two- to fourfold.
- Physical examination
  - – According to the American Academy of Sleep Medicine (AASM), features that suggest the presence of OSA include:
    - A neck circumference >17 inches for men and 16 inches for women.
    - Modified Mallampati score of 3 or 4 indicating a narrow airway as well as the presence of retrognathia, macroglossia, tonsillar hypertrophy, an enlarged uvula, high-arched/narrow hard palate, and nasal abnormalities.
      3. The narrower the airway is from any anatomic abnormality, the higher the likelyhood the airway will collapse and therefore a higher risk of sleep disordered breathing.

Pathogenesis

- Due to alterations in upper airway anatomy and neuromuscular control.
    - Patients with OSA have anatomic compromise, making them susceptible to pharyngeal collapse during sleep.
    - The upper airway during wakefulness is reduced in patients with OSA compared with subjects without OSA.
    - There is loss of volitional control of the upper airway; patients with sleep apnea experience no problems with their breathing or airway patency while awake as their consciousness does not allow for airway collapse.
        - This occurs because the wakeful state provides compensatory neuronal activation of dilator muscles in the anatomically compromised collapsible airway.
        - When asleep, this action is lost and patients with OSA experience obstructive events.
- Obesity contributes to upper airway narrowing by deposition of fat around the neck, resulting in increased extraluminal pressure predisposing it to collapse.
    - Central adiposity leads to reduction in lung volumes, resulting in loss of parenchymal traction on the trachea, making the airway more prone to collapse.
- Hormonal contribution
    - Leptin is an adipocyte-derived factor whose role is not only to induce satiety and increase metabolism but also to act as a respiratory stimulant.
    - Leptin levels are increased in obesity and OSA; obese individuals present a degree of leptin resistance.
- Age
    - As the patient ages, changes in the control of breathing at the onset of sleep increase the prevalence of sleep apnea.
        - However, no studies of sleep-related changes in chemosensitivity have been fruitful.
        - The loss of central control is a theory, but the central control of breathing has been shown to be relatively stable in older people.

- Another theory about the increased prevalence of sleep apnea in older people is that the comorbidities associated with sleep apnea predispose an individual to sleep apnea.
    1. In those with diabetes and renal failure there is a high prevalence of sleep apnea, which is increased in older people. This relationship does not imply causality, only association.
- The increase in OSA may be due to a decrease in the size of the upper airway lumen in older people, especially males.
    2. Changes in anatomy with respect to the dimensions of the upper airway include pharyngeal airway lengthening in both males and females.
    3. As a person ages the hyoid bone descends, with resultant increased pharyngeal resistance. In healthy elderly people, pharyngeal resistance is increased compared with that in younger people, indicating a predisposition to airway collapse.
- No one theory explains the increased incidence, but the evidence is compelling as to the strength of age as a risk factor for sleep disordered breathing.

Treatment of OSA

- Patients with OSA need treatment.
    - These patients have associated major comorbidities including daytime somnolence, impaired cognition, poor quality of life, and increased risk of motor vehicle accidents.
    - Obstructive sleep apnea has been identified as an independent risk factor for a number of cardiovascular diseases, including hypertension, stroke, congestive heart failure, atrial fibrillation, and coronary artery disease.
    - It has also been associated with a number of comorbid conditions, including type 2 diabetes and pulmonary hypertension. Identification and treatment of these patients is important for these reasons.

Medical and Surgical Options

- The most effective and reliable treatment for mild, moderate, and severe OSA remains continuous positive airway pressure (CPAP) (Figs. 13.3A and B).
  - Noninvasive positive airway pressure provides a pneumatic splint and keeps the upper airway open; it also can increase lung volumes as it can transmit this pressure into the lower airways.
  - Continuous positive airway pressure is delivered by an interface on the face and has been available since 1981.
  - The pressure needed to keep the airway patent is titrated during a PSG in the sleep laboratory or at home through an autotitrating device that determines the pressure through a complex algorithm.
    - In the laboratory a sleep technologist will adjust the pressure to eliminate apneas and hypopneas (Figs. 13.4A and B).
- Continuous positive airway pressure interfaces
  - Significant improvements have been made in the design of the masks and pressure-delivery systems to allow patients to be more comfortable with the interface.

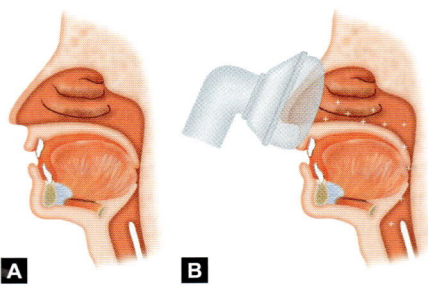

Figs. 13.3A and B: Nasal continuous positive airway pressure. (A) The airway is closed; (B) the addition of positive airway pressure opens the upper airway.

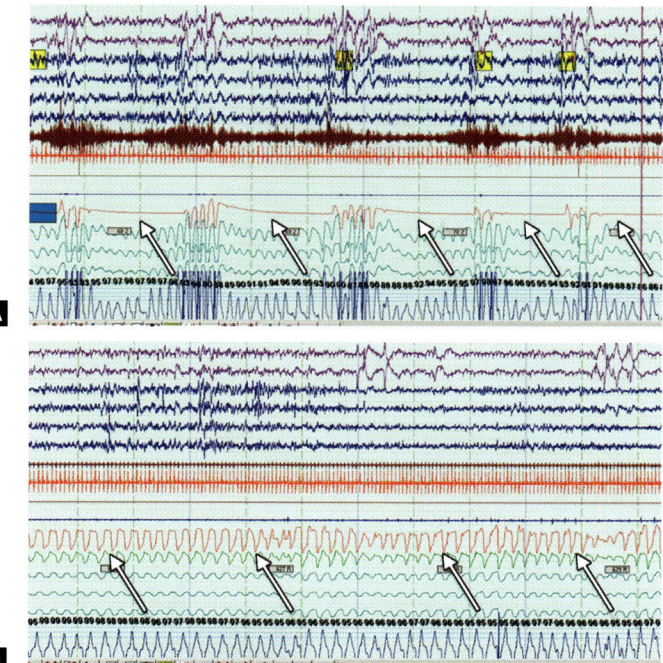

Figs. 13.4A and B: (A) A polysomnogram showing apneas (arrows). (B) A polysomnogram showing the use of noninvasive positive pressure ventilation. Arrows show the treatment eliminating the apneas.

- Nasal masks (Fig. 13.5), full face masks (Fig. 13.6), and nasal cannula-like interfaces (Fig. 13.7) all deliver a pressure that transmits through the upper airway and prevents upper airway collapse.
  – Positive airway pressure can be delivered by continuous CPAP, bilevel positive airway pressure (BiPAP), or autotitrating positive airway pressure (APAP) modes.

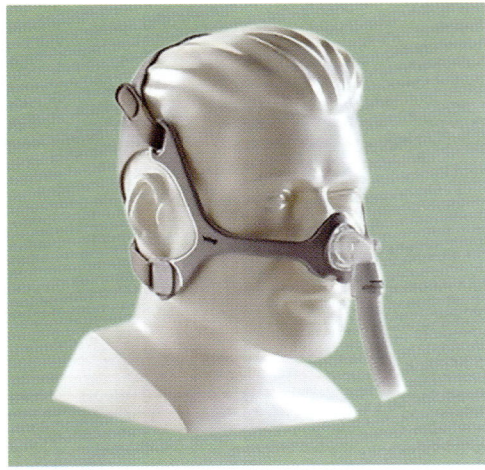

Fig. 13.5: Nasal mask.

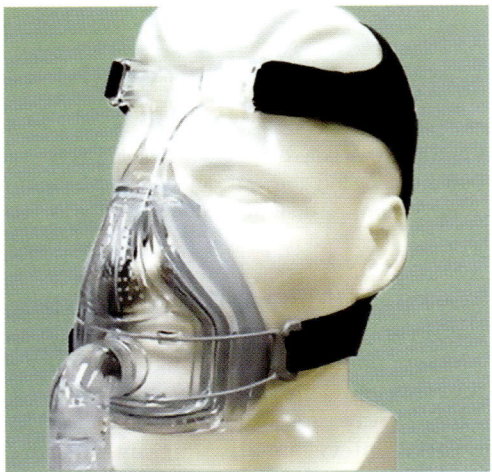

Fig. 13.6: Full-face mask.

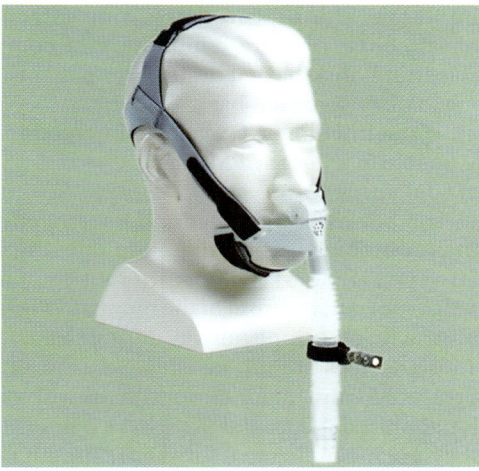

Fig. 13.7: Nasal pillows.

- Bilevel modes deliver a pressure during inhalation and then a lower pressure during exhalation to prevent upper airway collapse.
  - Patient comfort can drive the decision to use one mode over another.
  - One mode of support may not provide adequate pressure to eliminate sleep disordered breathing.
  - The use of CPAP, BiPAP, and APAP has been shown to be effective in eliminating obstructive events.
- Treatment of disordered breathing leads to improvement in daytime sleepiness, cognition, quality of life, and reduction of cardiovascular morbidity and mortality.
  - Adherence to CPAP, BiPAP, or APAP therapy can be poor.
  - Several studies demonstrate compliance rates of, at best, 50%.
    - Reasons for poor compliance with CPAP therapy include mask discomfort causing skin abrasion and

intolerance to the pressure. Side effects such as nasal congestion are common, and complaints of claustrophobia make it difficult for patients to use the machine on a regular basis.

- Alternative treatments for OSA have emerged for patients who are unable to tolerate CPAP therapy.
    - Oral appliances
        - Placed between the upper and lower teeth and slide the lower jaw forward, therefore opening the upper airway (Fig. 13.8). Others attempt to stabilize the tongue toward the front of the mouth to prevent it from obstructing the upper airway during sleep.
        - These devices are not as effective as positive airway pressure treatment for those patients with severe OSA. Randomized controlled trials have demonstrated that they are most effective for the treatment of mild-to-moderate OSA.

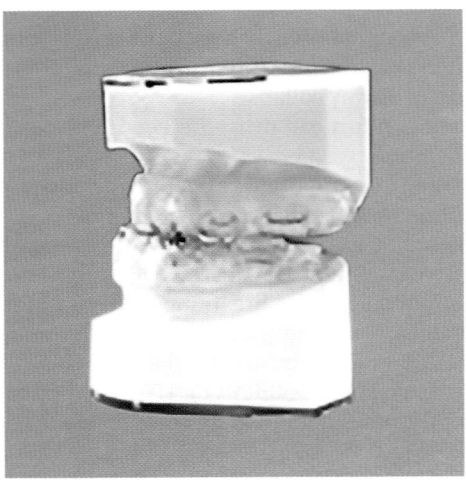

Fig. 13.8: Dental device.

- Positional therapy for positional OSA.
  - Positional OSA, where sleep-disordered breathing events occur predominantly in the supine position, is quite prevalent in patients with mild (50%) and moderate (19%) OSA. In these, a positional device can be employed (Fig. 13.9).
  - A study by Permut et al. demonstrated that positional therapy was equivalent to CPAP at normalizing the AHI, even in severe disease.
- Surgical intervention of the upper airway
  - Surgical options in adults with sleep disordered breathing include uvulopalatopharyngoplasty, laser-assisted uvulopalatopharyngoplasty, maxilla-mandibular advancement, palatal implants, radiofrequency ablation, and tracheostomy.
  - Discussion of the various techniques is beyond the scope of this chapter. Due to the lack of rigorous data

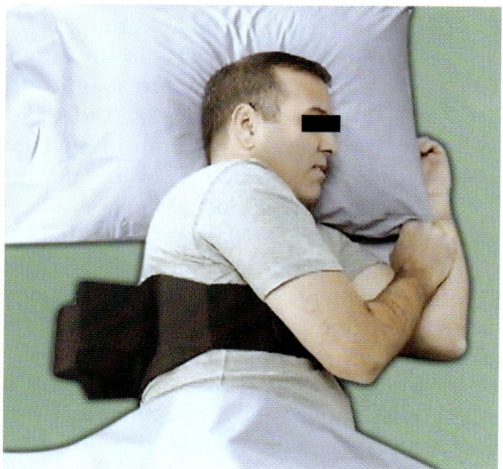

Fig. 13.9: Positional device.

evaluating surgical modifications of the upper airway, these procedures should be reserved for patients who have failed medical therapies. Parameters for the surgical approach of the upper airway for OSA have been published by the AASM.

- Lifestyle modifications
  - These changes in behavior should be encouraged for all patients and include the following:
    - Avoidance of alcohol as well as sedatives and narcotics, which can decrease upper airway tone and patency.
    - Weight loss
      1. Diet and exercise
      2. Bariatric surgery
         a. One randomized controlled trial looked at the effects of weight loss surgery versus conventional therapy in the management of OSA. The bariatric surgical group achieved a significantly greater mean weight loss of 27.8 kg at 2 years compared with 5.1 kg in the conventional weight loss group.
            i. Greater weight loss in the surgical group did not translate into significantly greater improvements in OSA. The AHI decreased by 14 events per hour in the conventional group and by 15.5 events per hour in the bariatric surgery group.
    - Although weight loss is associated with improvement in AHI, there is great variability in the individual effect. Therefore, patients should continue treatment for OSA even after significant weight loss until a repeat PSG confirms normalization of the AHI.
  - Other therapies exist that attempt to keep the upper airway patent, all with varying levels of success. Positive airway pressure remains the most effective, and as with any alternative therapy careful patient selection is key.

CONCLUSION

Sleep disordered breathing is a serious disease with some effective treatments. Eliciting a thorough history and appropriate physical examination can lead to quick diagnosis and effective therapy. Treatment should be individualized to find the most effective option for treatment. Appropriate treatment will improve quality of life and can affect mortality and morbidity.

SUGGESTED READING

1. Aurora RN, Casey KR, Kristo D, et al. Practice parameters for the surgical modifications of the upper airway for obstructive sleep apnea in adults. Sleep. 2010;33(10):1408.
2. Dempsey JA, Veasey SC, Morgan BJ, et al. Pathophysiology of sleep apnea. Physiol Rev. 2010;90 (1):47-112.
3. Dixon JB, Schachter LM, O'Brien PE, et al. Surgical vs conventional therapy for weight loss treatment of obstructive sleep apnea: a randomized controlled trial. JAMA. 2012;308(11):1142-9.
4. Epstein L, Kristo D, Strollo Jr P, et al. Clinical guideline for the evaluation, management and long-term care of obstructive sleep apnea in adults. J Clin Sleep Med. 2009;5(3):263-76.
5. Friedman M, Tanyeri H, La Rosa M, et al. Clinical predictors of obstructive sleep apnea. Laryngoscope. 2009;109(12):1901-07.
6. Gold AR, Schwartz AR. The pharyngeal critical pressure: the whys and hows of using nasal continuous positive airway pressure diagnostically. Chest J. 1996;110(4):1077-88.
7. Guilleminault C, Partinen M, Hollman K, et al. Familial aggregates in obstructive sleep apnea syndrome. Chest. 1995;107(6):1545-51.
8. Marin JM, Carrizo SJ, Vicente E, et al. Long-term cardiovascular outcomes in men with obstructive sleep apnoea-hypopnoea with or without treatment with continuous positive airway pressure: an observational study. Lancet. 2005;365(9464):1046-53.
9. Patil SP, Schneider H, Schwartz AR, et al. Adult obstructive sleep apnea: pathophysiology and diagnosis. Chest J. 2007;132(1):325-37.
10. Permut I, Diaz-Abad M, Chatila W, et al. Comparison of positional therapy to CPAP in patients with positional obstructive sleep apnea. J Clin Sleep Med. 2010;6(3):238.

11. Rosen CL, Auckley D, Benca R, et al. A multisite randomized trial of portable sleep studies and positive airway pressure autotitration versus laboratory-based polysomnography for the diagnosis and treatment of obstructive sleep apnea: the HomePAP study. Sleep. 2012;35(6):757-67.

Section
4

The Larynx

Section Editor: *Ahmed M S Soliman*

Chapter 14

Hoarseness (Dysphonia)

Resha S Soni, Ahmed M S Soliman

Chief Complaint
"My voice has been hoarse for several weeks now".

BACKGROUND

- Hoarseness (dysphonia) is characterized by an alteration in vocal quality, vocal effort, volume, or pitch that impairs communication or reduces voice-related quality of life.[1]
- It affects up to one third of the adult population at least once during their lifetime.[2]

BRIEF OVERVIEW OF LARYNGEAL ANATOMY AND PHYSIOLOGY

The main functions of the larynx are respiration, phonation, and lower airway protection.

Anatomy of the Larynx (Fig. 14.1)

- Laryngeal musculature:
  - *Cricothyroid*: Lengthening (tension) of vocal folds
  - *Posterior cricoarytenoid*: Abduction of vocal folds
  - *Lateral cricoarytenoid*: Adduction of vocal folds
  - *Interarytenoid*: Adduction of vocal folds; only unpaired muscle

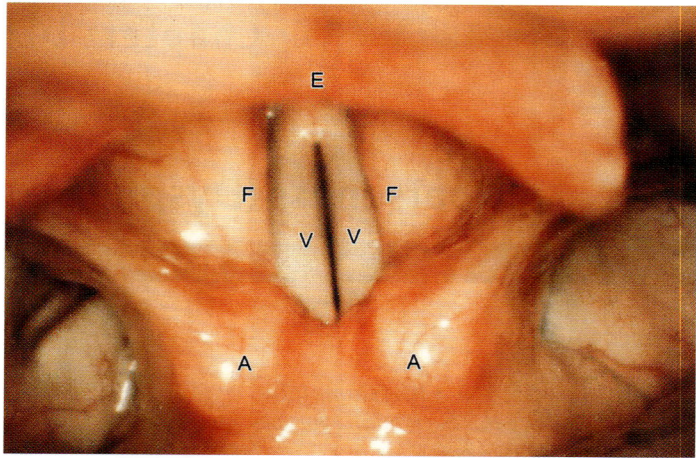

Fig. 14.1: Normal larynx in the surgical position.
(E: Epiglottis; F: False vocal fold; V: True vocal fold; A: Arytenoid).

- – *Thyroarytenoid*: Adduction of vocal folds; medial aspect called the *vocalis*
- Laryngeal cartilages:
  - – Hyaline cartilage
    - · Thyroid
    - · Cricoid
    - · Arytenoid
  - – Fibroelastic cartilage
    - · *Corniculate*: At the apex of arytenoid
    - · *Cuneiform*: Within aryepiglottic folds
- Laryngeal joints:
  - – Cricothyroid joint
  - – Cricoarytenoid joint
- Innervation—Vagus (CN X):
  - – Superior laryngeal nerve
    - · *External branch*: Motor input to cricothyroid muscle
    - · *Internal branch*: Sensory above the vocal folds

- Recurrent laryngeal nerve:
  - Motor supply to all internal muscles of larynx *except cricothyroid*; sensory below the vocal folds[3]

Physiology of Voice Production

- The true vocal fold consists of layers from superficial to deep:
  - Stratified, nonkeratinized squamous epithelium on the free edge; pseudostratified columnar epithelium on superior and inferior edges
  - Superficial lamina propria (Reinke's space)
  - Intermediate lamina propria
  - Deep lamina propria
  - Thyroarytenoid muscle complex (medial and lateral bellies)
- *Vocal ligament:* This is made up by the intermediate and deep lamina propria.
- The gelatinous superficial lamina propria along with the squamous epithelium moves freely over the underlying vocal ligament and muscle to produce vibrations; this is visualized using videostroboscopy or high-speed video and is referred to as the *mucosal wave.*

DIAGNOSTIC WORKUP

History

- Typical questions:
  - "When did the voice change begin? Sudden or gradual?"
  - "How long has it been going on?"
  - "Is it present upon awakening?"
  - "Does it worsen as the day goes on?"
  - "Do you experience wavering of the voice?"
  - "Is there a history of intubation?"
  - "Any surgeries or trauma?"
  - "Are you using oral inhalers, anticholinergic medications?"
  - "Profession or hobby that requires excess voice use"

- Assess for associated symptoms:
  - Was the voice change preceded by an upper respiratory tract infection? (Think: viral or vocal fold paresis)
  - Cough?
  - Dysphagia? Odynophagia? Referred otalgia? (Think: malignancy)
  - Heartburn?
  - Dyspnea?
  - Hemoptysis?
- Assess for constitutional symptoms:
- Fever? Unintentional weight loss? Night sweats?
- Smoking status? Alcohol consumption?
- Caffeine intake?

Physical Examination

- Assess for quality of voice:
  - *Maximum phonation time*: This is the length of time a patient can vocalize after taking a deep breath; <10 seconds is abnormal.
  - *Pitch* (Hz): This is related to the frequency of vocal fold vibration.
  - *Volume* (decibels): This is related to the intensity or loudness of the voice.
  - *Quality* (timbre): This is the character of the voice as related to synchronicity of vocal fold vibration.
  - GRBAS scale is an auditory perceptual scale often used by voice clinicians to objectively assess voice with ratings of 0–3 (0 is normal, 1 is a slight degree, 2 is a medium degree, and 3 is a high degree).
  - *Grade*: overall global impression of the voice.
    - *Roughness*: Raspy or rattling voice (mass lesions of the vocal folds).
    - *Breathiness*: Whispering voice (unilateral vocal fold motion impairment, vocal atrophy).
    - *Asthenia*: Small, weak voice (psychogenic dysphonia and myasthenia gravis).

- *Strain*: Tight, effortful voice (adductor spasmodic dysphonia, vocal paresis with compensatory hyperfunction)
- Assess for quality of respirations.
- Focused head and neck examination:
  - Cranial nerve and complete neurologic examination.
  - Nasal cavity/nasopharynx/oropharynx: Look for mucosal lesions.
  - Neck examination with palpation for lymphadenopathy, masses; look for scars.
  - *Indirect mirror if possible or flexible fiberoptic laryngoscopy*: Assess vocal fold mobility, erythema, edema, masses, lesions, glottic competence.
  - *Videostroboscopy*: This provides visualization of mucosal vibration.
- *Voice handicap index and voice-related quality of life surgery*: These are widely used validated quality of life questionnaires used to assess psychosocial burden of voice disorder.[4]
- *Laryngeal electromyography*: This aids in evaluating the laryngeal neuromusculature.
- Chest radiograph ± computed tomographic (CT) neck with contrast indicated if initial workup reveals a paralyzed vocal fold without a known cause, to identify vascular abnormalities and/or mass lesions.[5]

DIFFERENTIAL DIAGNOSIS

- Congenital:
  - *Laryngeal web*: This is rare in adults but more commonly found in the pediatric population.
- Infectious:
  - *Viral, bacterial, fungal infections of the larynx*: These are treated with anti-inflammatories, voice rest, antimicrobials, and antifungal medications, respectively.
- Inflammatory:
  - *Laryngopharyngeal reflux (LPR)*: Symptoms include hoarseness, throat clearing, globus sensation, and

cough. Laryngoscopy is notable for erythema and edema of the postcricoid region as well as vocal fold edema and endolaryngeal mucus. Using questionnaires such as the reflux symptom index and reflux findings score may be helpful in making diagnosis. Treatment is done with proton pump inhibitors and dietary modifications. Refractory cases are evaluated with dual port pH probe with impedance and manometry.

– *Allergic rhinitis*: Patients may have associated nasal symptoms and findings of congestion, rhinorrhea, and thick postnasal discharge. Inhaled corticosteroids may cause a fungal overgrowth of the pharynx and larynx. Environmental irritants such as cleaning solutions may cause nonspecific erythema and edema of the nose, pharynx, and larynx; history is important in making this diagnosis.

– *Reinke's edema*: The superficial layer of the lamina propria is susceptible to fluid accumulation in smokers and in hypothyroidism; check thyroid function tests; smoking cessation; consider microlaryngoscopy with removal of gelatinous material in cases that have not resolved after 6–12 months.

– Benign vocal fold lesions:[6]

  • *Vocal fold nodules*: Bilateral lesions on the free edge at the junction of the anterior and middle one third of the vocal fold. Normal or minimal impairment of vibratory mucosa, usually soft at first but may become fibrous with time; associated with voice overuse, particularly in young boys and adult women; usually respond to voice therapy.

  • *Vocal fold polyp*: This is typically unilateral, exophytic, and can be translucent or hemorrhagic, on the free edge with normal or minimal impairment of vibratory mucosa, responds to voice therapy; rough voice quality; risk factors include voice overuse, particularly, a sudden brief burst. Surgical excision is warranted if voice therapy is ineffective.

- *Vocal fold cyst*: This is typically unilateral, encapsulated lesions with impairment of vibratory mucosa; may be mucoid or epidermoid; the latter is less common. Symptoms may be longstanding (>1 year). Surgical excision is required if voice therapy is ineffective.
- *Vocal fold granuloma*: This appears on the medial aspect of vocal process of the arytenoids; associated with orotracheal intubation or chronic reflux and throat clearing; often bilateral when caused by intubation; may be associated with throat and ear pain; voice therapy, botulinum toxin injection, and antireflux therapy are often effective. Surgical excision alone often results in rapid recurrence if underlying mucoperichondrium is exposed.
- *Pseudocyst*: Subepithelial lesion associated with chronic glottic incompetence, fluid underneath a thinned epithelium; mucosal wave is usually intact; surgical excision is warranted if voice therapy fails.

- Trauma:
  - *Arytenoid dislocation*: This presents as unilateral vocal fold motion impairment after intubation; many resolve spontaneously; endoscopic relocation is often unsuccessful; may represent injury to the posterior cricoarytenoid (PCA) branch of the recurrent laryngeal nerve rather than true dislocation; high-resolution fine-cut CT scan through the larynx may help make diagnosis.
  - *Vocal hematoma*: This may be as a result of acute phonotraumatic event or instrumentation of the larynx. Most will resolve spontaneously; some may require surgical evacuation and sealing of the feeding vessels if recurrent.
  - *Caustic inhalation injuries*: These are uncommon but may result in edema of the vocal folds; supportive care with humidified air and steroids is considered as appropriate.
- Neoplastic:
  - *Laryngeal papilloma*: Wart-like appearance of examination; may be single or diffuse; caused by human

papilloma virus types 6 and 11. Juvenile onset more likely to be diffuse; excision with CO_2 or preferably potassium-titanyl-phosphate or pulse dye laser usually required; microdebrider is useful for excision of bulky lesions; adjuvant therapies include Avastin, cidofovir, and interferon. Malignant transformation is rare but possible.

- *Carcinomas*: Squamous cell type is most prevalent in the larynx. Supraglottic and subglottic lesions present with hoarseness later than glottis lesions in which hoarseness is the primary symptom. A history of tobacco and alcohol use is typical but not always present.

- Neuromuscular and psychiatric:
  - *Unilateral vocal fold paralysis*: Patients present with a breathy dysphonia; may be idiopathic or iatrogenic; thyroid surgery, anterior cervical spine surgery, carotid endarterectomy, cardiac, and neurosurgery are common causes of the latter; early vocal fold injection will improve voice and may obviate need for additional therapy in some patients.
  - *Multiple sclerosis*: This is usually present with articulatory problems but also pitch perturbation; managed primarily with voice therapy.
  - *Myasthenia gravis*: Dysarthria, vocal fatigue, lack of pitch control, hypophonia; treated with voice therapy and pharmacologic management of myasthenia gravis.
  - *Muscle tension dysphonia*: This is due to hyperfunction of the false vocal folds. It is usually secondary to underlying glottic insufficiency; treatment of this is essential to improvement. Voice therapy to break behavior is often necessary.
  - *Spasmodic dysphonia*: Focal dystonia affecting intrinsic laryngeal muscles; this is present with an action-induced hyperfunction of the affected muscle. Adductor type (more common—95%) is present with strangled quality to voice; abductor type (less common—5%) is present with breathy voice. Treatment with botulinum toxin injection

into the affected muscle is effective. Surgical procedures are rarely necessary.

– *Presbyphonia*: Vocal fold bowing due to muscle atrophy in the elderly population

– *Psychogenic dysphonia*: This usually presents with a breathy dysphonia with a whisper-like quality to the voice upon phonation; laughing, coughing, and crying will produce voiced sounds. Involvement of mental health professionals is often necessary in the treatment of this patient population.

- Systemic diseases:
  – Hypothyroidism, sarcoidosis, inflammatory arthritis, pubescence.

GENERAL MANAGEMENT OF DYSPHONIA

Management is dependent on the underlying cause!

- *Vocal hygiene*: This encompasses education in environmental, behavioral, vocal habit, and dietary modification.
  – Humidification of air.
  – Avoid smoke and dust and alcohol consumption.
  – Avoid frequent throat clearing.
  – Avoid habitually speaking loudly for prolonged periods.
  – Increase fluid intake.
  – Avoid excessive caffeine intake due to its dehydrating effect.
  – Avoid spicy foods or large meals late at night.
- *Voice therapy*: In association with speech–language pathologists, the goal is to modify harmful vocal behaviors.
  – It is often used as the first-line treatment for vocal nodules, polyps, cysts, and functional dysphonias.[4]
  – It has been used to improve outcomes after surgical intervention for dysphonia.
- *Antireflux medications*: They have demonstrated effectiveness in treating laryngeal inflammation from LPR, although use as empiric therapy remains controversial.[5] Use should be for a

short, fixed duration due to risk of long-term complications, including renal disease and osteoporosis.

- *Vocal fold injection*: This is typically used as a temporizing measure in unilateral vocal fold immobility. It is also used for vocal fold atrophy, paresis, and presbylarynx. Injection materials include fat, collagen, carboxymethylcellulose (Prolaryn Gel), hydroxyapatite (Prolaryn Plus), hyaluronic acid (Restylane), micronized Alloderm (Cymetra).[4]
- Laryngoplasty (thyroplasty):[4]
  - *Type I*: Medialization by inward lateral compression of vocal fold with an implant placed via a thyroid cartilage window.
  - *Type II*: Lateralization of the vocal fold by lateral expansion of the thyroid cartilage used in adductor spasmodic dysphonia.
  - *Type III*: Posterior relaxation of vocal folds; it is used to lower pitch in puberphonia or as part of gender reassignment surgery.
  - *Type IV*: Anterior tensing of vocal folds used to increase vocal pitch.
- Reinnervation procedures: These are indicated for unilateral permanent vocal fold paralysis. Ansa cervicalis has similar nerve fiber composition to the recurrent laryngeal nerve and is used for grafting.

REFERENCES

1. Schwartz SR. Clinical practice guideline: hoarseness (dysphonia). Otolaryngol Head Neck Surg. 2009;141(3 Suppl 2):S1-31.
2. Keesecker SE, Murry T, Sulica L. Patterns in the evaluation of hoarseness: time to presentation, laryngeal visualization, and diagnostic accuracy. Laryngoscope. 2015;125(3):667-73.
3. Feierabend RH, Shahram MN. Hoarseness in adults. Am Fam Physician. 2009;80(4):363-70.
4. Syed I, Daniels E, Bleach NR. Hoarse voice in adults: an evidence-based approach to the 12 minute consultation. Clin Otolaryngol. 2009;34(1):54-8.

5. Chang JI, Bevans SE, Schwartz SR. Evidence-based practice: management of hoarseness/dysphonia. Otolaryngol Clin North Am. 2012;45(5):1109-26.
6. Rosen CA, Gartner-Schmidt J, Hathaway B, et al. A nomenclature paradigm for benign midmembranous vocal fold lesions. Laryngoscope. 2012;122(6):1335-41.

Chapter 15

Dysphagia

Gary Linkov, Barbara Ebersole, Nausheen Jamal

> ### Chief Complaint
> *"I am having difficulty swallowing".*

DEFINITIONS

Dysphagia: Symptom indicating abnormal passage of food or liquid bolus from mouth to stomach.

Odynophagia: Painful swallowing in the mouth, throat, or esophagus.

Globus: Sensation of a foreign body caught in the throat.

RELATED TERMS

- *Aspiration*: When food, liquid, or saliva passes below the vocal folds and into the trachea.
- *Penetration*: When food, liquid, or saliva enters the laryngeal vestibule but does not go below the vocal folds. Penetration can be transient (enters the larynx and is promptly evacuated) or residual (enters and remains in the larynx). Residual penetration carries an increased risk of delayed aspiration.

ANATOMY AND PHYSIOLOGY IN NORMAL SWALLOWING

- Normal swallowing involves more than 30 nerves and muscles.

- The swallow is a pressure-driven mechanism regulated by valving structures and dependent on speed, force, and co-ordination of movements.
- *Six valves*: Lips, glossopalatal, glossopharyngeal, velopharyngeal, larynx, upper esophageal sphincter (UES).
- Driving force (pressure generators that direct food from oral cavity to esophageal inlet): Oral tongue, base of tongue, and pharyngeal constrictors.
- *Airway protection*: Glottic and supraglottic closure in combination with excursion of the hyolaryngeal complex (upward and anterior movement).
- Respiration pre/postswallow is most commonly expiratory, with a swallow apnea duration ranging from 0.77 to 1.32 seconds.
- Swallow speed and force decline with increasing age.
- *Three main phases of swallowing*: Oral, pharyngeal, and esophageal (according to the location of bolus).
- Liquid and solid mechanics differ in oral phase; oral stage is subdivided into oral preparatory and oral propulsive.
- Oral phase of swallowing is under voluntary control.
- Pharyngeal and esophageal phases are reflexive and involuntary.
- Swallow reflex is an innate, semiautomatic reflex movement elicited by mechanical, chemical, and/or thermal stimulation.
- It is initiated by cerebral cortex; organized by swallowing central pattern generator in the medulla.

INTRODUCTION AND KEY POINTS OF DYSPHAGIA

- *Medical history*: Key features include the following:
  - Location of symptoms
  - Types of foods and/or liquids that cause symptoms
  - Progressive or intermittent
  - Duration of symptoms
  - Context of onset (i.e. preceding upper respiratory infection, intubation, and prior surgery)
  - Associated signs and symptoms (i.e. odynophagia, cough, hoarseness, heartburn, dyspnea, globus, and weight loss)

- History of pneumonia
- Diet and lifestyle (i.e. caffeinated beverages and cigarettes)
- Prior studies, treatments, or procedures (chest X-ray, barium swallow studies, endoscopies).

- *Classification*: Dysphagia is most commonly categorized into one or both of the following categories (it can be differentiated on the basis of careful history alone in about 80% of cases):
  - *Oropharyngeal dysphagia*: Localized to mouth and/or throat:
    - *Frequent accompanying symptoms*: Choking, coughing, sensation that food gets caught, nasal regurgitation, halitosis, abnormal mastication, oral pocketing, or expectoration of food/liquid.
    - *Associated possible neurological findings*: Weakness of cranial nerves 7–12, tongue fasciculations, hemiparesis, ptosis of eyelid, end-of-day weakness (myasthenia gravis), Parkinson's disease, etc.
  - *Esophageal dysphagia*: Difficulty transporting food through the esophagus secondary to structural or neuromuscular defects in the smooth muscle portion of the esophagus:
    - *Frequent accompanying symptoms*: Globus, bolus regurgitation, delayed coughing after eating, frequent belching.
    - If occurs equally with solids and liquids, it will usually include an esophageal motility problem.
    - If progressive to solids, consider peptic stricture or carcinoma.

DISEASE BURDEN AND EPIDEMIOLOGY

- Incidence of dysphagia is reported to be as high as 20% in the general population.
- It occurs in all age groups but prevalence increases with age.
- The cause of dysphagia is different among various age groups and geographic locations.

- Dysphagia may lead to medical complications, including aspiration, pneumonia, possible airway obstruction, weight loss, malnutrition.

CAUSES AND TREATMENT OF DYSPHAGIA

The goal is to identify and treat the underlying cause.

- Oropharyngeal:
  - Mechanical and obstructive:
    - Zenker's diverticulum.
    - *History*: Older adults, male, initially transient dysphagia, aspiration pneumonia, foul breath, gurgling in throat, regurgitation of food into mouth, stasis, and weight loss.
    - *Findings*: Diverticulum on barium swallow at level of hypopharynx (path of least resistance), neck mass (rare).
    - *Treatment*: Endoscopic diverticulotomy, open diverticulectomy:
    - Cricopharyngeal spasm:
      - *History*: Globus sensation, aggravated with stress.
      - *Findings*: Cricopharyngeal bar on barium swallow, manometry with elevated UES pressures.
      - *Treatment*: Botulinum toxin injection, dilation, cricopharyngeal myotomy.
    - Head and neck malignancies:
      - *History*: Weight loss, trismus, hemoptysis, otalgia.
      - *Findings*: Neck mass, oral cavity, oropharyngeal, or laryngeal lesion.
      - *Treatment*: Surgery, radiation and/or chemotherapy, dysphagia therapy during and after treatment.
    - Head and neck cancer treatment:
      - *History*: Surgical, chemotherapy/radiation therapy for advanced stage cancers of the oral cavity, pharynx, or larynx.
      - *Findings*: Anatomic surgical defect, fibrotic changes, muscle weakness, xerostomia, diminished

pharyngeal, or laryngeal sensation, hypopharyngeal stricture.
- ○ *Treatment*: Dysphagia therapy, stricture dilation, palatal prosthetics.
- Cervical osteophytes:
  - ○ *History*: Older adults, worse with solids, aspiration symptoms with oral intake, slowly progressive.
  - ○ *Findings*: Anterior cervical bony spurring, epiglottic dysfunction during the swallow (limited retroflexion).
  - ○ *Treatment*: Conservative (diet modification), surgery (anterior cervical osteophyte resection); partial epiglottidectomy.
- *Other causes*: Infections, thyromegaly, lymphadenopathy, and reduced muscle compliance (myositis and fibrosis).
  - Neuromuscular:
    - Stroke:
      - ○ *History*: Aspiration pneumonia, associated cranial nerve, or extremity weakness.
      - ○ *Findings*: Incomplete oral clearance, reduced oral competence, facial, tongue and/or palatal weakness or asymmetry, pharyngeal weakness, dysarthria.
      - ○ *Treatment*: Dysphagia therapy, dietary modifications, cricopharyngeal myotomy, medialization if indicated.
    - Parkinson's disease:
      - ○ *History*: Rest tremor, bradykinesia, rigidity.
      - ○ *Findings*: Oral stage deficits, xerostomia from high levodopa dosage.
      - ○ *Treatment*: Disease medication management, dysphagia therapy.
    - Cranial nerve palsy:
      - ○ *History*: Hoarseness, choking with liquids, additional cranial nerve palsies.
      - ○ *Findings*: Vocal fold paralysis.

- ○ *Treatment*: Injection laryngoplasty (for vocal fold paresis or paralysis), dysphagia therapy.
- Myasthenia gravis:
  - ○ *History*: Fluctuating muscle weakness, worse later in day or after exercise.
  - ○ *Findings*: Ptosis, fatigable chewing, nasal regurgitation due to palatal weakness.
  - ○ *Treatment*: Disease medication management, plasmapheresis, dysphagia therapy.
- Multiple sclerosis:
  - ○ *History*: Relapsing remitting.
  - ○ *Findings*: Sensory symptoms in limbs or face, visual loss, motor weakness.
  - ○ *Treatment*: Disease medication management (immunosuppressive), dysphagia therapy.
- *Other causes*: Amyotrophic lateral sclerosis and muscular dystrophy.
  - – Other
    - Poor dentition (worse with solids).
    - Oral ulcers.
    - *Xerostomia*: difficulty with dry foods → use moist foods and liquid wash; cevimeline hydrochloride; pilocarpine.
    - *Medications*: Anticholinergics, diuretics.
    - *Cognitive impairment*: Typically involves oral (volitional) stage; hallmark symptom is bolus holding.
    - *Respiratory dysfunction* (*e.g. advanced chronic obstructive pulmonary disease or congestive heart failure*): Associated with abnormal respiratory coordination during swallowing, leading to laryngeal penetration and/or aspiration.
- Esophageal:
  - – Mucosal:
    - Peptic stricture secondary to gastroesophageal reflux
    - Rings and webs
    - Esophageal tumors

- Chemical injury
- Radiation injury
- Infectious esophagitis
- Eosinophilic esophagitis
- *Treatment options*: Dilation, medical management, dietary modification, open reconstruction.
  - Mediastinal:
    - Tumors (lung and lymphoma)
    - Infections (tuberculosis and histoplasmosis)
    - Inflammatory (sarcoid)
    - Cardiovascular (vascular compression).
  - Neuromuscular:
    - Achalasia
    - Scleroderma
    - Postsurgical (postfundoplication).

CLINICAL EVALUATION (FLOWCHARTS 15.1 TO 15.4)

- Bedside swallow evaluation, the following way should be considered:
  - Perceptual evaluation without visualization of swallow structures
  - *Diagnostician*: Speech-language pathologist
  - Food administered to a patient in various textures
  - *Subjective clues used to assess for penetration and aspiration*: Throat clear, cough, "wet" voice
  - Inexpensive, no radiation exposure, no transportation required
  - Not sensitive for silent penetration and aspiration episodes.
- Barium swallow (esophagram):
  - *Diagnostician*: Radiologist
  - Assessment of esophageal dysphagia
  - Patient swallows suspension of barium with concurrent radiography of the neck and thorax
  - Inexpensive, noninvasive.

Flowchart 15.1: Oral stage symptoms only.

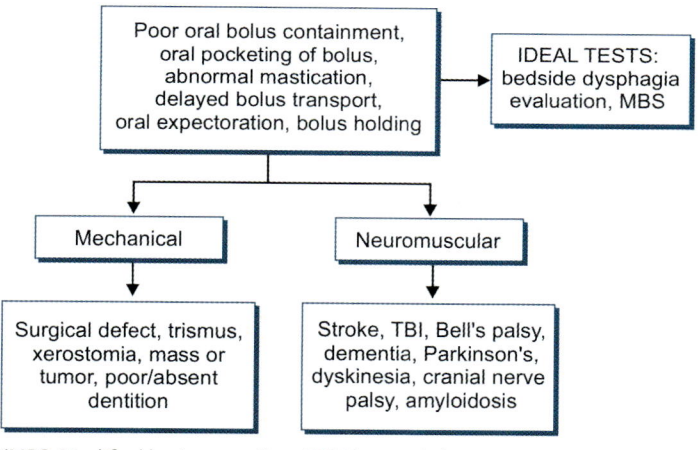

(MBS: Modified barium swallow; TBI: Traumatic brain injury).

Flowchart 15.2: Pharyngeal stage symptoms only.

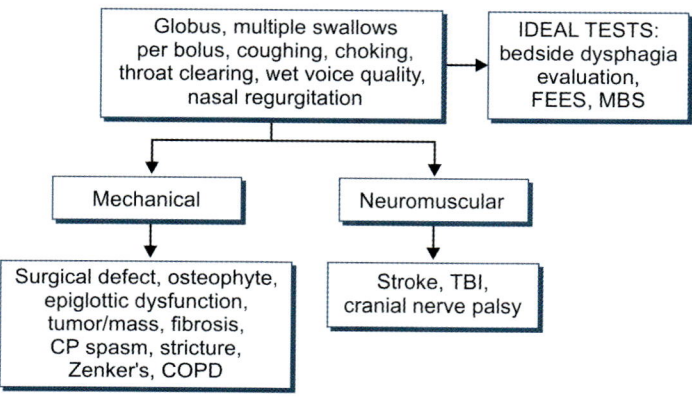

(FEES: Fiberoptic endoscopic evaluation of swallowing; CP: Cricopharyngeal; COPD: Chronic obstructive pulmonary disease; TBI: Traumatic brain injury).

Flowchart 15.3: Both oral and pharyngeal stage symptoms.

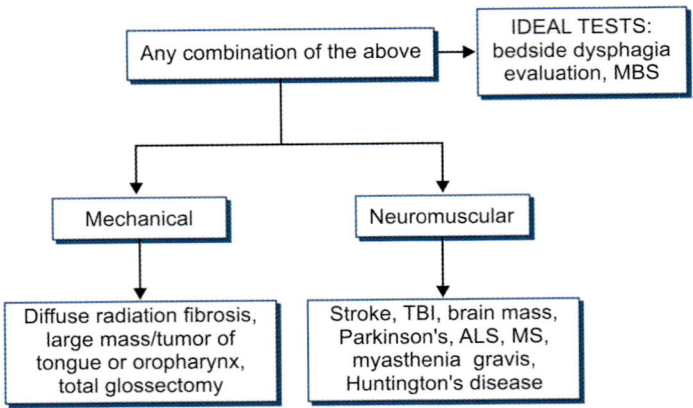

(ALS: Amyotrophic lateral sclerosis; MS: Multiple sclerosis; MBS: Modified barium swallow; TBI: Traumatic brain injury).

Flowchart 15.4: Esophageal stage symptoms.

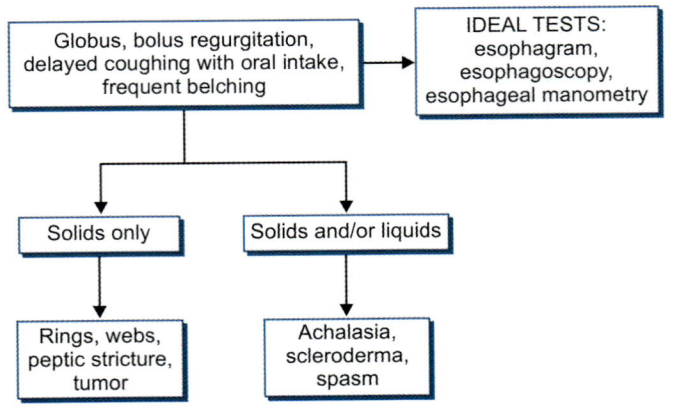

- Modified barium swallow (videofluoroscopic swallow study):
  - *Diagnostician*: Speech-language pathologist ± radiologist
  - Assessment of oropharyngeal dysphagia
  - Requires the presence of both a speech-language pathologist and a radiologist trained in swallowing
  - Barium-coated food is given to the patient in varying consistencies
  - Dynamic view of deglutition from oral cavity to lower esophageal sphincter
  - Requires transportation of the patient to appropriate facility for testing.
- Fiberoptic endoscopic evaluation of swallowing ± sensory testing:
  - *Diagnostician*: Otolaryngologist and/or speech-language pathologist
  - Portable study incorporating flexible fiberoptic laryngopharyngoscopy to assess dynamic swallowing abnormalities, assess sensation, and aspiration
  - No radiation, accurate anatomical information
  - Limited ability to detect penetration aspiration during the swallow
- Esophageal manometry:
  - *Diagnostician*: Gastroenterologist
  - For achalasia, scleroderma, esophageal spasm.
- Esophagoscopy:
  - *Diagnostician*: Gastroenterologist or otolaryngologist
  - Direct visualization for structural causes
  - Ability to biopsy and treat
  - It can be done transnasally as an in-office procedure without sedation.

SUGGESTED READING

1. Hiss SC, Treole K, Stuart A. Effects of age, gender, bolus volume, and trial on swallowing apnea duration and swallow/respiratory phase relationships of normal adults. Dysphagia. 2001;16(2): 128-35.

2. Malagelada JR, Bazzoli F, Elewaut A, et al. World Gastroenterology Organisation Practice Guidelines: Dysphagia. Milwaukee, WI: World Gastroenterology Organization; 2007.

3. Matsuo K, Palmer JB. Anatomy and physiology of feeding and swallowing—normal and abnormal. Phys Med Rehabil Clin N Am. 2008;19(4):691-707.

4. Schindler JS, Kelly JH. Swallowing disorders in the elderly. Laryngoscope. 2002;112(4): 589-602.

5. Vaezi MF. The esophagus: anatomy, physiology, and diseases. In: Flint PW, Haughey BH, Lund VJ, et al (Eds). Cummings: Otolaryngology Head and Neck Surgery, 5th edition. Philadelphia, PA: Elsevier; 2010. pp. 955-6.

Chapter 16

Chronic Cough

Resha S Soni, Nausheen Jamal

> **Chief Complaint**
> *"I have had a cough for several months now".*

BACKGROUND

- Prevalence of cough is up to 33% worldwide regardless of age group.
- Higher incidence in women.
- Associated with a high incidence of psychosocial burden and increased rates of anxiety, depression, and social isolation. Patients also report insomnia, urinary incontinence, headaches, emesis, throat pain, and rib pain.[1]

DEFINITIONS

Acute cough: Lasting < 3 weeks.
Subacute cough: Lasting 4–8 weeks.
Chronic cough: Lasting > 8 weeks; it is pathologic.

RELEVANT ANATOMY

Nasal vestibule → nasal cavities → nasal choana → nasopharynx → oropharynx
Oral cavity → oropharynx → hypopharynx → supraglottic larynx → glottis → subglottis → trachea → lungs

BRIEF PHYSIOLOGY OF THE COUGH REFLEX

- Cough is a protective reflex that serves to clear the airway of excessive secretions and debris.
  - *Neurosensory arc*: Afferent sensory limb → central processing (nucleus tractus solitarius of medulla) → efferent limb.
- Cough can occur reflexively (limited conscious involvement) or behaviorally (requiring higher cortical processing).
- The cough reflex has recently been hypothesized as having neuroplasticity, so that a hypersensitive response is elicited over time by the cough itself, causing chronic inflammation and tissue remodeling.[2]
  - This abnormally sensitive cough reflex has been termed *cough hypersensitivity syndrome.*

CHRONIC COUGH AND AIRWAY REMODELING

- Biopsies of the airway in patients with chronic cough reveal basement membrane thickening, increased numbers of mast cells, hyperplasia of goblet cells, and subepithelial fibrosis.
  - Increased mast cells and neutrophils in bronchoalveolar lavage fluid.
  - Increased level of inflammatory biomarkers: histamine, prostaglandin D2 and E2, tumor necrosis factor alpha, interleukin 8, thromboxane.
- Eosinophils in the airway mucosa are considered the hallmark of chronic airway inflammation.[2]

DIAGNOSTIC WORKUP (FLOWCHART 16.1)

History

- Patients' perception of where the cough anatomically originates has little correlation with the actual origin of the cough.[1]
- Consider using a journal log, cough quality of life questionnaire, or cough severity index to quantify cough severity.[2,3]

Flowchart 16.1: Basic algorithm for chronic cough.

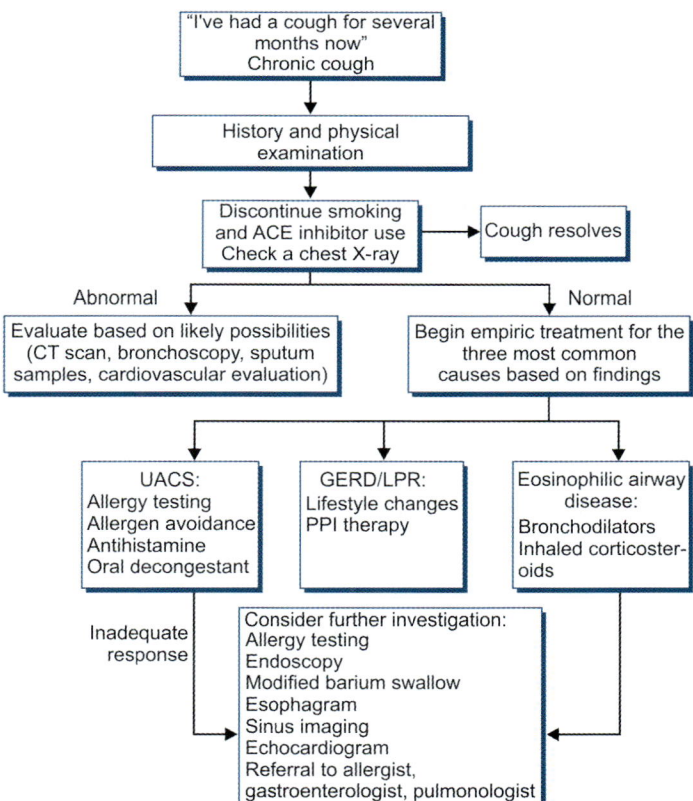

(ACE: Angiotensin converting enzyme; CT: Computed tomography; UACS: Upper airway cough syndrome; GERD: Gastroesophageal reflux disease; LPR: Laryngopharyngeal reflux; PPI: Proton pump inhibitor).

- Assess qualitative cough severity, overall duration, frequency of attacks, subjective triggers, any alleviating/exacerbating factors, as well as constitutional symptoms.

- Typical questions need to be answered?
  - "When did the cough first begin? Was it preceded by an upper respiratory tract infection?"
  - "Is there any history of intubation?"
  - "Is it constant or intermittent?"
  - "How does the cough affect your daily functioning?"
  - "Is it productive? Do you have a history of pneumonia?" (Think: pulmonary)
  - "Is it worse at night?" (Think: reflux, cough-variant asthma)
  - "What do you believe triggers the cough? Does it occur during meals?" (Think: laryngeal sensory neuropathy, laryngeal penetration/aspiration)
- Assess for associated symptoms:
  - "Do you experience frequent throat clearing, a choking sensation or globus sensation?"
- Dysphagia? Odynophagia?
  - Dyspnea?
  - Dysphonia?
  - Hemoptysis? (Think: cancer, tuberculosis)
- Assess for constitutional symptoms:
  - Fever? Unintentional weight loss? Night sweats?
- Smoking status?
- Angiotensin converting enzyme inhibitor (ACE-I) use?
- Geographic location? Occupational exposures? (Think: noxious fumes/chemical exposure, endemic mycoses)

Physical Examination

- Assess for quality of voice/hoarseness.
- Assess for quality of respirations.
- Focused head and neck examination:
  - Cranial nerve examination.
  - Anterior rhinoscopy for mucosal edema, erythema, turbinate hypertrophy.
  - Oral cavity/oropharynx for exudates or cobblestoning of mucosa.

- Neck examination with palpation for lymphadenopathy, jugular venous distension.
- *Mirror examination*: Assess vocal fold mobility, pooling of secretions, erythema, edema, masses, lesions, mucus stranding.
- Perform flexible fiberoptic laryngoscopy if mirror examination is not tolerated or inadequate.
- Evaluate subglottis and upper trachea for evidence of stenosis.
- *Further workup*:
  - Chest radiograph is the *first, most important step*![4]
- *Stroboscopy and medical speech evaluation*: Assess vocal fold mobility, mucosal vibration, vocal quality, and pitch.
- *Flexible endoscopic evaluation of swallowing with sensory testing*: Assess for degree of dysphagia and for laryngeal penetration, and aspiration that could be contributing to cough; assess for decreased laryngeal sensation.
- *Transnasal endoscopy*: Assess for esophageal lesions, ulcerations, and masses, all of which can present with cough.
- Office spirometry detects airway obstruction.
  - Exhaled nitric oxide (NO) measurements help diagnose asthma and eosinophilic bronchitis.
  - An elevated exhaled NO level predicts response to corticosteroids.[5]
- Sputum culture.
- May supplement with chest/sinus computed tomography (CT), modified barium swallow study, esophagogastroduodenoscopy, barium esophagram, and/or allergy testing as clinically indicated.

POTENTIAL CAUSES OF CHRONIC COUGH

- Common:
  - *Airway irritants*: Tobacco smoke, chemicals, noxious fumes
  - *Medications*: ACE inhibitors, β-blockers
  - Upper airway cough syndrome (postnasal drip)

- – *Esophageal*: Gastroesophageal reflux disease, laryngopharyngeal reflux
  - – Asthma
  - – Chronic obstructive pulmonary disease
- Less common:
  - – *Infectious*: Viral, fungal, mycobacterial, pertussis
  - – Interstitial lung disease
  - – Congestive heart failure
  - – Primary lung cancer
  - – Airway stenosis
- Uncommon:
  - – *Tumors*: Benign and malignant involving the proximal and the distal airway
  - – *Neurologic*: Sensory receptor irritability, vagal neuropathy, maladaptive behaviors
  - – Chronic irritation to external auditory canal
  - – Sarcoidosis
  - – Aspiration
  - – Foreign body
- Chronic cough is typically multifactorial.
- Coordinated care among primary care physicians and specialists in otolaryngology, gastroenterology, pulmonology, and allergy is essential.

APPROACH TO MOST COMMON CAUSES OF CHRONIC COUGH

- Empiric treatment of the three most common causes is typically more practical and cost-effective than extensive testing.[4]

Upper Airway Cough Syndrome (Postnasal Drip)

- A combination of criteria is used to diagnose as there are no specific pathognomonic findings:
  - – Anterior rhinorrhea
  - – Nasal congestion

- – Nasal obstruction
- – Sneezing
- – Subjective dripping sensation into oropharynx
- – Frequent throat clearing
- Physical examination reveals nasal mucosal erythema, edema, and clear or mucoid discharge.
- Nasopharyngolaryngoscopy confirms above and may show mucus in nasopharynx and hypopharynx; larynx is without significant abnormality.
- Patients can have reactivity to allergens tested via the skin-prick test.
- Recommend allergen avoidance.
- Empiric therapy with antihistamine and oral decongestant should be considered for initial management.
- Alternative therapies include intranasal corticosteroids, nasal anticholinergics, nasal saline irrigation, and mast cell stabilizers.
- Regular use of topical decongestants should be avoided, as these can cause atrophic rhinitis (*rhinitis medicamentosa*).
- Patients typically respond within 2 weeks; however, it may take several months of therapy before adequate therapeutic response is achieved.[5]

Gastroesophageal Reflux Disease and Laryngopharyngeal Reflux

- Symptoms typically include the following:
  - – Heartburn
  - – Regurgitation
  - – Dysphagia
  - – Positional cough
- Laryngopharyngeal reflux is when the acidic contents of the upper digestive tract reflux beyond the upper esophageal sphincter. This occurs in the upright position. Typical associated symptoms are globus sensation, throat clearing, hoarseness, and cough.

- Laryngoscopy findings include postcricoid edema, interarytenoid edema and inflammation, contact granulomas, pseudosulcus, pachydermia, mucus stranding, ventricular obliteration.
- *Gold standard for diagnosis*: 24-hour dual port pH impedance monitoring
- Lifestyle changes are recommended first: Avoid late-night meals, tight-fitting clothing, and foods that are known to exacerbate symptoms (e.g. caffeine, chocolate, spicy foods, greasy foods, and citrus products); weight loss.
- Proton pump inhibitor (PPI) therapy for at least 3–6 months, with or without use of H2 blockers or prokinetic agents.
- Proton pump inhibitor therapy twice daily is more effective than once daily; this should be taken 30–60 minutes before meals.
- Symptoms may take up to 2 months to begin to improve.
- Antireflux surgery may be considered in refractory cases.
- Consider referral to a gastroenterologist.

Eosinophilic Airway Disease

- Typically manifested by wheezing, chest tightness, dyspnea, and phlegm production.
- *Asthma*:
    - Airway hyper-responsiveness.
    - + Bronchodilator response.
    - Atopy.
    - + Mast cells.
- Cough-variant asthma:
    - Usual features of dyspnea and wheezing are absent.
    - + Bronchodilator response.
- Nonasthmatic eosinophilic bronchitis:
    - Increased sputum eosinophilia (>3% eosinophils on induced sputum sample).
    - Normal results on spirometry and methacholine challenge test.

- Chronic obstructive pulmonary disease.
- Obtain chest X-ray.
- Empiric trial of inhaled corticosteroids and bronchodilators may be initiated.
- Referral to a pulmonologist.

Neurogenic Cough

- Typically a diagnosis of exclusion.
- Cough is typically preceded by a sensation in the throat described as a "tickle."
- Patients will often describe specified triggers: cold air, certain smells, etc.
- *Neuromodulator therapy*: Amitriptyline, nortriptyline, and gabapentin are among the preferred choices.[6]

REFERENCES

1. Terasaki G, Paauw DS. Evaluation and treatment of chronic cough. Med Clin North Am. 2014;98 (3):391-403.
2. Chung KF. Approach to chronic cough: the neuropathic basis for cough hypersensitivity syndrome. J Thorac Dis. 2014;6(Suppl 7):S699-707.
3. Shembel AC, Rosen CA, Zullo TG, et al. Development and validation of the cough severity index: a severity index for chronic cough related to the upper airway. Laryngoscope. 2013;123(8):1931-6.
4. Irwin RS, Baumann MH, Bolser DC, et al. Diagnosis and management of cough executive summary: ACCP evidence-based clinical practice guidelines. Chest. 2006;129(1 Suppl):1-23S.
5. Iyer VN, Lim KG. Chronic cough: an update. Mayo Clin Proc. 2013;88(10):1115-26.
6. Jeyakumar A, Brickman TM, Haben M. Effectiveness of amitriptyline versus cough suppressants in the treatment of chronic cough resulting from postviral vagal neuropathy. Laryngoscope. 2006; 116(12):2108-12.

Chapter 17

Dyspnea

Norman Chan, Ahmed M S Soliman

> ***Chief Complaint***
> *"I have difficulty breathing".*

DEFINITIONS

Stridor: High-pitched sound produced by turbulent airflow through a partially obstructed airway. Inspiratory stridor usually results from supraglottic obstruction. Lower airway obstruction typically produces expiratory stridor. Biphasic stridor is associated with obstruction at the level of the glottis or a fixed anatomic obstruction at any level.

Stertor: Low-pitched snorting or wet, gurgling noise due to partial obstruction involving areas above the larynx.

RELEVANT AIRWAY ANATOMY

Nasal vestibule → nasal cavities → nasal choana → nasopharynx → oropharynx

Oral cavity → oropharynx → hypopharynx → supraglottic larynx → glottis → subglottis → trachea → bronchi

CAUSES OF AIRWAY OBSTRUCTION

Congenital Causes

Please refer to Chapters 33 and 37.

Infectious Causes

Peritonsillar Abscess

a. *Symptoms*: Sore throat, unilateral otalgia, dysphagia, odynophagia, and dyspnea are typical associated complaints.

b. *Diagnosis*: Medial displacement of the ipsilateral tonsil, contralateral uvular deviation, and ipsilateral soft palate effacement along with trismus may be seen on physical examination.

c. *Treatment*: Antibiotics and either needle aspiration or incision and drainage of the abscess.

Retropharyngeal Abscess

a. *Symptoms*: Sore throat, dysphagia, fever, and dyspnea are frequent complaints.

b. *Diagnosis*: A bulge in the posterior pharyngeal wall may be seen. Lateral neck X-ray or computed tomography (CT) scan of the neck with intravenous (IV) contrast are diagnostic.

c. *Treatment*: Intravenous antibiotics followed by prompt incision and drainage, either intraorally or via a transcervical approach are indicated because delay can lead to spread of infection into the mediastinum.

Epiglottitis

This condition is increasingly rare because of routine *Haemophilus influenza* type B vaccination in children.

a. *Symptoms and physical signs*: Affected children usually have a high fever, rapid progression of symptoms, drooling, odynophagia, and assume a tripod position.

b. *Diagnosis*: Usually clinical diagnosis. Lateral neck X-ray classically demonstrates the "thumb" sign.

c. *Treatment*: In children, securing the airway in the operating room with endotracheal intubation or tracheotomy is critical. Blood cultures followed by antibiotics are indicated. In adults, the most common organism is *Streptococcus* and the presentation is often more insidious. Only 20% or fewer will require airway intervention. Serial laryngoscopy is prudent to assess progression of airway edema.

Laryngotracheobronchitis (Croup)

Croup is the most common infectious cause of stridor in children. The most common cause is parainfluenza virus type 1. It most commonly occurs in children of ages 6 months to 3 years.

a. *Symptoms*: The typical clinical course is that of initial upper respiratory infection symptoms that progress to include a barking cough and inspiratory stridor.
b. *Diagnosis*: Anteroposterior soft tissue neck X-ray may show the classic "steeple" sign that results from subglottic narrowing.
c. *Treatment*: It includes corticosteroids, nebulized racemic epinephrine, humidification, and supplemental oxygen. Patients diagnosed with recurrent croup warrant direct laryngoscopy and bronchoscopy to evaluate for an underlying airway abnormality.

Tuberculous Laryngitis

This condition is rare and accounts for <1% of all cases of tuberculosis. It may be mistaken for laryngeal carcinoma, chronic laryngitis, or laryngeal candidiasis. This laryngitis may not be associated with active pulmonary tuberculosis.

a. *Diagnosis*: A biopsy of the lesion that reveals acid fast bacilli is diagnostic.
b. *Treatment*: Antitubercular drugs are required for treatment.

Traumatic Causes

Penetrating Injuries

Damage inflicted by bullets depends on their velocity and yaw. Gunshot wound severity depends on weapon model, projectile size, and distance from the target with greater damage inflicted at closer ranges. Exsanguination is the most common cause of death.

a. *Classification*: Injuries are classified by location in the neck.

    i. Zone I is located below the level of the cricoid and is partially protected by the clavicles and sternum.

    ii. Zone II is located between the level of the cricoid and the angles of the mandible. It is the most commonly injured zone.

    iii. Zone III is located between the angles of the mandible and the skull base. Zones I and III are difficult to access surgically.

b. *Principles of management*: Initial steps in management include securing the airway, maintaining adequate perfusion, and assessing the severity of wounds.

    i. Intubation should only be performed if the larynx and trachea are intact and in direct continuity, and the airway can be visualized. Direct transcervical tracheal intubation is safer than nasotracheal or orotracheal intubation when upper airway visualization is inadequate or when there is significant disruption of laryngotracheal anatomy.

    ii. Cervical spine immobilization is likely unnecessary in low-velocity penetrating neck trauma unless there is neurologic deficit or high suspicion of spinal injury.

    iii. Hemodynamically unstable patients should undergo immediate surgical exploration regardless of zones involved. Stable patients with zone I and III injuries should undergo angiography. Management of zone II injuries is an area of debate with some advocating surgical exploration in all cases. More recently, however, selective management with the use of multidetector CT, CT angiography, and endoscopy has become more common.

    iv. If digestive tract injuries are suspected, esophagoscopy can be performed. Rigid endoscopy is less likely to miss injuries at and above the level of the cricopharyngeus compared to flexible esophagoscopy, which is better for evaluating the distal esophagus. In the case of a confirmed esophageal injury, the patient should be kept NPO and IV antibiotics should be initiated. Small, contained injuries in stable patients may be managed with observation. Similarly, patients with delayed presentation and no signs of sepsis may be managed with observation. Patients with larger tears or signs of sepsis will require neck exploration with primary repair, use of local flaps and drainage. If there is extensive damage, esophageal diversion and delayed repair will often be necessary.

v. Direct laryngoscopy and bronchoscopy should be performed to assess the severity and extent of laryngotracheal injuries. Small, shallow laryngeal mucosal lacerations and nondisplaced cartilage fractures can be observed. Significant laryngeal mucosal lacerations should be repaired within 24 hours, if possible, usually with stenting and tracheotomy. Displaced laryngeal cartilage fractures require open repair.

Blunt Neck Injuries

These can have a delayed presentation.

a. *Principles of management*: If a patient has arterial hemorrhage, cervical bruit, expanding cervical hematoma, focal neurologic deficit, discrepancy between neurologic examination and imaging findings, ischemic stroke on secondary head CT, cervical spine fracture, diffuse axonal injury with Glasgow Coma Scale <6, LeFort II or III fracture, basilar skull fracture with carotid canal involvement, or near hanging with anoxic brain injury, an urgent CT angiography should be performed.

b. *Biffl Grading Scale* for blunt carotid injuries
   i. *Grade I injury*: Vessel wall irregularity or dissection with <25% luminal stenosis
   ii. *Grade II injury*: Intraluminal thrombus or raised intimal flap, or dissection or intraluminal hematoma with >25% luminal stenosis

   iii. *Grade III injury*: Pseudoaneurysms
   iv. *Grade IV injury*: Vessel occlusion
   v. *Grade V injury*: Complete vessel transection

c. *Blunt cerebrovascular injury* treatment includes anti-coagulation regardless of severity. Grade II and III injuries may benefit from endovascular stenting. Carotid cavernous fistula should be embolized with metallic coils. All patients with blunt cerebrovascular injury should have repeat CT angiography 7–10 days later to assess for possible complications such as pseudoaneurysm formation.

d. *Blunt laryngotracheal trauma* may result in airway edema, hematoma, or laryngeal framework instability that may progress to airway obstruction. Flexible fiberoptic laryngoscopy and CT imaging are useful diagnostic modalities.

   i. Endolaryngeal edema, hematoma, contusion, abrasion, most nondisplaced fractures, and small lacerations can be observed and may benefit from steroids and cool mist inhalation.

   ii. Displaced laryngeal fractures should be repaired with 2-point fixation within 24 hours or as soon as possible.

   iii. Mucosal lacerations involving two or more anatomic sites or the free margin of the vocal folds require repair.

   iv. Anterior commissure injuries, injuries with risk of synechia obliterating the laryngeal lumen, and severely comminuted and unstable skeletal fractures will require stenting.

Intubation Trauma

Injury may occur anywhere along the path that was used to insert the endotracheal tube. Laryngeal trauma occurs in up to 6% of cases. Vocal fold lacerations or hematoma, arytenoid dislocation or subluxation, vocal fold paralysis, and granuloma formation may occur. Ulceration of the posterior larynx and posterior glottic stenosis are more likely with the use of large endotracheal tubes and prolonged intubation. Risk is further increased in agitated patients with concomitant nasogastric tubes and gastroesophageal reflux.

a. *Treatment*: Steroids, proton pump inhibitors, and removal of granulations, repair of lacerations, adequate sedation, early tracheotomy when indicated.

Laryngotracheal Stenosis

a. *Etiology:* An inflated cuff of an endotracheal tube or tracheostomy tube that exceeds capillary perfusion pressure can cause tissue necrosis that heals with scarring resulting in stenosis. Use of overly large endotracheal tubes, tracheotomy, and prolonged intubation can also result in tracheal stenosis.

b. Diagnosis:

  i.   Patients will present with stridor, which is often progressive over 1–2 months after extubation or decannulation.

  ii. Flexible laryngoscopy may reveal vocal fold immobility or visible subglottic narrowing in cases of posterior glottic or subglottic stenosis, respectively, but may be normal in cases of tracheal stenosis. A high index of suspicion based upon the history and the presence of stridor is necessary to make the correct diagnosis.

c. Treatment:

  i.   Humidified oxygen, heliox, and systemic corticosteroids may temporarily improve symptoms until definitive treatment is possible.

  ii. Surgical options include direct laryngoscopy and bronchoscopy with steroid injection, laser incision, dilation, and application of mitomycin-C. If these options fail, open laryngotracheal reconstruction or cricotracheal resection can be pursued. In life-threatening acute presentations or when there are contraindications to the above, tracheotomy to bypass the obstruction may be necessary.

Caustic Ingestion

It is usually accidental in children and is associated with suicide attempts in adolescents and adults. Acids result in coagulative necrosis. Alkali solutions cause liquefactive necrosis that results in more damage. The esophagus is most likely to be injured at the gastroesophageal junction and areas externally where there is compression: cricopharyngeus, aortic arch, and left main stem bronchus. Superficial esophageal burns usually heal without complication. Deeper burns can result in fibrosis and stricture formation. Circumferential injuries are more likely to result in strictures. Complications include gastric outlet obstruction, autovagotomy, and esophageal carcinoma.

a. *Esophageal burns*:
   i. Classification
      1. *First degree*: Mucosal erythema
      2. *Second degree*: Erythema and non-circumferential exudate
      3. *Third degree*: Circumferential exudate
      4. *Fourth degree*: Circumferential exudate with esophageal wall perforation.
   ii. Treatment
      1. Orotracheal intubation, if necessary, should be performed under direct visualization to prevent further mucosal injury and edema.
      2. Steroids can reduce airway edema.
      3. Avoid emetics, gastric lavage or attempts at neutralization.
      4. The decision to perform endoscopy is based on type, concentration, and amount of caustic substance ingested and patient signs and symptoms. It is safest within 24 h.
      5. Contraindications to endoscopy include radiologic evidence of perforation, third-degree hypopharyngeal burn, and significant airway edema.

6. First-degree burns can be observed.

7. Second-degree burns require measures to prevent and treat strictures. Prophylactic dilation is not indicated.

8. Management of third-degree burns also revolves around stricture prevention and treatment. Stricture prevention methods include prophylactic dilations and the use of sucralfate and antireflux medications. Use of corticosteroids is controversial. If used, antibiotics should be given as well. Esophageal stents can also be employed in certain cases. If strictures are present, they can be treated with balloon and bougie dilation. Retrograde dilation through a gastrostomy is safest for multiple strictures. If they are refractory to dilation, local resection with end-to-end reanastomosis, colon patch esophagoplasty, or esophageal stricture bypass with a colonic conduit can be attempted. Third-degree injuries require close observation because progression to fourth-degree burn is possible. Broad spectrum antibiotics may be indicated. Fourth-degree burns require esophagectomy.

Aerodigestive Tract Foreign Bodies

Aerodigestive tract foreign bodies are most commonly found in toddlers. A high index of suspicion is necessary because of possible unwitnessed ingestion or aspiration.

Airway Foreign Bodies

There are three associated clinical phases. Choking, gagging, and coughing occur immediately after ingestion or aspiration of the foreign body. An asymptomatic phase follows after fatigue of protective reflexes. The last clinical phase involves symptoms related to complications including pneumonia, abscess formation, esophageal erosion or perforation, mediastinitis, and tracheoesophageal fistula.

a. Symptoms include dyspnea, stridor, hoarseness, and aphonia.
b. Laryngeal and tracheal foreign bodies are the least common, except in children under 1 year old.
c. Most are located in the right main stem bronchus.
d. Foreign body irritation can lead to edema and complete airway obstruction.
e. Vegetable matter can swell while in the airway. Prompt removal is indicated.

Esophageal Foreign Bodies

a. Symptoms include vomiting, dysphagia, odynophagia, and excessive salivation.
b. The most common location is just below the cricopharyngeus.
c. Large foreign bodies can cause airway obstruction.
d. Coins are the most commonly encountered esophageal foreign bodies.
e. Button batteries can cause very rapid esophageal perforations and must be removed immediately.

Evaluation

a. Evaluation of airway, breathing, and circulations (ABCs).
b. Complete head and neck physical examination and auscultation of the lungs
c. PA and lateral neck and chest X-rays.
d. Abdominal X-rays can demonstrate if an ingested foreign body has passed into the stomach or beyond.
e. Lateral decubitus inspiratory and expiratory chest X-rays evaluate for air trapping and hyperinflation on the obstructed side for airway foreign bodies.
f. In patients with high suspicion, negative radiologic studies are not adequate to rule out foreign bodies.

Treatment

Patients with suspected or confirmed aerodigestive foreign bodies should undergo rigid laryngoscopy, bronchoscopy, and/or esophagoscopy with removal.

Neoplasms

Tumors of the airway can cause varying degrees of airway obstruction depending on their size and location. Please refer to the chapters in Section 5 for more information on malignant tumors.

a. *Recurrent respiratory papillomatosis (RRP)*: Affected patients have exophytic airway lesions caused by human papilloma virus types 6 and 11. They are the most common benign laryngeal neoplasms in children. Recurrent respiratory papillomatosis is difficult to treat because of its tendency to spread and recur. The lesions most often occur at the interface between ciliated and squamous epithelium such as the vestibule, nasopharyngeal surface of the epiglottis, the upper and lower margins of the ventricle, the undersurface of the vocal cords, the carina and at bronchial spurs. Juvenile onset RRP is more aggressive than adult onset RRP. There can be vertical transmission from mother to child. Spontaneous remission occurs in some patients. Airway obstruction can be severe and require frequent endoscopic resection. Tracheotomy should be avoided because of the risk of distal spread of the papilloma. Surgical management is the primary treatment. Adjunctive treatments include local injections of cidofovir or Avastin, and IV interferon.

b. *Subglottic hemangioma*: It accounts for 1.5% of all congenital anomalies of the larynx. This will present primarily in children. It undergoes a proliferative and an involutional phase. It can potentially be fatal due to airway compromise. There is no universally accepted treatment approach. Close observation may be sufficient for small lesions. Systemic and intralesional corticosteroids, laser ablation, and surgical excision are some options. Propranolol used as a first-line agent may help patients avoid surgery.

Systemic Etiologies

Anaphylaxis

a. This is a potentially deadly immunologic reaction that occurs when a subject is re-exposed to an antigen to which they have been previously sensitized.

b. True anaphylaxis results from the release of histamine and other mediators when crosslinking of immunoglobulin E (IgE) antibodies or complement proteins occurs on the surface of mast cells or basophils.

c. Common antigens include foods, latex, medications, and insect stings.

d. Anaphylactoid reactions resemble anaphylactic reactions but are not mediated by IgE crosslinking or activation of the complement cascade. Instead, there is direct activation of mast cells. Radiology contrast material, vancomycin, and morphine can cause anaphylactoid reactions.

e. Exercise-induced anaphylaxis, food- and exercise-induced anaphylaxis, and idiopathic anaphylaxis are three other types of anaphylaxis. Anaphylaxis has a 1% mortality rate.

f. Peanuts, tree nuts, shellfish, milk, eggs, and bisulfite additives cause the majority of food allergies. Peanut, tree nut, and seafood allergies are usually lifelong while sensitivity to other foods may disappear if the causative food is avoided for 2 years.

g. Patients with a history of anaphylaxis to the venom of insects in the Hymenoptera order, including bees and wasps, can reduce their risk of repeat anaphylactic reaction with immunotherapy.

h. Exercise-induced anaphylaxis and food- and exercise-induced anaphylaxis are treated by the avoidance of very vigorous activity and food triggers.

i.   Allergy skin testing and immunotherapy shots are common triggers of anaphylactic reactions. Most of these anaphylactic reactions occur within 20 minutes of antigen exposure.

j.   Approximately 2%–3% of hospitalized patients have an allergic drug reaction. Penicillins are the most common cause.

k.   Treatment:
   i.   Airway, breathing, and circulation.
   ii. Administer epinephrine 1:1,000 concentration, 0.3–0.5 cc I M or SC.
   iii. The pediatric epinephrine IM or SC dose is 0.01 mg/kg.
   iv. Preferred site of administration is the thigh.
   v.   Epinephrine can be administered every 10 minutes as needed.
   vi. Vasopressors, bronchodilators, H1 and H2 receptor blockers, steroids, and heparin can be administered as necessary.
   vii. If a patient is taking beta-blockers, the initial epinephrine dose should be given as above and blood pressure should be carefully monitored for possible severe hypertension. Repeat doses should be reduced by half.

l.   Prevention is the best management strategy. Complete avoidance of triggers of allergic and anaphylactic reactions is necessary but is difficult to achieve. Patients with a history of anaphylaxis should wear a necklace or bracelet listing their allergies. Beta-blockers should be avoided by such patients whenever possible because they render epinephrine ineffective if an anaphylactic reaction should occur.

Angioedema

Angioedema is asymmetric, nonpitting, nontender edema that can affect any part of the body but commonly affects the head, neck, gastrointestinal and genitourinary tracts. Patients can present with angioedema alone or with concurrent urticaria. Angioedema can cause potentially life-threatening airway compromise.

a. *Symptoms*: Dyspnea, dysphagia, odynophagia, globus, hoarseness, stridor, pruritus, and abdominal pain.

b. *Classification*: Angioedema is broadly classified into mast-cell-mediated types and bradykinin-mediated types. The mast-cell-mediated types are typically associated with urticaria and pruritus and include the allergic IgE-dependent mast-cell degranulation, nonallergic direct mast-cell degranulation, and leukotriene-mediated mast-cell degranulation types.

   i. The bradykinin-mediated types are associated with increased production or decreased breakdown of bradykinin. Hereditary angioedema (HAE) has three types. Type I is associated with decreased amount and function of C1 inhibitor protein (C1INH). Type II is associated with decreased function of C1INH with a normal quantity of the protein. Type III is also known as hereditary angioedema with normal C1INH. These patients have normal quantities of functional C1INH. Diagnosis of hereditary angioedema requires that patients have a history of recurrent angioedema without urticaria, no history of taking a medication associated with angioedema, the positive family history of angioedema, and is refractory to treatment with chronic high-dose antihistamine or has a factor XII mutation.

   ii. Acquired angioedema results from rapid consumption of C1 inhibitor and/or the loss of inhibition of the complement cascade. Type I acquired angioedema is associated with paraneoplastic or lymphoproliferative processes. Type II is due to autoimmune diseases.

   iii. Drug-induced angioedema can be associated with numerous types of medications including angiotensin-converting enzyme (ACE) inhibitors, angiotensin receptor blockers, beta-blockers, calcium-channel blockers, diuretics, nonsteroidal anti-inflammatory drugs, antibiotics, and proton pump inhibitors. Idiopathic angioedema is defined as three or more episodes of angioedema in a 6–12-month period with no etiology after thorough workup.

c. *Diagnosis*: Complement C4 levels, C1 inhibitor protein levels and function, and C1q antibodies can help to differentiate among the types of angioedema.

   i. *Type I HAE*: Decreased C4 level, decreased C1INH quantity/function, C1q normal.

   ii. *Type II HAE*: Decreased C4 level, C1INH protein level normal, decreased C1INH protein function, C1q normal.

   iii. *Hereditary angioedema with normal C1INH*: C4 levels and C1INH quantity and function are normal.

   iv. *Acquired angioedema types I and II*: Decreased C4 level, decreased C1INH quantity and function, decreased C1q.

   v. *Drug-induced angioedema*: C4 levels and C1INH quantity and function are normal.

   vi. *Idiopathic angioedema*: C4 levels and C1INH quantity and function are normal.

d. *Treatment*: In all cases of angioedema, assessment of airway status is most important. Flexible fiberoptic laryngoscopy is critical. It allows the determination of the need for airway control and is the best method to do so. Edema involving the tongue and larynx will often require fiberoptic nasal intubation. In cases of severe laryngeal edema, awake tracheotomy will be necessary.

e. *Additional treatment*

   i. *Type I and II HAE*: Icatibant (competitive, selective bradykinin B2 receptor antagonist), Berinert (pasteurized and nanofiltered C1INH concentrate), Cinryze (nanofiltered plasma-derived C1INH), ecallantide (selective inhibitor of kallikrein receptor) and recombinant C1INH can all be used to treat acute attacks. Partial or complete prevention can be attained with C1INH replacement therapy. Attenuated androgens and tranexamic acid can be used for prophylaxis.

   ii. *Hereditary angioedema with normal C1INH*: Icatibant and C1INH concentrate may be used for treatment of acute episodes; danazol, progesterone, and tranexamic acid can be used as prophylaxis.

iii. *Acquired angioedema*: C1INH concentrate, icatibant, and ecallantide can be used to treat acute attacks. Tranexamic acid and attenuated androgens can be used prophylactically.

iv. *Drug-induced angioedema*: Discontinue the offending agent. For ACE inhibitor-related angioedema, H1 and H2 blockers, corticosteroids, and epinephrine are widely used although their effectiveness has not been confirmed by double-blind randomized controlled trials. Patients with ACE-inhibitor-related angioedema may experience progression of their angioedema despite prompt administration of these medications. Close observation in a monitored unit is prudent. However, patients with angioedema isolated to the lips are unlikely to have progression.

v. *Idiopathic angioedema*: Daily second-generation H1 antihistamines, such as fexofenadine, loratadine, and cetirizine, are used as first line for prophylaxis. Other antihistamines and leukotriene receptor antagonists can be added as needed. Corticosteroids can be used for acute episodes.

Granulomatosis with Polyangiitis (Wegener Granulomatosis)

This is a necrotizing, granulomatous, small and medium vessel vasculitis associated with upper and lower respiratory tract granulomas and glomerulonephritis. Most patients are Caucasian and usually present in the fifth decade of life. Up to 23% of patients develop significant subglottic stenosis and will require laryngoscopy with dilation and steroid injection. Cricotracheal resection is reserved for patients who fail this therapy and have inactive disease. The presence of cytoplasmic antineutrophil cytoplasmic antibody aids in diagnosis. Treatment involves use of immunosuppressant drugs such as corticosteroids, cyclophosphamide, azathioprine, and methotrexate.

Sarcoidosis

The onset is usually in the third to fifth decades of life. It is more common in women and African Americans. This systemic, idiopathic disease involves formation of noncaseating granulomas, most commonly in the lungs. The yellow submucosal nodules or polyps of sarcoidosis can appear anywhere in the upper respiratory tract. Laryngeal sarcoid is characterized by a diffusely enlarged, pale-pink, turban-like epiglottis. It may also involve the subglottis and present with hoarseness and stridor. The usual treatment of sarcoidosis is oral corticosteroids. Local steroid injections into the glottis and subglottis have also been used successfully, usually with dilation in the latter site.

DIAGNOSTIC WORKUP

For any patient presenting in acute respiratory distress, attention should be directed to evaluating the ABCs first. The history and remainder of the physical examination can be completed when the patient's condition is more stable.

History

"When did you start having difficulty breathing?"

"What were you doing when you started having difficulty breathing?"

"Did you suffer any trauma to your head or neck?"

"Did you start taking any new medications or encounter any new chemicals recently?"

"What did you have to eat before you started having difficulty breathing?"

"Do you have a history of heart, lung, or autoimmune disease?"

"Have you recently been around anyone who has been sick and had similar symptoms?"

"Have you recently had any surgery?"

"Do you have any of the following symptoms: fever, chills, night sweats, sore throat, difficulty swallowing, pain with swallowing, difficulty opening your mouth, hoarseness, runny nose, stuffy nose, nose bleeds, or cough?"

"Have you ever had to have a breathing tube placed in your throat? If so, how long was it kept in place?"

Physical Examination

Complete head and neck examination should be performed with attention to the nasal cavity, nasopharynx, oral cavity, oropharynx, and larynx. Flexible fiberoptic laryngoscopy is essential in evaluating the upper aerodigestive tract. However, its usefulness is limited in patients who are intubated.

Ancillary Tools

Imaging studies, including plain films, CT scans and magnetic resonance imaging (MRI), can help to delineate the nature and extent of a lesion obstructing the airway. Plain films and CT scans are rapidly obtained whereas MRI is reserved for stable patients because it requires considerably more time.

Direct laryngoscopy and bronchoscopy and esophagoscopy can aid in diagnosis by direct visualization and the ability to take biopsies.

SUGGESTED READING

1. Bork K. An evidence based therapeutic approach to hereditary and acquired angioedema. Curr Opin Allergy Clin Immunol. 2014;14(4):354-62.
2. Boston, M. Neonatal respiratory distress. In: Johnson JT, Rosen CA (Eds). Bailey's Head and Neck Surgery: Otolaryngology, 5th edition. Philadelphia, PA: Lippincott Williams and Wilkins; 2014. pp. 1328-37.
3. Burgess CA, Dale OT, Almeyda R, et al. An evidence based review of the assessment and management of penetrating neck trauma. Clin Otolaryngol. 2012;37(1):44-52.
4. Dohar JE, Anne S. Stridor, aspiration, and cough. In: Johnson JT, Rosen CA (Eds). Bailey's Head and Neck Surgery: Otolaryngology, 5th edition. Philadelphia, PA: Lippincott Williams and Wilkins; 2014. pp. 1338-55.
5. Hom DB, Maisel RH. Penetrating and blunt trauma to the neck. In: Flint PW, Haughey BH, Lund VJ, et al (Eds). Cummings

Otolaryngology: Head and Neck Surgery, 5th edition. Philadelphia, PA: Elsevier; 2010. pp. 1625-35.

6. Kost, K. Advanced airway management—intubation and tracheotomy. In: Johnson JT, Rosen CA (Eds). Bailey's Head and Neck Surgery: Otolaryngology, 5th edition. Philadelphia, PA: Lippincott Williams and Wilkins; 2014. pp. 908-44.

7. Liang T, Tso DK, Chiu RY, et al. Imaging of blunt vascular neck injuries: a review of screening and imaging modalities. AJR Am J Roentgenol. 2013;201(4):884-92.

8. Schaefer SD. Management of acute blunt and penetrating external laryngeal trauma. Laryngoscope. 2014;124(1):233-44.

9. Sher J, Davis-Lorton M. Angioedema with normal laboratory values: the next step. Curr Allergy Asthma Rep. 2013;13(5):563-70.

10. Weissbrod PA, Merati AL. Upper airway stenosis: evaluation and management. In: Johnson JT, Rosen CA (Eds). Bailey's Head and Neck Surgery: Otolaryngology, 5th edition. Philadelphia, PA: Lippincott Williams and Wilkins; 2014. pp. 879-95.

Section

5

The Head and Neck

Section Editor: Jeffrey C Liu

Chapter 18

Thyroid and Parathyroid Glands

Jennifer R Cracchiolo

THYROID EMBRYOLOGY

The thyroid is derived from endoderm of first and second pharyngeal pouches—*foramen cecum.*

Ventral diverticulum forms at 4 weeks and descends inferiorly through mesenchymal tissue, anterior to hyoid to its pretracheal position at 7 weeks.

Parafollicular C cells (secrete calcitonin): These cells are derived from neural crest cells of fourth pharyngeal pouch, migrate and infiltrate into superior thyroid lobes.

Pathology of Abnormal Development

- *Athyreosis*: Congenital absence of thyroid.
- *Ectopic thyroid*: Aberrant thyroid that presents anywhere along the path of embryonic descent. It may present as a base of tongue mass in the case of a lingual thyroid.
- *Thyroglossal duct cyst*: This results from incomplete obliteration of the thyroid duct (*see* Chapter 33).

Surgical Anatomy

Thyroid gland (shield) is made of two lobes connected by an isthmus (Fig. 18.1). It is located approximately at the level of C4–5 vertebrae.*

Vascular Anatomy

The arterial and the venous supply are meticulously dissected and ligated during thyroid surgery. Attention to hemostasis is important to avoid postoperative hematoma.†

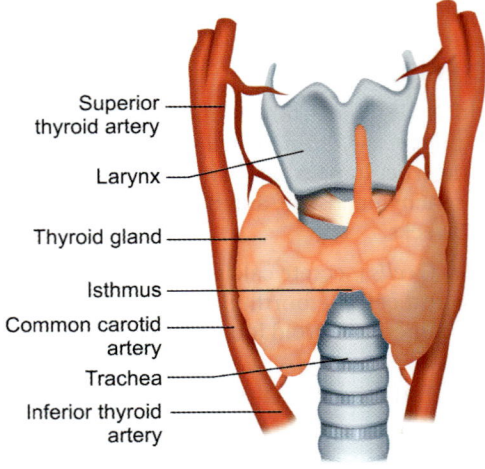

Fig. 18.1: Anatomy of the thyroid gland.

---

*The pyramidal lobe is a superior extension of the remnant embryonic thyroglossal tract. In total thyroidectomy, following the pyramidal lobe to its superior extent needs to be included in dissection to assure complete removal of thyroid tissue.

†Postoperative hematoma after thyroid surgery is a surgical emergency requiring evaluation and possible intervention at the bedside. Given the close proximity of the surgical bed to the airway, the patient may be in respiratory distress, which resolves with hematoma evacuation.

Arterial Supply

- External carotid artery (ECA) → Superior thyroid artery (first branch off ECA)
- Thyrocervical trunk → Inferior thyroid artery
- *Unpaired thyroid ima artery*: It may arise from innominate artery, carotid artery, or directly off aortic arch.*

Venous Supply

- Paired superior, middle, and inferior veins.

Nerve Anatomy

- Identification and preservation of the nerves arising from the vagus nerve requires the knowledge of anatomy as well as surgical skill.

External Branch of Superior Laryngeal Nerve[†]

- *Innervates*: Cricothyroid muscle
- Cernea classification[1]
- Type 1 nerves cross >1 cm above the upper border of the thyroid gland.
- Type 2a nerves cross within 1 cm of the upper border of the thyroid.
- Type 2b nerves cross below the upper border of the gland.

Recurrent Laryngeal Nerve (RLN)

- The RLN innervates all intrinsic muscles of larynx except *cricothyroid muscle*[‡]

---

*Thyroid ima artery may be a source of significant bleeding during *tracheostomy or thryoidectomy.* Control of bleeding may be difficult as the artery can retract into mediastinum.

[†]External branch of superior laryngeal nerve is at risk for injury during ligation of the superior thyroid vascular pedicle. Type 2b is most at risk. Patients with injury to external branch of superior laryngeal nerve during thyroidectomy will complain of inability to yell or "hit a high note."

[‡]Entry point of RLN is a fixed point. Stretch injury when retracting the thyroid medially during surgery can occur at this point.

- It ascends in tracheoesophageal groove, then enters larynx at cricothyroid joint.

Ligaments

- *Anterior suspensory ligament*: This arises from anterior aspects of tracheal rings and inserts on the posterior aspect of the thyroid isthmus Avascular plane.
- *Posterior suspensory ligament (ligament of Berry)*: This is the condensation of thyroid capsule that connects the posterior-medial aspect of the gland to the tracheal rings and cricoid cartilage.

THYROID PHYSIOLOGY

Table 18.1 presents hormones of thyroid homeostasis.

Table 18.1: Hormones of thyroid homeostasis.

Hormone	Produced from	Target organ/Effects	Affected by thyroid hormone
Thyrotropin-releasing hormone	Hypothalamus	Anterior pituitary increase production of thyroid-stimulating hormone	No
Thyroid-stimulating hormone	Anterior pituitary	Thyroid stimulates iodine uptake, thyroid growth, release of thyroid hormone	Yes
Thyroid hormone Tri-iodothyronine (T3) active form thyroxine (T4): 90% of thyroid output	Thyroid	Neurologic and skeletal growth and development, calorie utilization, catecholamine utilization	NA

Laboratory Tests in Thyroid Disease

- *Thyroid-stimulating hormone (TSH)*: Most sensitive in diagnosis of hypothyroidism or hyperthyroidism.
- *Total T4*: Measures bound + free T4.
- *Free T4*: More specific in diagnosis of hypothyroidism or hyperthyroidism.
- *Total T3*: Measures bound + free T3, useful for *hyperthyroid patients*, toxic nodules, and multinodular goiters, and rarely helpful to hypothyroid patients as it is the last test to become abnormal.
- *Thyroxine-binding globulin (TBG)*: The protein that *binds thyroid* hormone (TH) in circulation.
- *Resin T3 Uptake (RT3U)*: The indirect measure of TBG, measures binding capacity of TBG. *Increased RT3U* represents *decreased total TBG* such as in low-protein states (anabolic steroid use). *Decreased* RT3U represents *increased total TBG states* (pregnancy and oral contraception use).
- *Thyroglobulin (Tg)*: The protein produced by normal thyroid cells and also thyroid cancer cells, and used in patients after total thyroidectomy in cancer surveillance to monitor the presence of Tg-producing cells after treatment, *not* as thyroid function test or for diagnosis of cancer.
- *Thyroid antibodies*: These are used in the diagnosis of autoimmune thyroiditis or in assessing the reliability of following Tg in cancer surveillance (Table 18.2).

Pharmacology in Thyroid Disease

- *Beta blockers*: These are used in patients with hyperthyroidism to block effects of peripheral TH. Do not alter thyroid pathogenesis.
- *Thinamides*: *Propylthiouracil* and *methimazole* block TH synthesis and prevent conversion of T4 to T3 in periphery. There is a risk of agranulocytosis and parotitis. Propylthiouracil is associated with liver failure. Methimazole contraindicated in pregnancy (teratogen).

Table 18.2: Antibodies involved in thyroid disease.

Thyroid antibody	Disease state	Comments
Thyroid peroxidase antibody	Hashimoto's thyroiditis	
Thyroid-stimulating hormone (TSH) receptor antibody	Graves' disease	Autoantibody binds to TSH receptor, mimicking TSH activity, resulting in hyperthyroidism
Thyroglobulin antibody	Hashimoto's thyroiditis	Also used in cancer surveillance; presence of antibody renders measurements of thyroglobulin less reliable

- *Levothyroxine: Levothyroxine* is a synthetic form of T4. Titrate to TSH levels.
- *Cytomel*: *Liothyronine* is a synthetic form of thyroid hormone (T_3). It has shorter half-life than levothyroxine. Shorter half-life is utilized during TH withdrawal in preparation for radioactive iodine treatment.
- *Thyrogen*: This is the recombinant form of human TSH used as an adjunctive diagnostic tool for serum Tg testing with or without radioiodine imaging. It is also used in adjunctive treatment for radioiodine ablation of thyroid tissue remnants in patients who have undergone a total thyroidectomy for well-differentiated thyroid cancer and who do not have evidence of distant metastatic thyroid cancer. It is used in place of TH withdrawal.
- *Iodides: Lugol's solution.* Excess iodine inhibits organification and prevents TH release (*Wolff–Chaikoff effect*). It is transient and used preoperatively in patients with hyperthyroidism.

Diseases Resulting in Disrupted Thyroid Physiology

- Often patient history and physical examination will prompt further workup for functional thyroid diseases. Table 18.3 lists common presenting symptoms, laboratory findings, and differential diagnosis associated with TH abnormalities.

Table 18.3: Hyperthyroidism versus hypothyroidism.	
Hyperthyroidism characterized as low TSH and high TH	*Hypothyroidism characterized as high TSH and low TH*
Graves' disease, toxic nodule or goiter, acute or subacute thyroiditis, exogenous TH (iatrogenic, struma ovarii, patient induced), pituitary tumor (central)	Thyroiditis, iodine deficiency, postsurgical, drug induced (lithium), radiation induced
Weight loss, anxiety, insomnia, tremors, tachycardia, sweating, heat intolerance, proptosis, diarrhea, muscle weakness, thinning hair	Weight gain, fatigue, dry skin, hair loss, intolerance to cold, constipation, slow mentation, depression, hoarseness, bradycardia, hyporeflexia, thickened tongue

(TSH: Thyroid-stimulating hormone; TH: Thyroid hormone).

Graves' Disease

- Graves' disease is an autoimmune disease representing 60% of hyperthyroidism. It is more common in women 30–40 years old. Physical examination shows a diffusely enlarged gland. Bruit can often be appreciated over the thyroid gland secondary to *hypervascularity.**
- *Diagnosis*: Thyroid function tests (suppressed TSH, increased TH, + TSH receptor antibody, and radioactive iodine scan with diffuse uptake).
- *Treatment:* Radioactive iodine ablation, antithyroid medications (often not a long-term treatment), β blockers, and thyroidectomy.

Thyroiditis

Thyroiditis is an inflammatory process secondary to autoimmune disease or infection and often associated with a preceding period

---

*Exophthalmos secondary to inflammation and the accumulation of hydrophilic glycosaminoglycans in orbital tissues.

of hyperthyroidism followed by hypothyroidism. Table 18.4 summarizes some common forms of thyroiditis.

Hashimoto's Thyroiditis

This is an autoimmune disease, the most common cause of thyroiditis. Women are 5–10 times over men; reported prevalence in White women is in the 1–2% range.[2] It presents as painless, symmetrically enlarged goiter, thyroid peroxidase antibody present in 70–90% of patients. Histology shows lymphocytic infiltration with germinal centers.

- *Diagnosis*: Thyroid function tests (increased TSH, decreased TH)
- *Treatment*: Thyroid replacement hormone, surgery for large goiters

Syndromes Associated with Thyroid Disease

- *Pendred syndrome*: *Autosomal recessive,* bilateral sensorineural hearing loss, goiter.
- *Cowden's syndrome*: Mutations in phosphatase and tensin homolog hearing loss, multiple thyroid adenomas, follicular thyroid cancers, and craniofacial abnormalities.
- *Gardner syndrome (familial adenomatous polyposis)*: *Autosomal dominant*, cribriform variant of papillary thyroid cancer, colon polyps.
- *Carney complex*: Autosomal dominant, thyroid follicular adenomas, skin pigment abnormalities, myxomas, endocrine tumors, and schwannomas.
- Multiple endocrine neoplasia (MEN) 2: refer to the "Medullary Thyroid Cancer" section.

Management of Thyroid Nodules

For thorough evidence-based guidelines for workup and evaluation of thyroid nodules, refer to the American Thyroid Association (ATA) Guidelines.

Table 18.4: Causes of thyroiditis.

Thyroiditis	Onset	Thyroid hormone status	Symptoms	Findings	Treatment
Hashimoto's	Gradual	Hyper then hypo	Painless	Goiter	Thyroid replacement, surgery for large goiters
Subacute (de Quervain's)	Acute after viral illness	Hyper, then hypo	Painful	Painful to palpation	NSAIDs
Riedel's	Gradual	Hypo	Variable	"Woody" gland	Observation, thyroid replacement as needed
Acute suppurative*	Acute	Euthyroid	Severe pain	Painful, fever, toxic	Systemic antibiotics, I & D if needed

*Consider a brachial cleft anomaly (type 3) in young patients who present with thyroidal abscess or suppurative thyroiditis. (NSAIDs: Nonsteroidal anti-inflammatory drugs; I & D: Incision and drainage).

- *Thyroid nodules*: Discrete lesion within the thyroid gland that is distinct from the surrounding thyroid tissue parenchyma.

Prevalence

- Palpable thyroid nodules are found in ~5% of women and 1% of men living in iodine-sufficient parts of the world.
- High-resolution ultrasound (US) can detect thyroid nodules in 19–67% in the population.
- Thyroid cancer occurs in 5–15% of nodules depending on age, sex, radiation exposure, and family history.

Evaluation[3]

- Nodules >1 cm should be evaluated.
- Nodules <1 cm that require evaluation:
  - Associated lymphadenopathy
  - Higher risk, such as the history of head and neck irradiation or the family history of thyroid cancer in one or more first-degree relatives
  - Suspicious US findings (microcalcifications, hypoechoic, increased nodular vascularity, infiltrative margins, taller than wide on transverse view)
  - Found on position emission tomography scan (risk of malignancy in fludeoxyglucose-positive nodules is about 30% and the cancers may be more aggressive).[4]

Flowchart 18.1 presents an algorithm for evaluation of thyroid nodule. Table 18.5 presents the Bethesda criteria for thyroid nodules.[5]

Molecular Testing in Thyroid Nodule

Afirma

This is used in indeterminate nodules by fine needle aspiration (FNA; Bethesda III and IV) "rule out test" and takes into account messenger ribonucleic acid expression levels in a 164-gene

Flowchart 18.1: Algorithm for evaluation of thyroid nodule.

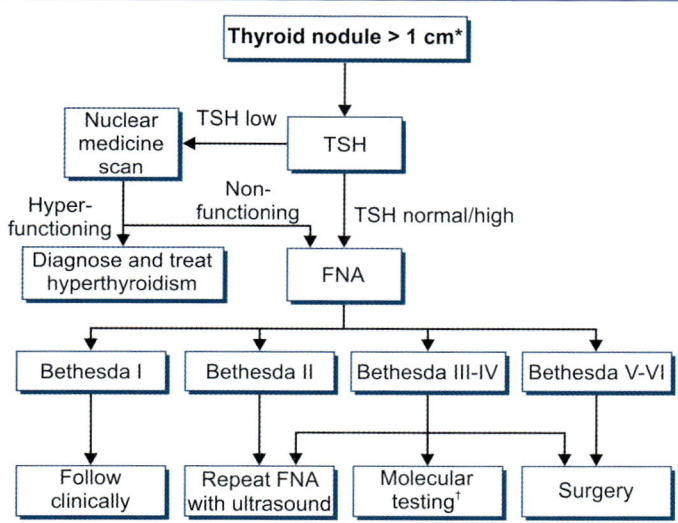

*See indications for nodules <1 cm that should be evaluated.
†See the "Molecular Testing in Thyroid Nodules" section.
(TSH: Thyroid-stimulating hormone; FNA: Fine-needle aspiration).

Bethesda criteria	FNA result	Chance of malignancy (%)
I	Nondiagnostic or unsatisfactory	1–4
II	Benign	0–3
III	Atypia of undetermined significance follicular lesion of undetermined significance	5–15
IV	Follicular neoplasm or suspicious for a follicular neoplasm	15–30
V	Suspicious for malignancy	60–75
VI	Malignant	97–99

Table 18.5: Bethesda criteria.

(FNA: Fine needle aspiration).

panel. The result is benign (<6%) or suspicious (40% chance of malignancy). The negative predictive value is of 94%.[6]

ThyroSeq—Thyroid Cancer Next-Generation Sequencing Panel

This is used in indeterminate nodules by FNA (Bethesda categories III–V) and malignant nodules when molecular testing is expected to affect the decision to perform surgery or extent of surgery. Mutations are detected by next-generation sequencing. It identifies mutations inthyroid-cancer-related genes and gene fusions. It may also be useful in clinical decision making with regard to administration of radioactive iodine, intensity of follow-up, and targeted therapies.[7]

MALIGNANT THYROID NEOPLASMS

Well-Differentiated Thyroid Carcinoma

Papillary Carcinoma

- This represents 70–80% of malignant thyroid neoplasms.*
- It is more common in women than in men, often seen in young patients.
- *Risk factors*: Radiation and family history
- *Mitogen-activated protein kinase (MAPK) pathway* central to pathogenesis. It is associated with *BRAF V600E* mutation resulting in constitutive activation of MAPK pathway.
- First site of metastasis is *lymph nodes.* Level 6 central compartment lymph nodes are often the first metastatic site, followed by lateral neck. Retropharyngeal lymph nodes are also at risk.
- *Histopathology:* "Orphan Annie" eye appearance, prominent nucleoli, grooved nuclear margins, large nucleoli.

---

*Papillary carcinoma should be considered with cystic nodal disease in the neck or mediastinum. Large cystic nodal metastases can be seen with microcarcinomas. Bulky lymphadenopathy is common at presentation in pediatric population. Cystic fluid is often "rusty" in color secondary to hemorrhage into cyst.

- *Diagnosis*: Fine needle aspiration, lateral neck US to assess lateral neck lymph node status preoperatively.

Histological subtypes with clinical relevance:
- *Tall cell, sclerosing, columnar*: Unfavorable characteristics, more likely to have extrathyroidal extension, and may be radioactive iodine resistant.
- *Cribriform*: It is associated with Gardner's syndrome.
- *Follicular variant*: When encapsulated, slow growing, it behaves more like follicular adenoma.

Follicular Carcinoma

- It is more likely in women and older patients.
- Follicular carcinoma is well differentiated but lacks the characteristics of papillary thyroid carcinoma. It is *less likely* to spread to the lymph nodes and *more likely* to have *distant metastases.*
- *Histopathology:* Solid sheets of cells, *extracapsular spread*, and *vascular invasion* that differentiates from follicular adenoma.

Histological Subtypes with Clinical Relevance

- *Hurthle cell carcinoma*: It is more aggressive, has higher rate of distant metastases, and is more often radioactive iodine resistant.

Prognosis

Overall, well-differentiated thyroid cancer has an excellent prognosis. Factors affecting prognosis have been reported in Table 18.6.[8-10]
- *Treatment*: Surgery ± radioactive Iodine represents the mainstay of treatment. Total thyroidectomy is required if radioactive iodine is planned and allows for surveillance by measuring Tg levels. Central neck dissection and lateral neck dissection are indicated for structural disease. Elective neck dissection is controversial. *Sorafenib* (tyrosine kinase

Table 18.6: Schemas of well-differentiated thyroid cancer.

Lahey clinic[8]	Mayo clinic[9]	MSKCC[10]
A—age	M—metastasis	G—grade of the tumor
M—metastasis	A—age	A—age
E—extent	C—completeness of	M—metastasis
S—size	surgical resection	E—extrathyroidal extension
	I—invasion	S—size
	S–size	

(MSKCC: Memorial Sloan Kettering Cancer Center)

inhibitor) has been approved for locally recurrent or metastatic, progressive, differentiated thyroid carcinoma refractory to radioactive iodine treatment.
- For latest treatment recommendations, please refer to the ATA Guidelines.[3]

Medullary Thyroid Cancer

This is derived from neuroendocrine parafollicular C cells. It is often found at superior poles secondary to higher concentration of C cells, which release calcitonin, carcinoembryonic antigen (CEA), gastrin, adrenocorticotropic hormone, substance P.*

- Sporadic and inherited (autosomal-dominant) forms. It is associated with RET proto-oncogene.
- MEN 2a presents in the third decade associated with pheochromocytoma, hyperparathyroidism.
- MEN 2b presents in first and second decades associated with pheochromocytoma, mucosal neuromata, marfanoid habitus.
- Familial nonmultiple endocrine neoplasia presents in the fourth decade.
- *Histopathology*: Small round cells, spindle-shaped neoplastic cells, and amyloid stroma.

---

*Calcitonin and CEA doubling time are used in management, surveillance, and follow-up of medullary thyroid cancer.

Management
- Screen for germline mutations in RET.

American Thyroid Association Guidelines recommend the following:[11]
- Children with *ATA-D mutations (MEN 2b)* should undergo prophylactic total thyroidectomy as soon as possible and within the first year of life.
- Children with *ATA-C mutations (Codon 634)* should undergo prophylactic total thyroidectomy before the age of 5 years.
- Children with *ATA-A* and *ATA-B RET mutations*, prophylactic total thyroidectomy, may be delayed beyond the age of 5 years in the setting of a normal annual basal stimulated serum calcitonin.
- Patients with MEN syndrome should be evaluated for other associated diseases.
- Total thyroidectomy and prophylactic central neck dissection in the setting of clinically detected medullary thyroid cancer is recommended.

The US Food and Drug Administration has approved two kinase inhibitors for metastatic disease, cabozantinib and vandetanib.

Anaplastic Thyroid Cancer
- Anaplastic thyroid cancer is hypothesized to be a terminal dedifferentiation event from differentiated thyroid cancer.
- It is uniformly fatal.
- *Histopathology*: "Bizarre cells," giant cells with high areas of necrosis and high mitotic rate.

Management
- The utility of surgical treatment is often limited. Palliative external beam radiation and chemotherapy (doxirubicin) are sometimes utilized.*

---

*In a rapidly growing thyroid malignancy, consider anaplastic thyroid cancer or lymphoma. Lymphoma must be ruled out as treatment and prognosis are significantly different in lymphoma versus anaplastic thyroid cancer.

PARATHYROID

Most commonly, four parathyroid glands exist at the posterior aspect of the thyroid gland and are responsible for calcium regulation. These glands are encountered during thyroid surgery where they are identified, meticulously dissected, and preserved. Alternatively, in the case of disease such as parathyroid adenomas, hyperplasia, and, very rarely, carcinoma, the pathologic glands are identified and removed. Uniquely, management of parathyroid disease requires not only an in-depth knowledge of anatomy but also an understanding of physiology and embryology.

Anatomy and Embryology

Superior parathyroid glands ("deep" parathyroids) are derived from the fourth branchial pouch. These glands exist "deep" to the RLN anatomically. This relationship can change when retracting the thyroid medially during surgery.[*]

Inferior parathyroid glands ("superficial" parathyroids) are derived from the third branchial pouch. These glands exist superficial to the RLN and are more variable in location.[†]

Calcium Physiology

Parathyroid hormone (PTH) is produced by chief cells within parathyroid glands and regulates calcium levels. Under normal physiologic conditions, this is secreted in response to low calcium levels. Parathyroid hormone increases serum calcium levels and decreases serum phosphate.

PTH Target Organs

- Bowel increases absorption of calcium and phosphate in intestine indirectly, following an increase in vitamin D.

---

[*]Classic relationship: Superior gland is located 1 cm above the intersection of the RLN and inferior thyroid artery.

[†]Thymus is also derived from the third branchial pouch, which is why inferior parathyroids are sometimes located in the anterior mediastinum within the thymus.

Kidney increases renal calcium resorption and phosphate excretion, and increases conversion of vitamin D to active form.
- Bone mobilizes calcium from bone. Parathyroid hormone acts on osteoblasts, which subsequently drive osteoclast activity.

Calcitonin, produced by *C cells,* works to *decrease serum levels of calcium*, inhibits calcium reabsorption from bone, and increases kidney reabsorption of calcium and phosphate.

HYPERCALCEMIA

Symptoms of Hypercalcemia

- *Neurologic*: Confusion, fatigue, depression, memory changes
- *Gastrointestinal*: Constipation and abdominal pain
- *Genitourinary*: Kidney stones, polyuria
- *Musculoskeletal*: Bone pain, arthritis, osteopenia, osteoporosis
- "Stones, bones, abdominal groans, and psychiatric moans"

Differential Diagnosis of Hypercalcemia*

- C: Calcium supplementation
- H: Hyperparathyroidism
- I: Iatrogenic (drugs such as thiazides)
- M: Milk alkali syndrome
- P: Paget disease of the bone
- A: Acromegaly and Addison's disease
- N: Neoplasia (common cause)
- Z: Zollinger–Ellison syndrome (MEN Type I)
- E: Excessive vitamin D
- E: Excessive vitamin A
- S: Sarcoidosis

---

*Hyperparathyroidism is the most common cause of hypercalcemia.

TYPES OF HYPERPARATHYROIDISM

Primary Hyperparathyroidism

- Elevated PTH → It results in elevated calcium.

Etiologies include the following:

- Benign adenoma; it represents 85% of cases.
- About 2–10% present with double adenomas.
- Four gland hyperplasia, 10% of cases, can be sporadic or associated with MEN 1 or MEN 2a syndrome.
- *Treatment*: Parathyroidectomy.

Secondary Hyperparathyroidism

- Hypocalcemia → Increased PTH → Compensatory parathyroid hyperplasia
- Etiologies include the following: chronic renal failure, ontogenesis imperfecta, Paget's disease, and multiple myeloma.
- *Treatment*: Correct underlying condition.

Tertiary Hyperparathyroidism

- Persistent elevated PTH in the environment of normal to increased calcium → PTH response becomes autonomous, persists after correction of underlying pathology.
- *Treatment*: Three and a half gland parathyroidectomy.

Evaluation of Hyperparathyroidism

Diagnosis of primary hyperparathyroidism is frequently biochemical, often driven by an abnormal laboratory value. The patient's symptoms can often be vague and subtle. In some cases, the diagnosis of primary hyperparathyroidism offers the link between signs and symptoms that span multiple organ systems. Table 18.7 summarizes laboratory patterns associated with elevated PTH.

Table 18.7: Laboratory patterns in disorders with elevated parathyroid hormone.

Diagnosis	PTH	Serum calcium	24-hour urine calcium	Vitamin D levels
Primary hyperparathyroidism	Elevated	Elevated	High	Low to normal
Familial hypocalciuric hypercalcemia	Elevated	Elevated	Low	Variable
Vitamin D deficiency	Elevated	Low to normal	Normal to high	Low

(PTH: Parathyroid hormone).

Laboratory Findings

When a patient presents with an elevated PTH, there are important pathologies to rule out. These represent diseases with elevated PTH that are nonsurgical diseases. These laboratory tests should be ordered before surgery.

Imaging Localization Studies

- *Sestamibi scan*: Technetium 99m is useful if planning a unilateral parathyroid exploration and to rule out aberrant parathyroid glands.
- *Hybrid single-photon emission computed tomography/ computed tomography:* It provides functional and anatomic information and is useful in re-explorations.
- *Ultrasound*: US may provide location of adenoma. Preoperative US also allows for evaluation of thyroid nodules that my require workup before surgery. If planning a neck exploration for parathyroid disease, suspicious thyroid nodules should be evaluated to avoid a second operation.

National Institutes of Health Indications for Surgical Treatment of Asymptomatic Primary Hyperparathyroidism[12]

- Serum calcium >1.0 mg/dL of upper limit of normal.
- *Bone density*: Dual-energy X-ray absorptiometry: T score 2.5 at lumbar spine, total hip, femoral neck, or distal one third of the radius or vertebral fracture.
- *Creatinine clearance*: 60 cc/min, 24-hour urine for calcium 400 mg per day (10 mmol per day), presence of *nephrolithiasis* or *nephrocalcinosis.*
- *Age* less than 50.
- Patients for whom medical surveillance is neither desired nor possible and in patients opting for surgery.

Parathyroid Carcinoma

Carcinoma should be considered in patients with extremely high preoperative calcium levels (>14). PTH levels may be 3–10 times above the upper limit of normal. There may be a palpable mass or vocal cord paralysis at presentation.

Postoperative Hypocalcemia

Hypocalcemia can be a surgical complication of total thyroidectomy or four-gland parathyroidectomy. Patients at risk include those with hyperthyroidism, large goiter, preoperative vitamin D deficiency, central neck dissection, and invasive cancers with significant dissection required.

- *Early symptoms*: Perioral and extremity numbness and tingling.
- *Late signs*: Seizures, laryngospasm, bronchospasm, cardiac failure, frank tetany, QT prolongation, and altered mental status.
- *Chvostek's sign*: Facial twitching elicited when tapping over proximal facial nerve.
- *Trousseau's sign*: Carpal spasm occurs when the upper arm is compressed by a tourniquet.

- Parathyroid hormone assay after thyroidectomy has been shown to accurately predict the trend of serum calcium postoperatively.[13]
- *Treatment for mild symptoms*: Oral calcium and vitamin D. Correct magnesium.
- Intravenous calcium gluconate for severe signs or symptoms.

REFERENCES

1. Cernea CR, Ferraz AR, Nishio S, et al. Surgical anatomy of the external branch of the superior laryngeal nerve. Head Neck. 1992;14(5):380-3.
2. Weetman AP. Thyroid disease. In: Rose MR, Mackay IR (Eds). The Autoimmune Diseases. Philadelphia: Elsevier; 2006.
3. American Thyroid Association (ATA) Guidelines Taskforce on Thyroid Nodules and Differentiated Thyroid Cancer, Cooper DS, Doherty GM, et al. Revised American Thyroid Association management guidelines for patients with thyroid nodules and differentiated thyroid cancer. Thyroid. 2009;19(11):1167-214.
4. Kang KW, Kim SK, Kang HS, et al. Prevalence and risk of cancer of focal thyroid incidentaloma identified by 18F-fluorodeoxyglucose positron emission tomography for metastasis evaluation and cancer screening in healthy subjects. J Clin Endocrinol Metab. 2003;88(9):4100-4.
5. Cibas ES, Ali SZ, The Bethesda System for Reporting Thyroid Cytopathology. Thyroid. 2009;19 (11):1159-65.
6. Alexander EK, Kennedy GC, Baloch ZW, et al. Preoperative diagnosis of benign thyroid nodules with indeterminate cytology. N Engl J Med. 2012;367(8):705-15.
7. Nikiforov YE, Carty SE, Chiosea SI, et al. Highly accurate diagnosis of cancer in thyroid nodules with follicular neoplasm/suspicious for a follicular neoplasm cytology by ThyroSeq v2 next-generation sequencing assay. Cancer. 2014;120(23):3627-34.
8. Cady B, Rossi R. An expanded view of risk-group definition in differentiated thyroid carcinoma. Surgery. 1988;104(6):947-53.
9. Hay ID, Bergstralh EJ, Goellner JR, et al. Predicting outcome in papillary thyroid carcinoma: development of a reliable prognostic scoring system in a cohort of 1779 patients surgically treated at one institution during 1940 through 1989. Surgery. 1993;114(6):1050-7; discussion 1057-8.

10. Shaha AR. Implications of prognostic factors and risk groups in the management of differentiated thyroid cancer. Laryngoscope. 2004;114(3):393-402.

11. American Thyroid Association Guidelines Task Force, Kloos RT, Eng C, et al. Medullary thyroid cancer: management guidelines of the American Thyroid Association. Thyroid. 2009;19(6):565-612.

12. Bilezikian JP, Brandi ML, Eastell R, et al. Guidelines for the management of asymptomatic primary hyperparathyroidism: summary statement from the Fourth International Workshop. J Clin Endocrinol Metab. 2014;99(10):3561-9.

13. Noordzij JP, Lee SL, Bernet VJ, et al. Early prediction of hypocalcemia after thyroidectomy using parathyroid hormone: an analysis of pooled individual patient data from nine observational studies. J Am Coll Surg. 2007;205(6):748-54.

Chapter 19

Salivary Glands

Jennifer R Cracchiolo

EMBRYOLOGY

The parotid, submandibular, and sublingual glands are all derived from the following:
- Ectoderm
- The first pharyngeal pouch
- At 5.5–8 weeks of gestation
- *Order of development*: Parotid → Submandibular → Sublingual

ANATOMY OF SALIVARY GLANDS (FIG. 19.1)

Parotid Gland

The parotid gland is the largest salivary gland, lies at the lateral aspect of the face, and is bordered (1) *anteriorly* by the masseter, (2) *posteriorly* by the sternocleidomastoid muscle, (3) *superiorly* by the zygomatic arch, and (4) inferiorly by the upper border of the posterior belly of the digastric.

The parotid gland is divided into a superficial lobe (80% of total volume) and deep lobe (20% of total volume) by the facial nerve.
- The deep lobe of the parotid gland exists in the parapharyngeal, prestyloid space.*

---

*Tumors involving the deep lobe of the parotid gland can often be visualized in the oropharynx.

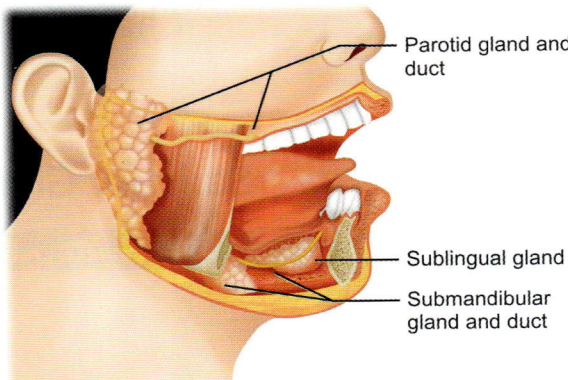

Fig. 19.1: Anatomy of the salivary glands.

- The gland is encased in parotid fascia, which is continuous with the superficial layer of the deep cervical fascia.
- *Stensen's duct* travels over masseter muscle and enters oral cavity adjacent to second molar.*

Blood Supply

Arterial: External carotid courses deep to the gland and divides into maxillary artery and superficial temporal artery.

Venous drainage: Maxillary vein + Superficial temporal vein → Retromandibular vein → Internal jugular vein

Surgical Neural Anatomy

Facial nerve: The facial nerve divides the superficial and deep lobes of the parotid gland. This is identified and preserved during

---

Accessory parotid gland: In patients presenting with a midcheek, infrazygomatic or buccal submucosa mass, an accessory parotid neoplasm should be included in the differential diagnosis.

parotidectomy. Landmarks for facial nerve identification include the following:

1. *Tragal pointer*: About 1 cm inferior and deep to this structure.
2. *Tympanomastoid suture line*: About 6–8 mm from the inferior aspect of the fissure.
3. *Posterior belly of digastric*: Insertion point marks depth of the nerve.
4. Retrograde via distal branches allows safe dissection of the nerve, if the position is distorted by pathology.

    Great auricular nerve: Sensory nerve to ear; posterior branch may be preserved during parotidectomy.*

Lymph Nodes

- These are *within* the content of the parotid gland.
- Intraparotid lymph nodes often represent the first draining nodal bed for cutaneous malignancies of the face and scalp.
- In pediatric patients, enlarged lymph nodes more commonly represent infection or inflammation.

Histology

Serous acinar cells; they produce *serous saliva*.

Submandibular Gland

The submandibular gland sits within the *submandibular triangle* with the following:
- *Superior margin* at the inferior edge of the mandible.
- *Inferior margin* at the level of the anterior and posterior digastric.

---

*It may also be used as a cable graft if the nerve is sacrificed; the cut end is a common source of postoperative neuroma, as considered in patients presenting with tender subcutaneous nodule after parotidectomy.

The submandibular gland is separated from the parotid gland by the thickened *parotid-masseteric fascia* that extends from the most anterior edge to the most inferior tip of the parotid.

Blood Supply

Facial artery arises from external carotid artery and courses deep to posterior belly of the digastric. It then travels lateral to the muscle through the gland and indents the inferior edge of the mandible.*

Facial vein lies lateral to the gland.† Dividing and retracting the vein superiorly protects the *marginal division of the facial nerve.*

Surgical Neural Anatomy

- *Lingual nerve*: Sensory nerve lies superficial to duct in the floor of the mouth.‡
- *Hypoglossal nerve*: Motor function to the tongue; it lies *medial* to *digastric* that lies *medial* to submandibular gland.
- *Submandibular ganglion*: Suspended from the *lingual nerve* by two filaments from the inferior aspect of the lingual nerve.§
- *Marginal mandibular nerve*: Provides motor function to muscles of facial expression (depressor labii inferioris, depressor anguli oris, mentalis), runs just deep to platysma

---

*Submandibular gland excision may require division of the facial artery twice.

†*Facial vein* represents one of two surgically relevant structures that lie superficial to the *anterior belly of the digastric*. The other is the *marginal division of the facial nerve.*

‡Understanding of this relationship is essential in submandibular gland excision via a cervical approach when the *duct is ligated* and the *lingual nerve is preserved*, and during excision of floor of mouth lesion (e.g. ranula) through the oral cavity.

§Ganglion is clamped, tied, and ligated during submandibular gland excision; a small blood vessel runs with the ganglion, which can retract under the mandible at the time of ligation.

lateral to the submandibular gland within the submandibular gland fascia.*

Warthin's Ducts

They open just lateral to lingual frenulum at the floor of mouth just posterior to incisors.[†]

Histology

Contains predominantly serous acinar cells with 10% mucous cells.

Sublingual Gland

Paired gland, separated by *lingual frenulum*, exists within the submucosal content of the floor of mouth.[‡] It is attached *anteriorly* to the mandible at the *sublingual fossa,* which lies *superior* to *mylohyoid.*

Drainage via multiple ducts at the floor of mouth through *Rivinus ducts.* It can also drain via submandibular duct through communication via *Bartholin duct.*[§]

Histology

It contains predominantly mucous cells.

Minor Salivary Glands

These glands are located throughout the oral cavity and upper airway but are concentrated in the *oral cavity.*[‖]

---

*The *marginal mandibular nerve* is one of two surgically relevant structures that run *superficial* to the *anterior belly of the digastric* muscle. The other is the *facial vein.*

[†]During excision of lesions involving the floor of the mouth, the duct can be cannulated and preserved. If disruption of the duct is required, marsupialization with or without ductoplasty should be performed.

[‡]Removal of sublingual gland off mandible within the sublingual fossa is required for complete resection of sublingual gland lesions.

[§]Mucocele of sublingual gland presents as ranula (see the "Benign Tumors of the Salivary Gland" section).

[‖]Neoplasms from minor salivary glands present as *submucosal* masses in the oral cavity, larynx, or hypopharynx.

Histology

These glands contain the highest percentage of *mucous* acinar cells and produce mucinous saliva.*

SALIVARY GLAND FUNCTION

Humans secrete about 1 L of saliva a day, which is 99.5% water and also contains lubricates (glycoproteins), amylase, buffers (bicarbonate), and antimicrobial proteins (immunoglobulin A, mucins, lysozyme, histamine, and lactoferrin). It protects against dental caries.

- *Parotid gland:* Gustatory and olfactory—*stimulated.*
- Submandibular, sublingual, minor salivary glands: Basal rate of flow—unstimulated.
- It is controlled by autonomic nervous system—*parasympathetic* dominant.

Pathways

Parotid Gland

Inferior salivatory nucleus (medulla) → Glossopharyngeal nerve → Lesser superficial petrosal nerve → Otic ganglion (synapse) → Auriculotemporal nerve (postganglionic parasympathetic fibers) → *Parotid gland*

Submandibular and Sublingual Glands

Superior salivary nucleus (pons) → Nervus intermedius (cranial nerve VII) → Chorda tympani → Submandibular ganglion (synapse) → Postganglionic parasympathetic fibers → *Submandibular and sublingual glands*

Salivary Gland Dysfunction

- Excessive saliva: *Sialorrhea*
- Drooling: *Ptyalism*

---

*Exception: Ebner's glands are minor salivary glands at the base of the tongue, serous acini only.

Etiology

- *Neurologic*: Cognitive and physical disabilities, cerebral palsy, Parkinson's disease, stroke, epilepsy, and Wilson's disease.
- *Hypersecretion*: Medication-induced gastroesophageal reflux disease.
- *Anatomic*: Oral incompetence, macroglossia, significant malocclusion.
- *Toxins*: Heavy metal poisoning (autonomic nervous system dysfunction).
- *Dysphagia* can result in ptyalism, secondary outlet obstruction.

Management

- Speech pathology should evaluate swallowing function.*

Medical:
- *Anticholinergic medications*: Glycopyrrolate, scopolamine, botox.

Surgical:
- *Duct rerouting*: Duct is rerouted to the posterior oral cavity.
- *Chorda tympani neurectomy*: Transtympanic procedure, short-lived result; it must be repeated secondary to nerve regrowth.
- Parotid duct ligation and submandibular gland excision represent the gold standard.†

Impaired Saliva Production

- Xerostomia
- Primary salivary disorder
- Sjögren's disease (see "Salivary Gland Pathology in Systemic Disease")

---

*Neurologically normal children with sialorrhea or ptyalism should be evaluated for *heavy metal poisoning*.
†Fistula and sialocele are possible complications.

- Dehydration
- Iatrogenic
- Medication
  - Psychotropic, beta blockers, general anesthesia
- Radiation
  - Irreversible damage seen at observed at 25 Gy
  - Preferential damage of *acinar cell* with sparing of *ductal cells*

Treatment

- Address underlying pathology.
- Aggressive dental care with fluoride treatments.
- Artificial saliva.
- Frequent small drinks.
- Pilocarpine (nonselective muscarinic receptor agonist).

SALIVARY GLAND PATHOLOGY

Diffuse Salivary Gland Enlargement

Acute Sialadenitis

Acute sialadenitis presents with unilateral, painful, preauricular facial swelling. Patients will sometimes complain of foul taste in mouth secondary to draining purulent saliva from Stensen's duct.

Pathophysiology

- *Salivary stasis*: This may be secondary to decreased salivary flow related to hydration status (more common in parotid gland) or from obstruction, i.e. calculi (more common in submandibular gland).
- Chronic infection or calculi can result in scarring, duct stenosis, and diminished secretory function resulting in *chronic sialadenitis*. Chronic sialadenitis of the *submandibular gland* with heavy lymphoid infiltration results in a *Kuttner's tumor*.

- *Most common bacteria*: *Staphylococcus aureus* (the most common), *Streptococcus viridans*, and anaerobes.*

Diagnosis

- Clinical diagnosis; identify pus from Stensen's duct and culture.

Treatment

- Antibiotics treatment with coverage for *Staphylococcus, Streptococcus,* and anaerobes
- Hydration
- Sialogogues
- Massage
- Warm compresses

Mumps

Consider in a 4- to 6-year-old child with *bilateral* parotid gland enlargement who was not vaccinated with measles, mumps, and rubella vaccine.

Diagnosis

- Clinical and serologic

Management

- Supportive

Granulomatous Diseases

Granulomatous diseases should be considered in patients with human immunodeficiency virus (HIV), immigrants, and patients

---

Classic patient: Nursing home or elderly patient, elderly postsurgical patient, patient with congestive heart failure, the medicine service is "running dry." Consider methicillin-resistant *S. aureus* in nursing home patients.

with inflammatory salivary lesions that do not respond to first-line antibiotic treatments.

Possible ideologies include tuberculosis, atypical mycobacteria, actinomycosis, cat scratch disease, and toxoplasmosis.

SALIVARY GLAND PATHOLOGY IN SYSTEMIC DISEASE

Sarcoidosis

- *Noncaseating* granulomatosis systemic disease that involves salivary glands.
- *Heerfordt disease* involves acute parotitis, uveitis, facial nerve paralysis.
- Serum angiotensin-converting enzyme levels are often elevated.

Sjögren's Syndrome

- Systemic *autoimmune disease* with destruction of acinar and ductal cells results in parotid hypertrophy. Patients will often present with dry eye as well as xerostomia.*
- Anti Ro (SSA) and anti La (SSB) antibodies are present and are useful in the diagnosis.
- *Minor salivary gland biopsy* is the gold standard for diagnosis.
- Supportive treatment for xerostomia (see above).

Sialoadenosis

- Recurrent noninflammatory, non-neoplastic salivary gland swelling secondary to underlying nutritional, endocrine, or metabolic disease, seen in cirrhosis, diabetes, malnutrition, and pancreatic insufficiency.

---

*Patients are at a higher risk of B-cell lymphoma, specifically mucosa-associated lymphoid tissue.

HIV

- Patients with HIV have salivary gland enlargement that may be secondary to lymphoid hyperplasia, infection, or malignancy.
- Solid masses carry a *40%* risk of *malignancy.*
- *Lymphoepithelial cysts* represent degeneration of parotid lymph nodes, a benign process that can become enlarged and cosmetically deforming. Patients presenting with numerous unilateral or bilateral cystic masses of the parotid gland should be tested for HIV.
- It has higher risk for infectious etiologies such as toxoplasmosis and tuberculosis.

WORKUP OF SALIVARY PATHOLOGY

FNA

Routine fine-needle aspiration is not always performed as it does not affect the indication for surgery or the extent of surgery. It is useful in ruling out inflammatory lesions, identifying systemic disease, ruling out metastases, and evaluating lesions in patients who are poor candidates for surgery. It also provides useful information that may be helpful in preoperative patient consultation.

Imaging

Imaging of salivary gland pathology aids in treatment planning. Ultrasound, computed tomography (CT), and magnetic resonance imaging (MRI) can be used and offer unique benefits depending on the pathology.

Ultrasound

It is cost effective without radiation exposure and often used in pediatric patients.

Computed Tomography

With and *without contrast*, it is a commonly used preoperative imaging modality for evaluation of salivary calculi, neoplasms, tumor size, and surrounding anatomy, especially bony anatomy.

- *Calculi*: Submandibular gland *80% radiolucent*, parotid gland *20% radiolucent*.

Magnetic Resonance Imaging

- Anatomic assessment with evaluation of *perineural spread* in malignancy.
- Salivary masses often hypointense on T1 imaging.
- Benign and low-grade tumors (less cellular) are often hyperintense on T2.

NEOPLASMS OF THE SALIVARY GLANDS

Benign Tumors of the Salivary Gland

Pleomorphic Adenoma (Benign Mixed Tumor)

- Pleomorphic adenoma is derived from intercalated duct cells.
- It is the most common salivary neoplasm, 85% present in parotid gland.
- Histologically, it is a "mixed tumor" with three components:
  - Myoepithelial
  - Epithelial
  - Stromal
- It can undergo malignant transformation; estimated 25% of untreated cases.[1]

Warthin's Tumor (Papillary Cystadenoma Lymphomatosum)

- Warthin's tumor is derived from striated duct cells.
- It is almost exclusively in parotid.
- It can present as cystic mass.
- It has 10% bilateral masses.

- It is more common in smokers.
- Warthin's tumor can become inflamed, painful, and infected. Given its clonal nature by polymerase chain reaction and its clinical symptoms, this lesion may represent an inflammatory process rather than a true neoplasm.
- Histologically, it contains cystic spaces, papillary architecture, lymphoid stroma, and oncocytic epithelium.

Lipomas

- Characteristic MRI and CT scan findings often make the diagnosis.

Postsurgical Neuroma

Patients will present with a history of past surgery and a painful, mobile, superficial mass, often in area of sacrificed great auricular nerve. It is treated with local excision after ruling out recurrent salivary neoplasm.

Ranula

- Retention cyst of the sublingual gland.
- It can be retained in the sublingual space or extend deep to the mylohyoid (*plunging ranula*).

Mucocele

- This is a pseudocyst of minor salivary glands, often seen on the lower mucosal lip of children from biting trauma.

Malignant Tumors of the Salivary Gland

- In patients who present with a salivary gland mass and complain of *pain, rapid growth, or paralysis,* malignant neoplasm must be ruled out.
- Parotid gland mass tumors are less likely to be malignant, whereas submandibular, sublingual, and minor salivary gland tumors are more likely to be malignant.

- Prior exposure to *ionizing radiation* appears to substantially increase the risk of developing malignant neoplasms of the major salivary glands, particularly *mucoepidermoid carcinoma* (*see* "Mucoepidermoid Carcinoma" below).
- *Metastatic disease*, specifically cutaneous malignancies of the face, ear, and scalp, should always be in the differential diagnosis of salivary masses. This most commonly involves the parotid gland, which contains intraglandular lymph nodes.

Primary Salivary Gland Malignant Tumors

Mucoepidermoid Carcinoma

- Mucoepidermoid carcinoma is derived from excretory ductal cells.
- It is the most common salivary gland malignancy in adults and children.
- Mucoepidermoid carcinomas are graded as low, intermediate, and high.
- Low grade can be cystic.
- Tumors involving minor salivary glands show a strong predilection for the lower lip.

Adenoid Cystic Carcinoma

- Adenoid cystic carcinoma is derived from intercalated ductal cells.
- It is the most common malignant tumor of the submandibular, sublingual, and minor salivary glands, the second most common overall.
- Propensity for perineural invasion.
- Three histologic types: cribriform (best prognosis), solid (worst prognosis), tubular.
- Distant failure is most common mode of failure. This can often occur > 5 years after treatment of the primary tumor.*

---

*Patients with adenoid cystic carcinoma must have prolonged follow-up as they can present with distant metastasis 10–15 years after the treatment of primary tumor; the most common site of distant recurrence is the *lungs*.

Acinic Cell Carcinoma

- This is derived from *acinic cells.*
- It is a low-grade tumor that can sometimes occur bilaterally.

Polymorphous Low-Grade Adenocarcinoma

- This is derived from intercalated ductal cells.
- It often presents in the oral cavity, specifically in the hard palate.
- It is a low-grade tumor with high rate of perineural invasion.

Salivary Duct Carcinoma

- Salivary duct carcinoma is a high-grade, aggressive tumor with high prevalence of early regional and distant metastasis.
- Given early regional metastasis, elective neck dissection should be considered in this salivary malignancy.

Carcinoma Ex Pleomorphic Adenoma

- This arises from longstanding pleomorphic adenoma.
- It should be considered in any longstanding salivary tumor that begins to grow rapidly.

Lymphoma

- Lymphoma most often involves the *parotid gland.*
- Mucosa-associated lymphoid tissue lymphomas are most common.
- It can occur in patients with *Sjögren's syndrome.**

Treatment of Malignant Salivary Gland Disease

Surgical treatment represents the mainstay of management of salivary malignancies. This includes complete superficial

---

*It is important to make diagnosis of lymphoma as it is treated with systemic therapies rather than surgery; core or excisional biopsy may be required.

parotidectomy and/or total parotidectomy if the deep lobe is involved.

Modified radical neck dissection should be completed in patients with clinically positive disease. Elective neck dissection of levels 1–3 should be considered for tumors of high grade or stage.

- *Enucleation* of tumor from within the parotid bed results in unacceptably *high recurrence rates.*
- *Adjuvant radiation* is utilized for high-grade or high-stage lesions. Perineural invasion is a relative indication for postoperative radiation.[2]

REFERENCES

1. Thackray AC, Lucas R. Tumors of the Major Salivary Glands: Atlas of Tumor Pathology. Washington, DC: Armed Forces Institute of Pathology; 1983.
2. Armstrong JG, Harrison LB, Spiro RH, et al. Malignant tumors of major salivary gland origin. A matched-pair analysis of the role of combined surgery and postoperative radiotherapy. Arch Otolaryngol Head Neck Surg. 1990;116(3):290-3.

SUGGESTED READING

1. Califano J, Eisele DW. Benign salivary gland neoplasms. Otolaryngol Clin North Am. 1999;32:861-74.
2. Cummings C, Harker L, et al (Eds). Otolaryngology—Head and Neck Surgery, 5th edition, Vol. 2, Section 2. Philadelphia: Elsevier; 2010.
3. Rice DH. Malignant salivary gland neoplasms. Otolaryngol Clin North Am. 1999;32(5):875-86.

Chapter 20

Reconstruction

Christopher E Fundakowski

There are no hard and fast rules when it comes to reconstruction of head and neck defects. Each clinical/operative scenario needs to be considered on a case-by-case basis. One of the overarching principles of reconstruction is to begin by considering the most simple option and working toward the more complex, contemplating the pros and cons of each. The concept is frequently referred to as "the reconstructive ladder" (Table 20.1).

SECONDARY INTENTION

This is a means of tissue healing where the wound is intentionally left open and given the opportunity to heal from within secondary to granulation and contracture.

Table 20.1: The reconstructive ladder: simple to complex.

Secondary intention: Least complex
Primary intention
Skin graft (split thickness)
Skin graft (full thickness)
Local random flaps
Local axial flaps
Regional pedicled flaps
Free flaps: Most complex

- *Pros/Cons*: It is the most simple/rapid option, may be useful for contaminated/infected wound, is likely to yield suboptimal cosmetic result; lengthened healing time is required.

PRIMARY INTENTION

This is the direct closure of wound by approximation of edges.

- *Pros/Cons*: It has immediate closure, improved cosmetic appearance over secondary intention; it must consider implications of defect size/depth/location as high-tension closure may distort surrounding anatomy (e.g. ectropion when closing cheek defect); may not be an option for large defects.
- *Skin graft*: Harvesting various thickness and dimensions of skin in order to reconstruct defects.
- *Split thickness graft*: Epidermal/partial dermal autograft (it can vary in thickness depending on the use and preference; typically 10–30 mm).
  - *Pros/Cons*: It is quickly harvested with dermatome; it is able to harvest large grafts from multiple donor sites; donor site heals spontaneously; higher rate of success/take compared to full-thickness grafts; it may not have ideal color match; it may experience more contraction.
  - *Common uses*: Oral cavity mucosal defects, tongue, cutaneous defects (face and scalp).
- *Full thickness graft*: Epidermal/full dermis autograft
  - *Pros/Cons*: It has improved color match and texture, less contraction; higher failure rate requires closure of donor site.
  - *Common uses*: It is used in skin defects on face/nose.
- Skin graft healing phases:
  - *Imbibition*: It takes 24–48 hours; graft survives by passively absorbing nutrients by diffusion.
  - *Inosculation*: It takes 48–72 hours; capillary buds from recipient tissue bed connect to graft vessels.

- *Neovascularization*: It takes 72 hours and more and forms new vessels.
- *Dermal regeneration template (Integra)*: This is a porous scaffold where dermal cells can regenerate, allowing placement of a split-thickness skin graft at a later date; it is commonly used in burns and to increase the thickness of tissue bed.
- *Acellular dermis (Alloderm)*: This is the acellular dermal matrix derived from cadaveric skin; it provides additional dermal layer for soft tissue defects.
- *Flap*: This is the tissue that is mobilized to a defect (recipient site) while maintaining its own blood supply.
  Classification can be complex—terminology is based on blood supply, tissue type, and location/movement.

CLASSIFICATION BY BLOOD SUPPLY

- *Random flap*: Soft tissue where vascularity is based on perfusion by subdermal plexus and no named vessel.
  Example: Bilobed flap, rhomboid, advancement, rotation, transposition, island flap, and note flap.
- *Axial flap*: Soft tissue based on perfusion by named blood vessel in an anatomically defined vascular territory.
  Example: Paramedian forehead flap, melolabial flap, and buccinator flap.

CLASSIFICATION BY TISSUE TYPE

- Cutaneous: It contains skin, subdermal plexus, and subcutaneous fat.
  Example: Local (random) flaps, rotation flaps, advancement flaps, and transposition flaps.
- Composite: It contains multiple tissue types.
  Example: Fasciocutaneous (radial forearm free flap), osseocutaneous (fibula free flap), and myocutaneous (rectus abdominus free flap).

CLASSIFICATION BY LOCATION

- *Local flap*: Here, tissue is transferred into a defect from an adjacent area; also it can be described by the type of movement; commonly single stage, it may be affected by vascular disease and used for smaller defects.
- *Rotation flap*: This is a random flap of various sizes based on subdermal plexus, which rotates along an arch (Figs. 20.1A and B); it requires wide undermining and relatively long incision.
- *Transposition flap*: This is also a random flap of various sizes based on subdermal plexus, which takes the place of adjacent tissue.
- *Z-plasty*: This is used to lengthen and redirect contracted scars; increased length can be achieved by increasing the angle of flaps:
  - 30°: 25% gain in length
  - 45°: 50% gain in length
  - 60°: 75% gain in length
- *Bilobed flap*: This is a double transposition flap that allows increased movement compared to a single transposition flap (Figs. 20.2A and B).
- *Rhomboid flap (Limburg)*: This uses 60° and 120° angles to remove tension from defect (Figs. 20.3A and B).
- *Interpolated flap*: This is a flap of tissue that travels over/under a bridge of intact tissue, separating the donor site from the defect (it may require delayed division of pedicle), e.g. paramedian forehead flap and subcutaneous island flap.

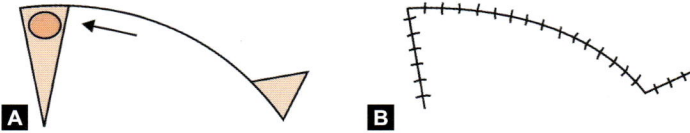

Figs. 20.1A and B: (A) Defect and anticipated rotation/advancement. (B) Closed wound. Example: cervicofacial rotation flap; commonly used for midface/cheek defects.

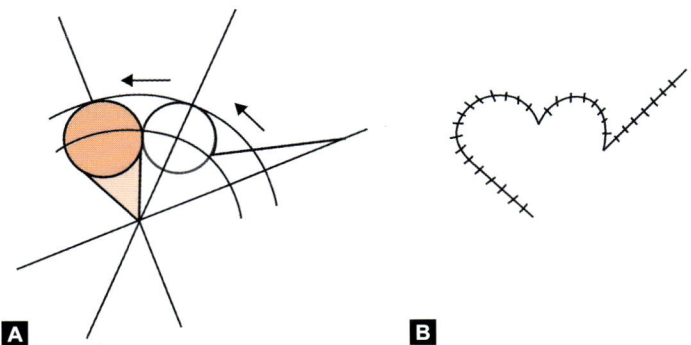

Figs. 20.2A and B: (A) Defect and anticipated bilobed flap. (B) Closed wound. Example: commonly used for nasal tip defects that are 1.5 cm or less.

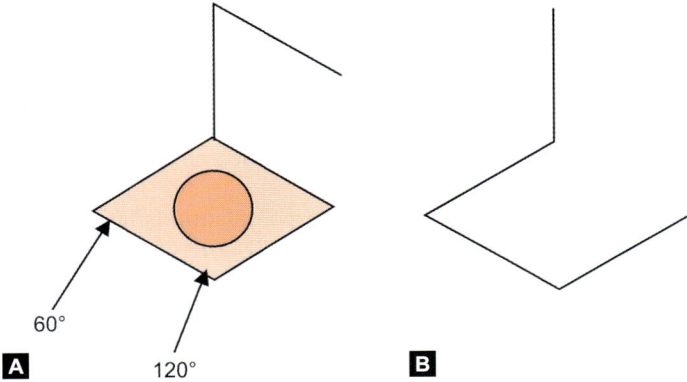

Figs. 20.3A and B: (A) Defect and anticipated rhomboid flap. (B) Closed wound. Example: commonly used for cheek/midface defects.

- *Paramedian forehead flap*: Based on supratrochlear artery, commonly used for nasal defects, pedicle recommended to be 1.5 cm in diameter, pedicle commonly divided at 2-3 weeks postoperation (depending on risk factors such as smoking history and vascular disease).

- *Advancement flap*: A random flap based on subdermal plexus that can be unilateral or bilateral (Figs. 20.4A and B); length/width ratio should not exceed 3:1; it commonly requires excision of Burrow's triangles to avoid standing cone deformity.
- *Regional/distant flap*: Here, the harvested tissue is from a noncontiguous anatomic site.
- *Pedicled flap*: Tissue harvested for reconstruction retains the original blood supply.
- *Pectoralis major*: Based on thoracoacromial artery, easy to harvest and close primarily, it is used for external (neck, cheek, and ear) and internal (oral cavity, pharyngeal, and laryngeal) defects; it can be harvested as myocutaneous or myofascial.
- *Supraclavicular artery island flap*: Fasciocutaneous, based on supraclavicular artery; used for similar defects as pectoralis, but is thinner and more pliable; it must have transverse cervical vessels available (careful after previous neck dissection).
- *Submental artery island flap*: Based on submental musculocutaneous perforator, it is used commonly for oral cavity defects.
- *Temporoparietal fascia flap*: Based on superficial temporal artery, it can be fascia only, or with skin; can be used for mastoid cavity, paranasal sinus, and intraoral defects.

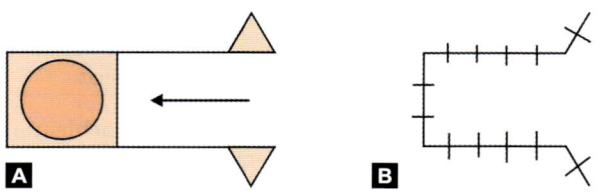

Figs. 20.4A and B: (A) Defect and anticipated advancement flap. (B) Closed wound. Example: commonly used for forehead and chin defects.

- *Buccinator flap*: Myomucosal, based on either buccal artery, proximal, or distal facial artery, and used for various intraoral defects.
- *Trapezius flap*: Musculocutaneous; can be harvested as superior (based on occipital and paraspinal perforators), lateral (based on superficial transverse cervical artery), or inferior island (most common, based on descending branches of transverse cervical artery), and commonly used for posterior neck/scalp.
- *Latissimus dorsi flap*: Musculocutaneous; based on thoracodorsal artery; commonly used for large lateral neck/face defects, also commonly harvested as a free flap.
- *Deltopectoral flap*: Fasciocutaneous, based on the second to fourth intercostal perforators; contraindicated if the patient has a history of prior cardiac bypass surgery utilizing internal mammary.
- *Free flap*: Tissue is harvested from original blood supply and will be anastomosed to both artery and vein at the recipient site.
- *Radial forearm free flap*: Fasciocutaneous, fascia only, or osteofasciocutaneous; is based on radial artery; innervated by lateral antebrachial cutaneous (branch of musculocutaneous nerve); can harvest approximately 12 cm of bone; extremely versatile flap for both internal and external defects; donor site covered with split thickness skin graft; it performs preoperative Allen's test to assess for adequate collateral ulnar circulation.
- *Anterolateral thigh free flap*: Musculocutaneous/septocutaneous; has variable thickness depending on patient habitus and harvest technique; is based on lateral circumflex femoral vessels; is innervated by lateral femoral cutaneous nerve; has multiple uses, particularly when needing more bulk/tissue than that the forearm can provide.
- *Fibula free flap*: Osseous or osseocutaneous; based on deep peroneal vessels, innervated by lateral sural cutaneous nerve; flap of choice for large bony defects where additional

soft tissue paddle is of benefit; uses computed tomographic angiography preoperatively to assess for aberrations in vascular anatomy (approximately 10%).

- *Scapula free flap*: Harvested as osteocutaneous or fasciocutaneous; based on circumflex scapular vessels, can harvest two separate skin paddles (scapular and parascapular), as well as two vascularized bone segments (lateral scapula and scapular tip based on angular artery); consider this flap for complex defects or when bone is needed and fibula anatomy is abnormal.
- *Rectus abdominus free flap*: Musculocutaneous, based on deep inferior epigastric vessels, able to provide a significant amount of tissue/bulk for large defects.
- *Iliac crest free flap*: Osseomyocutaneous, based on deep circumflex iliac artery, commonly used for large bony defects (mandible/maxilla, given natural curve of iliac crest); donor site morbidity to be considered.
- *Jejunal free flap*: Large segments can be harvested for pharyngoesophageal reconstruction, commonly based on second jejunal branch; jejunal flap will continue to provide secretions, which can assist with swallowing; donor site morbidity is to be considered.

SUGGESTED READING

1. Baker SR. Local Flaps in Facial Reconstruction, 3rd edition. Philadelphia, PA: Saunders; 2014.
2. Chim H, Salgado CJ, Seselgyte R. Principles of head and neck reconstruction: an algorithm to guide flap selection. Semin Plast Surg. 2010;24:148-54.
3. Hanasono MM, Matros E, Disa JJ. Important aspects of head and neck reconstruction. Plast Reconstr Surg. 2014;134:968-80.
4. Hayden RE, Nagel TH. The evolving role of free flaps and pedicled flaps in head and neck reconstruction. Curr Opin Otolaryngol Head Neck Surg. 2013;21:305-10.
5. Hurvitz KA, Kobayashi M, Evans GR. Current options in head and neck reconstruction. Plast Reconstr Surg. 2006;118:122-33.

6. Lohuis PJ, Godefroy WP, Baker SR, et al. Transposition flaps in nasal reconstruction. Facial Plast Surg Clin North Am. 2011;19:85-106.

7. Park CW, Miles BA. The expanding role of the anterolateral thigh free flap in head and neck reconstruction. Curr Opin Otolaryngol Head Neck Surg. 2011;19:263-8.

8. Pepper JP, Baker SR. Local flaps: cheek and lip reconstruction. JAMA Facial Plast Surg. 2013;15:375-82.

9. Rapstine ED, Knaus WJ, Thornton JF. Simplifying cheek reconstruction: a review of over 400 cases. Plast Reconstr Surg. 2012;129:1291-9.

10. Steiger JD. Bilobed flaps in nasal reconstruction. Facial Plast Surg Clin North Am. 2011;19:107-11.

11. Urken ML. Atlas of Regional and Free Flaps for Head and Neck Reconstruction: Flap Harvest and Insetting, 2nd edition. Philadelphia, PA: Lippincott Williams & Wilkins; 2011.

12. Wei F, Mardini S. Flaps and Reconstructive Surgery. Philadelphia, PA: Saunders; 2009.

Chapter 21

Oral Cavity and Oropharyngeal Cancer

Christopher E Fundakowski

In the United States in 2013, over 40,000 cases of oral cavity and oropharyngeal carcinoma were diagnosed, with approximately 8,000 deaths.[1]

The oral cavity and oropharynx are anatomic neighbors, but they behave as distinct diseases. Significant differences exist in patients' demographic and risk factor profiles, etiology, and prognosis, as well as in treatment.

ORAL CAVITY CANCER

Statistics

- About 264,000 cases of oral cavity cancer are diagnosed annually worldwide.[2]
- It is more common in men.
- Up to 66% of it is attributed to smoking.
- Incidence and etiology vary with countries (i.e. oral cavity cancer, secondary to smokeless tobacco, varies from 6% in the United States to 52% in India).

Risk Factors

- *Tobacco*: Both smoking and smokeless; smokers have up to 20-fold increased risk of oral cavity cancer.[3]

- *Alcohol*: Approximately fivefold increased cancer risk; synergistic effect of combined smoking/alcohol can increase cancer risk up to 50–80 times.[4]
- *Betal quid*: It is also known as *paan* areca nut and betal leaf.
- *Immunosuppression*: Acquired immune deficiency syndrome (AIDS), organ transplant, Fanconi anemia.
- *Sunlight/ultraviolet exposure*: It places lip at risk for malignancy.

Clinical Presentation

- *Precancerous lesions*: Cancer may develop from precursor lesions such as leukoplakia (3–33%, speckled or verrucous patterns, more commonly transform into cancer than homogeneous), erythroplakia (80–85%).
- *Cancerous lesions*: Quite variable, lesion may be white/red, may present with pain, otalgia (referred), bleeding, ill-fitting dentures, loose teeth, nonhealing tooth socket/ulcer, hypoesthesia (perineural invasion), trismus (pterygoid invasion), may also present with neck mass.
- *Neck*: About 20–30% occult cervical metastasis (16% will have "skip" metastasis).

Evaluation

- *Clinical history*: Comprehensive history plus relevant risk factors (*see* above).
- *Physical examination*: Assess for trismus, extent of lesion, cranial nerve examination, neck examination.
- Imaging:
  - *Primary lesion and neck*—Computed tomographic (CT) scan with contrast used most commonly, may benefit from magnetic resonance imaging when suspecting perineural or deep tongue invasion or iodine allergy.
  - *Metastasis evaluation*—May consider chest X-ray versus CT scan of the chest versus CT scan chest/abdomen/pelvis versus fluorodeoxyglucose–PET/CT (positron emission

tomography-computed tomography), depending on clinical suspicion for distant metastasis and equipment availability.

- *Biopsy*: May perform biopsy of suspect lesion, may perform fine-needle aspiration (FNA) of palpable neck mass.

Pathology

Common Histology

- Mostly squamous cell carcinoma (90–95%).
- Verrucous carcinoma (most common on buccal mucosa), rarely metastasizes.
- Basal cell carcinoma (common on lip).
- Minor salivary gland (<5%; i.e. mucoepidermoid carcinoma and adenocarcinoma).
- *Pseudoepitheliomatous hyperplasia*: It may be mistaken for squamous cell carcinoma (necrotizing sialometaplasia and granular cell tumor).

Genetics

- *Mutations*: Squamous cell carcinoma in Western (i.e. North/South America) countries commonly has TP53 mutations, whereas the same in Eastern countries (i.e. India and Southeast Asia) commonly has *ras* oncogene mutation.
  HPV16 is not thought to play a major role in pathogenesis in oral cancer (present in <3% of cases).

Anatomy

- *Subsites*: Lip, buccal mucosa, alveolus, retromolar trigone, hard palate, anterior two-thirds of the tongue (dorsal/ventral surfaces), and floor of the mouth.
  - The lip is the most common location of all subsites for oral cavity cancer; 90% of lip cancer located on lower lip; 90% squamous cell carcinoma; 90% 5-year survival if tumor is <2 cm; basal cell carcinoma located more

commonly on upper lip. Lower lip has bilateral lymphatic drainage versus upper lip with unilateral drainage (due to fusion planes).
–   The oral tongue is the second most common subsite in oral cavity for squamous cell carcinoma (lateral tongue is most common). Hard palate cancer may extend into nasal cavity via incisive foramen.

Staging

Staging of oral cavity tumors is presented in Table 21.1.
*   *Nodal staging*: Please refer to latest American Joint Committee on Cancer staging.
*   *Important prognostic features not incorporated in staging*: Tumor thickness, perineural invasion, lymphovascular invasion, and extracapsular nodal extension.

Treatment—Lip

Early Stage (1–2)

Surgical therapy (preferred) versus definitive radiation therapy to primary site; elective neck dissection in N0 not recommended; adjuvant therapy recommended in positive margin, perineural/lymphovascular invasion.

Table 21.1: Staging of oral cavity tumors.

T1	Tumor up to 2 cm in greatest dimension
T2	Tumor >2 cm and up to 4 cm in greatest dimension
T3	Tumor >4 cm in greatest dimension
T4a	Moderately advanced local disease *Lip*: Invasion through cortical bone, inferior alveolar nerve, floor of mouth, skin of face (chin and nose) *Oral cavity*: Invasion into adjacent structures only (cortical bone, into deep muscles of tongue, maxillary sinus, and skin of the face)
T4b	Very advanced local disease (commonly considered unresectable) Invades masticator space, pterygoid plates, skull base, internal carotid artery encasement

Advanced Stage (3–4)

Surgical therapy (preferred) versus definitive radiation or chemoradiation; ± neck dissection in N0 if treating surgically.

Treatment—Oral Cavity

Early Stage (1–2)

- Surgical therapy (preferred) ± ipsilateral neck dissection (guided by tumor thickness for tongue lesions) versus definitive radiation therapy.
- Recommended tumor thickness to advise neck dissection is 4 mm or greater (96% negative predictive value).[5]
- Bilateral neck treatment is considered in midline lesions (i.e. floor of the mouth).
- Staging neck dissection may serve both diagnostic and potentially therapeutic purposes as adjuvant radiation of the neck may be avoided if (1) nodes are negative or (2) one positive node exists without adverse features (i.e. extracapsular extension).[6]

Alternative to Staging Neck Dissection

Sentinel node biopsy may be utilized for clinically N0 patients to assess the need for therapeutic neck dissection; if the node is positive, then complete neck dissection is performed; there is a ~5% false negative rate; drainage patterns are not so predictable when the primary is located in the floor of the mouth; and overall results improve with the surgeon's experience.

Advanced Stage (3–4)

Surgical therapy with ipsilateral/bilateral neck dissection, followed, possibly, by radiation or chemoradiation versus multimodality clinical trial.

It is important to note that each of the subsites (as listed above) that encompass the oral cavity contributes to various degrees of function (i.e. speech and swallowing), and as a result, the decision for a particular intervention (whether surgical vs nonsurgical) must be specifically tailored to that site, and also must consider both prognosis and anticipated functional morbidity.

OROPHARYNGEAL CANCER

Recent discovery of the human papilloma virus (HPV) as a contributing factor has dramatically changed the approach to this cancer, as HPV status is now considered one of the most important clinical factors when treating these patients.

Statistics

- About 136,000 global cases of pharyngeal (naso-, oro-, hypo-) squamous cell carcinoma are reported annually.
- Approximately 40–90% of oropharynx cancer is HPV related. Human papilloma virus–associated oropharyngeal squamous cell carcinoma has increased 225% from 1988 to 2004 (approximately 5% per year from 2000 to 2004).
- Oropharyngeal cancer has a bimodal distribution (based on HPV status):
  - HPV+: Younger patients (median age for male patients is 58 years and that of female patients is 48 years)
  - HPV–: Older patients (median age is 62 years)
- Oropharyngeal cancer is more common in men (both HPV+ and HPV–).

Risk Factors

- *Human papilloma virus*: Up to 85% of adults may encounter exposure to HPV infection, although only a small percentage will develop malignancy (>90% HPV16 subtype); increased risk of cancer is associated with an increased number of oral sexual partners.[7]
- *Smoking*: Increased risk for squamous cell carcinoma.
- *Alcohol*: Increased risk for squamous cell carcinoma; effects are synergistic with smoking.

- *Immunosuppression*: AIDS, organ transplant, Fanconi anemia, dyskeratosis congenita (inherited bone marrow failure syndromes).

Clinical Presentation

HPV Negative

- Usually older, smoker, drinker, male; patients most commonly present with sore throat.
- Substance abuse driven with tobacco and alcohol as primary causes.
- Typically present with more advanced T stage relative to N stage.

HPV Positive

- Usually younger, male, nonsmoker, nondrinker/mild drinker; patients most commonly present with neck mass.
- Typically present with more advanced N stage relative to T stage.
- Neck nodes are commonly cystic.

Evaluation

- *Clinical history*: Comprehensive history plus relevant risk factors (*see* above).
- *Physical examination*: Assess for trismus, extent of lesion, cranial nerve examination, neck examination, fiberoptic examination to assess for potential airway compromise and tumor extent.
- Imaging:
  - *Primary lesion and neck*: Computed tomographic scan with contrast used most commonly.
  - Nodes are often cystic (may be confused with branchial cleft cyst).
  - *Metastasis evaluation*: May consider chest X-ray versus CT scan of the chest versus CT scan chest/abdomen/pelvis

versus FDG-PET/CT, depending on clinical suspicion for distant metastasis and equipment availability.
- *Biopsy*: May perform biopsy of suspect lesion (clinic vs OR), may perform FNA of palpable neck mass.

Pathology

Histology

- Squamous cell carcinoma (approximately 95% of oropharyngeal cancer)
    - *HPV positive*: Tumor histology often described as nonkeratinizing, poorly differentiated or with basaloid features.
    - *HPV negative*: Tumor histology often described as keratinizing, mild/moderately differentiated.
- Lymphoepithelioma (poorly differentiated subtype of oropharyngeal cancer).
- Lymphoma.

HPV

- Double-stranded deoxyribonucleic acid (DNA) virus with over 100 subtypes.
    - HPV16 responsible for over 90% of HPV+ oropharyngeal cancer.
- Proteins E6 and E7 play a major role in pathogenesis.
    - E6 inactivates/degrades p53 (tumor suppressor).
    - E7 binds to Rb (retinoblastoma, tumor suppressor).
- p16 will commonly be elevated in cancer cells that are infected with HPV, leading to its use as a surrogate clinical marker for an HPV-driven tumor.
- The presence of HPV DNA (highly specific, but not highly sensitive) does not equate to a tumor of HPV origin (the reason why p16 expression is needed).
- FNA performed on neck mass should have p16 protein (highly sensitive, but not highly specific) immunohistochemistry.

Outcomes

Patients with HPV+ oropharyngeal cancer will have approximately 25% improvement in overall survival and progression-free survival, and reduced risk for recurrence, compared to HPV-counterparts.[8]

This survival advantage is limited to HPV-associated tumors in the oropharynx, not other subsites.

HPV+ oropharyngeal cancer patients who smoke (>10 packs per year) have worse survival rate than HPV+ nonsmokers.[9]

Anatomy

- *Subsites*: Lateral pharyngeal wall (tonsil), posterior pharyngeal wall, soft palate, base of tongue.
- The tonsil/lateral pharyngeal wall is the most common location, followed by the base of the tongue (makes up 90% of all oropharyngeal squamous cell carcinoma).
  Posterior pharyngeal wall lesions are less common and with less metastatic potential.

Staging

Table 21.2 presents staging of oropharyngeal tumors. *Important prognostic features not incorporated in staging:* Perineural invasion, lymphovascular invasion, extracapsular nodal extension.

Table 21.2: Staging of oropharyngeal tumors.	
T1	Tumor up to 2 cm in greatest dimension
T2	Tumor >2 cm and up to 4 cm in greatest dimension
T3	Tumor >4 cm in greatest dimension
T4a	Moderately advanced local disease Tumor invades the larynx, extrinsic muscle of tongue, medial pterygoid, hard palate, or mandible
T4b	Very advanced local disease (commonly considered unresectable) Tumor invades lateral pterygoid muscle, pterygoid plates, lateral nasopharynx, or skull base, or encases carotid artery

Treatment

Early Stage (1–2)

- Definitive radiation versus resection of primary with staging ipsilateral/bilateral neck dissection.

Advanced Stage (3–4)

- Concurrent systemic chemoradiation versus resection of primary with neck dissection versus induction chemotherapy followed by radiation/chemoradiation.
- HPV+ oropharyngeal cancer is currently treated similar to site- and stage-matched HPV patients. Trials are underway aiming at de-escalating therapy.

Prevention

- Vaccines are available that target HPV6/11/16/18 (Gardasil, Merck) and 16/18 (Cervarix, GlaxoSmithKline).
- Recommended vaccination ages are 11–21 years for boys and 11–26 years for girls.
- Recommended vaccination ages in men who are immunocompromised, HIV+ are 22–26 years.
- Vaccine compliance is still low compared to other vaccines; reasons are multifactorial.
- Currently, there is no role for vaccination once patients are diagnosed with oropharyngeal cancer.
- HPV+ oropharyngeal squamous cell carcinoma is not contagious and cannot be transmitted.[10]

REFERENCES

1. Siegel R, Naishadham D, Jemal A. Cancer statistics, 2013. Cancer J Clin. 2013;63:11-30.
2. Ferlay J, Shin HR, Bray F, et al. GLOBOCAN2008 v2.0, Cancer Incidence and Mortality Worldwide: IARC cancerbase No. 10. Lyon (France); International Agency for Research on Cancer; 2010. [Online] Available from http://globocan.iarc.fr. [Accessed March 2015].

3. Boffetta P, Hecht S, Gray N, et al. Smokeless tobacco and cancer. Lancet Oncol. 2008;9(7):667-75.

4. Hashibe M, Brennan P, Chuang SC, et al. Interaction between tobacco and alcohol use and the risk of head and neck cancer: pooled analysis in the International Head and Neck Cancer Epidemiology Consortium. Cancer Epidemiol Biomarkers Prev. 2009;18(2):541-50.

5. Sparano A, Weinstein G, Chalian A, et al. Multivariate predictors of occult neck metastasis in early oral tongue cancer. Otolaryngol Head Neck Surg. 2004;131:472-6.

6. Fakih AR, Rao RS, Patel AR. Prophylactic neck dissection in squamous cell carcinoma of oral tongue: a prospective randomized study. Semin Surg Oncol. 1989;5:327-30.

7. Hemminki K, Dong C, Frisch M. Tonsillar and other upper aerodigestive tract cancers among cervical cancer patients and their husbands. Eur J Cancer Prev. 2000;9:433-7.

8. O'Rorke MA, Ellison MV, Murray LJ, et al. Human papillomavirus related head and neck cancer survival: a systematic review and meta-analysis. Oral Oncol. 2012;48:1191-201.

9. Rischin D, Young RJ, Fisher R, et al. Prognostic significance of p16INK4A and human papillomavirus in patients with oropharyngeal cancer treated on TROG 02.02 phase III trial. J Clin Oncol. 2010;28:4142-8.

10. Wu X, Watson M, Wilson R. Human papillomavirus-associated cancers—United States, 2004–2008. MMWR. 2012;61(15):258-61.

SUGGESTED READING

1. Ang KK, Harris J, Wheeler R, et al. Human papillomavirus (HPV) and survival of patients with oropharyngeal cancer. N Engl J Med. 2010;363:24-35.

2. Byers RM, Weber RS, Andrews T, et al. Frequency and therapeutic implications of "skip metastases" in the neck from squamous cell carcinoma of the oral tongue. Head Neck. 1997;19:14-9.

3. Cantrell SC, Peck BW, Li Q, et al. Differences in imaging characteristics of HPV-positive and HPV-negative oropharyngeal cancers: a blinded matched-pair analysis. AJNR Am J Neuroradiol. 2013;34:2005-9.

4. Chaturvedi AK, Engels EA, Pfeiffer RM, et al. Human papillomavirus and rising oropharyngeal cancer incidence in the United States. J Clin Oncol. 2011;29:4294-301.

5. Deschler DG, Richmon JD, Khariwala SS, et al. The "new" head and neck cancer patient—young, nonsmoker, nondrinker, and HPV positive. Otolaryngol Head Neck Surg. 2014;151(3):375-80.

6. Edge SB, Byrd DR, Compton CC, et al. (Eds). In: AJCC Cancer Staging Manual, 7th edition. New York: Springer; 2010. pp. 21-101.

7. National Comprehensive Cancer Network. NCCN Clinical Practice Guidelines in Oncology: Head and Neck Cancers. v.2.2014. [online] Available from www.nccn.org/professionals/physician_gls/pdf/head-and-neck.pdf. [Accessed March 2015].

8. Ragin CC, Taioli E. Survival of squamous cell carcinoma of the head and neck in relation to human papillomavirus infection: review and meta-analysis. Int J Cancer. 2007;121(8):1813-20.

Chapter 22

Larynx and Hypopharynx Cancer

Jeffrey C Liu

> ***Chief Complaint***
> *"My voice has changed".*

ANATOMY AND FUNCTION

- The larynx has many functions, including generating noise for speech, directing food/liquids/saliva into the esophagus, and directing air into the trachea. Prevention of aspiration is a major laryngeal function.
- The larynx is anatomically divided into three areas—the subglottis, glottis, and supraglottis. The three main cartilages are the cricoid, hyoid, and thyroid cartilages (Fig. 22.1).
- Broyle's tendon is the anterior attachment of the vocal ligament to the inner perichondrium of the thyroid. It consists of the vocal ligament, conus elasticus, thyroarytenoid ligament, and thyroid perichondrium.
- Paraglottic space—contiguous with pre-epiglottic space. Superior border: quadrangular membrane; inferior border—conus elasticus; lateral border: inner surface of the thyroid cartilage; medial border: ventricle.
- Pre-epiglottic space—superior border: hyoepiglottic ligament; anterior border: thyrohyoid membrane and

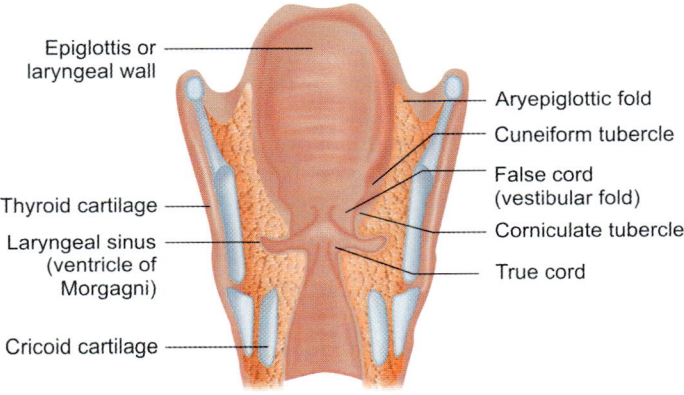

Fig. 22.1: The larynx.

    ligament; posterior border: anterior surface of the epiglottis and thyroepiglottic ligament.

- Hypopharynx—space behind the larynx. It is divided into four subsites: two piriform sinuses, postcricoid area, and posterior pharyngeal wall.
- The true vocal cord is made of stratified squamous epithelium, not respiratory epithelium.
- Lymphatic drainage is highly variable to different parts of the larynx. In general, the supraglottic and subglottic structures are rich in lymphatics; therefore, bilateral lymph node stations, specifically levels II/III/IV, are at risk when tumors arise from these areas.
- Glottic lymphatic drainage is minimal. Hence, regional lymphatics are not routinely addressed when treating early glottic cancer.
- There are multiple barriers to cancer spread in the larynx, including the conus elasticus, quadrangular membrane, and Broyle's tendon.
- Vocal cord fixation is usually a sign of paraglottic space invasion or arytenoid involvement.

EPIDEMIOLOGY

- Larynx cancer develops in approximately 6.2/100,000 men, with 12,200 new cases per year (National Cancer Institute, 2013).
- Despite advances in treatment over the last 30 years, overall survival of larynx cancer has changed little.[1]
- Within larynx cancer, glottic cancer makes up 59% and supraglottic cancer makes up 40%. Subglottic primary cancer is rare at 1%.
- Second primary cancers after larynx cancer arise in up to 20% of patients.
- This chapter is primarily about squamous cell carcinoma (SCC). Other pathologies exist that may have different management.

STAGING

- For up-to-date staging, please refer to the latest American Joint Committee on Cancer (AJCC) staging guidelines.
- Staging is divided into supraglottic, glottic, and subglottic subsites.
- The supraglottis is divided into five major subsites—false vocal cords, arytenoids, suprahyoid epiglottis, infrahyoid epiglottis, and aryepiglottic folds.
- Staging is structured by vocal cord function or extent of subsite involvement (supraglottis) or findings on radiographic imaging.
- For example, vocal cord fixation (functional) and pre-epiglottic space involvement (radiographic) are both indications for T3 stage.
- Extralaryngeal spread is the definition of T4. T4a tumors are conventionally resectable, but T4b are not conventionally resectable.
- Structures that are not conventionally resectable—prevertebral space, carotid artery, and mediastinal structures.

- Hypopharynx staging is by subsite involvement or size, resectability or extension.
- Nodal staging is the same for major head and neck cancer sites.

TREATMENT

Early Laryngeal Cancer

- Early laryngeal cancer: Defined as stage I/II. This means T1 or T2 tumors with N0 neck status.
- Single modality treatment with surgery or radiation alone is appropriate.

Early Glottic Cancer

- Early glottic cancer can be addressed either with primary radiation therapy or with primary surgery.
- Primary surgery may use the CO_2 laser (endoscopic) or cold knife. Open partial laryngectomy for early glottic cancers has largely fallen out of favor.
- As regional lymphatic spread is rare, these are not routinely addressed in oncologic management of early glottic cancer.
- Radiation strategy is usually with parallel opposing lateral portals.
- Both surgery and primary radiation have similar local control rates and rates of success.
- The 5-year local control for T1 with radiation is 93–94%.[2] For T1a treated with surgery, reports of 95% disease control.[3]
- Note, however, that surgical case outcomes are subject to selection bias.
- Voice outcomes have not favored one treatment modality over another.[4]

Supraglottic Cancer

- Supraglottic cancer can be addressed either with primary radiation therapy or with primary surgery.

- Bilateral regional lymphatic spread is a risk even for T1 tumors. Therefore, lymphatics must be addressed.
- Primary surgery is usually with the CO_2 laser (endoscopic). Open partial procedures have largely fallen out of favor. Bilateral neck dissection is considered for pathologic staging of lymphatics.
- Primary radiation therapy (RT) will include bilateral neck irradiation as well as addressing the primary lesion.
- A review of transoral laser endoscopic surgery of glottic/supraglottic cancers is beyond the scope of this chapter.

Advanced Laryngeal Cancer

- For advanced larynx cancer, multimodality therapy is favored for treatment. Advanced larynx cancer includes any T with N+ disease, or any T3/T4 disease regardless of N stage.
- Optimal management of advanced larynx cancer is a dense topic and an exhaustive review is beyond the scope of this chapter.
- All of the following treatment modalities have been explored in the literature for treatment of advanced larynx cancer: surgery with adjuvant (adj) RT, surgery with adj RT/chemo, induction chemo then RT alone, induction chemo then surgery with adj RT, induction chemo then chemo/RT, concomitant radiation and chemotherapy.
- Surgery in advanced larynx cancer can be endoscopic resection, or partial laryngectomy, or total laryngectomy.
- The options for partial laryngectomy techniques, either open or endoscopic, versus total laryngectomy are dependent on many factors. These include tumor-related factors such as location of tumor, patient-related factors such as lung function, and surgeon-related factors such as comfort and expertise with minimally invasive techniques.
- For a clearer delineation of choices of therapy, see National Comprehensive Cancer Network (NCCN) guidelines.
- Chemotherapy agents used in treatment of larynx cancer include cisplatin, carboplatin, taxol, and cetuximab.

- As a general rule, chemoradiation therapy for advanced larynx cancer uses cisplatin given at the same time as definitive RT. Concomitant chemoradiation is generally considered first-line nonsurgical management of advanced larynx cancer.
- As a general rule, total laryngectomy is recommended for significantly advanced T cancer (T4a) or for salvage after chemoradiation.

MAJOR TRIALS IN ADVANCED LARYNX CANCER

- *VA larynx trial*—a randomized control trial of advanced larynx cancer that examined two arms: either total laryngectomy with radiation or induction chemotherapy followed by definitive RT. Definitive therapy was chosen by response to induction chemotherapy. If patients had a partial or complete response after induction chemotherapy, they completed another cycle of chemotherapy and continued with definitive RT. Nonresponders went to immediate laryngectomy and RT.[5]
- There was no use of concomitant chemotherapy in this trial.
- About 65% of tumors were T3 tumors and were the most common tumor stage represented.
- Overall survival was the same in all arms.
- More than a third of chemotherapy patients still went on to total laryngectomy.
- *RTOG 91-11* trial was a randomized control trial of treatment of advanced larynx cancer. The three arms were induction chemotherapy followed by RT, RT alone, or concomitant chemoradiation therapy.[6]
- There was no surgical arm in the study.
- Larynx preservation was the primary study endpoint.
- The addition of chemotherapy increased treatment toxicity, primarily mucositis.
- Concurrent chemoradiation had the highest locoregional control.
- Overall survival was the same in all three arms.
- All 10-year data are now available for this study.[7]

VOICE REHABILITATION AFTER TOTAL LARYNGECTOMY

- There are three major approaches to voice rehabilitation after total laryngectomy: esophageal speech, electrolarynx usage, tracheoesophageal puncture (TEP).
- The air-insufflation test is used to evaluate candidacy for TEP. It is a functional test that looks at neopharyngeal function to determine whether TEP placement will be successful. It involves connecting a conduit, in the form of a catheter, from the tracheostoma, through the nose, and into the neopharynx/esophagus. The goal is to insufflate the neopharynx/esophagus at the level of TEP placement to look for phonation.
- The results are affected by many factors, including type or closure (primary vs flap), residual pharyngeal function, and whether a cricopharyngeal myotomy has been performed at the time of surgery. In general, unsuccessful production of voice is usually due to cricopharyngeal spasm. If lidocaine injection into the cricopharyngeus is successful at generating voice, this usually confirms cricopharyngeal spasm as the cause.

OTHER LARYNGEAL PATHOLOGIES

- The vast majority of larynx cancer focuses on management and treatment of SCC and is the focus of this chapter.
- Cartilage tumors are rarely seen in the larynx. Pathological differentiation of chondroma versus chondrosarcoma on biopsy can be difficult. Appropriate treatment should weigh the morbidity of resection, sometimes requiring total laryngectomy, against the risk of observation.
- Primary lesions of the cricoid can have a broad differential diagnosis, from SCC to salivary tumors to sarcoma. In general, it is difficult to resect these lesions and maintain the larynx. Single institutions have noted some success

with select patients.[8] Total laryngectomy is the conservative management when cricoid resection is necessary.

- Minor salivary gland tumors are occasionally seen in the larynx, such as adenoid cystic carcinoma and mucoepidermoid carcinoma. Resection with negative margins is the recommended approach, with adjuvant radiation as appropriate.
- Small cell neuroendocrine carcinoma is a rare and distinct tumor of the larynx. Total laryngectomy has not usually been successful at control, even with complete resection. Concomitant chemoradiation is the recommended modality for treatment.[9]

REFERENCES

1. Cosetti M, Yu GP, Schantz SP. Five-year survival rates and time trends of laryngeal cancer in the US population. Arch Otolaryngol Head Neck Surg. 2008;134(4):370-9.

2. Chera BS, Amdur RJ, Morris CG, et al. T1N0 to T2N0 squamous cell carcinoma of the glottic larynx treated with definitive radiotherapy. Int J Radiat Oncol Biol Phys. 2010;78(2):461-6.

3. Pradhan SA, Pai PS, Neeli SI, et al. Transoral laser surgery for early glottic cancers. Arch Otolaryngol Head Neck Surg. 2003;129(6):623-5.

4. Spielmann PM, Majumdar S, Morton RP. Quality of life and functional outcomes in the management of early glottic carcinoma: a systematic review of studies comparing radiotherapy and transoral laser microsurgery. Clin Otolaryngol. 2010;35(5):373-82.

5. Department of Veterans Affairs Laryngeal Cancer Study Group. Induction chemotherapy plus radiation compared with surgery plus radiation in patients with advanced laryngeal cancer. N Engl J Med. 1991;324(24):1685-90.

6. Forastiere AA, Goepfert H, Maor M, et al. Concurrent chemotherapy and radiotherapy for organ preservation in advanced laryngeal cancer. N Engl J Med. 2003;349(22):2091-8.

7. Forastiere AA, Zhang Q, Weber RS, et al., Long-term results of RTOG 91-11: a comparison of three nonsurgical treatment

strategies to preserve the larynx in patients with locally advanced larynx cancer. J Clin Oncol. 2013;31(7):845-52.

8. Zeitels SM, Burns JA, Wain JC, et al. Function preservation surgery in patients with chondrosarcoma of the cricoid cartilage. Ann Otol Rhinol Laryngol. 2011;120(9):603-7.

9. Ferlito A, Rinaldo A. Primary and secondary small cell neuroendocrine carcinoma of the larynx: a review. Head Neck. 2008;30(4):518-24.

Chapter 23

Skin Cancer

Jeffrey C Liu

INTRODUCTION

Skin cancer is the most common malignancy in humans. It is separated into two broad categories: melanoma and non-melanoma skin cancer (NMSC). Non-melanoma skin cancer includes multiple pathologies, including basal cell carcinoma (BCC), squamous cell carcinoma (SCC), and uncommon pathologies such as Merkel cell carcinoma (MCC), dermatofibrosarcoma protuberans, and microcystic adnexal carcinoma. This chapter is separated into melanoma and NMSC, with a primary focus on BCC and MCC.

NON-MELANOMA SKIN CANCER

Epidemiology

1. Skin cancer is the most common cancer.
2. About one million new cases a year; 10,000 patients die.
3. Basal cell carcinoma is the most common skin cancer, with about 33–39% of all Whites developing BCC at some point.
4. About 80% of NMSC are BCC and 16% are SCC.
5. Sun exposure—UV exposure is a major risk factor:
    a. Three time the rate of NMSC in Hawaii versus Midwest (Minnesota).

  b. Australians are particularly at high risk due to a combination of fair skin and significant sun exposure.

  c. Age is a surrogate for sun exposure: 55- to 70-year-old have 100 times the skin cancer risk of 20-year-old.

  d. Arsenic, tar, coal, paraffin, radiation are other exposure risk factors.

Staging

Please refer to American Joint Committee on Cancer (AJCC) staging manual for latest staging system. T stage is primarily defined by lesion size or invasion of critical structures in advanced T stage. Depth of invasion is currently not in the AJCC staging system for NMSC.

Basal Cell Carcinoma

Epidemiology

1. About 70% of BCC are in the head and neck and 25% on the trunk.
2. Median age at diagnosis is approximately 67 years.
3. Gorlin syndrome (basal cell nevus syndrome):
  a. It occurs between 1/57,000–256,000.
  b. Presentation of BCC, odontogenic keratocysts of jaw, palmoplantar pitting, skeletal abnormalities, and medulloblastoma.
  c. About 5% of patients have intellectual deficits.
  d. Autosomal dominant PTCH1 gene.

Subtypes

1. Nodular BCC ("pearly white telangiectasias") is the most common subtype.
2. Superficial (10%) is frequently on trunk and flatter, resembling eczema and slow growing.
3. Morpheaform (5%) is aggressive with ill-defined borders.

4. Morpheaform, micronodular, and infiltrative subtypes have indistinct borders with frequent incomplete resection—33–39%.
5. Basal cell carcinoma metastases are rare. Metastases are seen in 0.0028–0.1% of all cases.

Basic Science and Translational

Sonic hedgehog (SHH) pathway, including patched (PTCH) and smoothened, is now implicated in carcinogenesis. These genes were originally described in *Drosophila* patterning studies. Vismodegib is an SHH inhibitor now Food and Drug Administration approved for advanced BCC.[1]

Multiple strategies are available for treatment of BCC based on tumor size, location; see below for treatment options.

Cutaneous Squamous Cell Carcinoma

Epidemiology

1. About 200,000–300,000 new cases per year; 2,000 deaths per year.
2. *Risk factors*: In addition to the aforementioned risk factors of sun and chemicals, immunosuppression is a major risk factor.
3. Renal transplant patients have reported to have 18–36 times the risk for cutaneous squamous cell carcinoma (cSCC).
4. About 50% of skin cancers in organ transplant are cSCCs, whereas most NMSCs are usually BCC in immunocompetent patients.

cSCC Subtypes

1. These are graded as well, moderate, or poorly differentiated.
2. Verrucous—low grade and pushing borders.
3. Desmoplastic SCC—high-risk subtype. They have 10 times the local recurrence rate and 6 times the metastatic rate.

Defined High-Risk Features

1. Depth of invasion is >2 mm in thickness.
2. Invasion to Clark levels IV and V.
3. Perineural invasion.
4. Primary site is the ear or non-hair bearing lip.
5. Poorly differentiated or undifferentiated pathology.

Cutaneous Metastasis

1. Cutaneous metastasis is uncommon and occurs in about 5% of cSCC.
2. At-risk lymph nodes defined by cSCC primary site:
   a. Anterior to a vertical line through the external auditory canal: Parotid, neck levels II/III/IV at highest risk.
   b. Posterior to a vertical line through the external auditory canal: Occipital lymph nodes, neck levels II/III/IV/Va at highest risk.
   c. External jugular lymph node also at risk with cSCC.

Staging

1. Refer to AJCC NMSC staging system and the AJCC manual for latest staging.
2. Parotid basins are not formally in the AJCC staging system.
3. Depth of invasion is not in the staging, but > 2-mm thickness is considered high risk.
4. Nodal metastasis is a poor prognostic feature.

Treatment

There are multiple strategies for treatment of NMSC. The following are all accepted treatment strategies for appropriately sized lesions, with desiccation/curettage and topical therapy more commonly used in dermatologic practices.

1. Topical chemotherapy (5-fluorouracil cream)
2. Electrodesiccation and curettage
3. Photodynamic therapy

4. Surgical excision comes in two forms—Mohs surgery and standard surgical excision.

Mohs Surgery

Technique:
1. Mohs surgery creates a three-dimensional tumor map and all margins are examined.
2. Excision of main specimen is first done with 1- to 3-mm margins.
3. Prior to complete removal, wound edges are marked.
4. Specimen is divided, different sections are color-coded, and frozen sections are obtained for the entire margin.
5. The surgeon analyzes slides and identifies areas of residual tumor.
6. Additional excision, color-coding, and frozen sections are performed.
7. Tumor is excised in stages. It proceeds until negative margins are achieved.

Advantages:
1. All tumor margins are examined.
2. The procedure minimizes the loss of normal tissue.
3. It can be performed on an outpatient basis under local anesthesia.

Disadvantages:
1. This procedure is technically difficult for larger lesions.
2. It can take significant time due to multiple stages and frozen sections.
3. Specialized expertise is required for excision, orientation, and pathology slide interpretation.
4. Mohs surgery is primarily limited to BCC and SCC. It is difficult to perform on melanoma and other high-risk pathologies due to difficult interpretation of slides and lack of immunostaining of margins.

Outcomes:
1. Outcomes are highly favorable.

2. Leibovitch et al. compiled a 10-year history of Mohs surgery for cSCC. In 1,263 patients 61% were primary, 39% were recurrent, and 96.5% were head and neck. There was a 3.9% recurrence rate (15/381) after 5-year follow-up.[2]

Surgical Excision

1. En bloc excision.
2. Surgical excision with frozen section margins.
3. Depth of resection must be carefully considered preoperatively. Imaging is done as needed.
4. National Comprehensive Cancer Network (NCCN) 4–6-mm margin for low-risk lesions, 1-cm margin for high-risk lesions:
   a. High risk: >1-cm or >6-mm mask distribution, high grade, Clark's IV/V invasion, high-risk areas—scalp, eyelid, ears, nose, and lips.
5. Management of the neck:
   a. If nodes are positive, therapeutic lymphadenectomy or parotidectomy as appropriate.
   b. If nodes are at high risk, consider sentinel lymph node biopsy.
   c. Limited data on prophylactic neck dissection are available.
6. Adjuvant radiation is recommended for high-risk lesions, including the following:
   a. Bone invasion.
   b. Perineural invasion.
   c. Poorly differentiated SCC.
   d. Nodal metastasis.
   e. The role of adjuvant chemoradiation in cSCC has not been examined.

Outcomes (SCC):
1. Primary site cSCC recurrence rate is ~8% over 5 years.[3]
2. Depth of invasion associated with SCC recurrence and metastasis:[4]
   a. <2-mm thickness: 0.5% local recurrence, 1.9% metastasis.

    b. 2- to 6-mm thickness: 2.5% local recurrence, 4% metastasis.

    c. >6-mm thickness: 12.2% local recurrence, 16% metastasis.

Radiation alone:

1. This modality is generally reserved for poor-risk patients, palliative therapy, or unresectable lesions.
2. It has clinical efficacy against SCC and BCC, and can achieve cure.
3. Surgery is superior to radiation.

MALIGNANT MELANOMA (MM)

Epidemiology

1. While only 68,000 cases per year, as opposed to over 1 million NMSC cases, MM accounts for 75% of skin cancer deaths.
2. It is increasing in prevalence.
3. About 20% of MMs arise in the head and neck.
4. Risk factors:
   a. Acute, intense, intermittent sunburns are associated with an 80% increased risk of melanoma.[5]
   b. Immunosuppression.
   c. About 10% of MMs are hereditary syndrome.
   d. *Race*: Blacks have 1/20th the rate of melanoma as Whites.

Features and Subtypes

1. Asymmetry—one half is not like the other.
2. Borders irregular—scalloped, blending edges.
3. Color variegation—red, green, blue, black, and white.
4. Diameter—> 6 mm.
5. Elevation—elevation bad, flat better.
6. Superficial spreading:
   a. Most common (70%).
   b. Flat radial growth phase, 5–7 years.
7. Nodular:
   a. Constitute 15% of all MMs.
   b. Short radial growth phase, early vertical growth.

    c. Acral lentiginous.

    d. About 2–8%, palms, soles, nail beds.

    e. Equal among Whites/Blacks.

    f. Aggressive, early vertical growth.

8. Lentigo maligna:

    a. 10%, prolonged radial growth—10 years.

    b. Arises from premalignant areas, also known as Hutchinson freckle.

    c. Proclivity for the dermal–epidermal junction and tends to follow hair follicles.

    d. About 5% risk of transformation to invasive MM.

9. Desmoplastic:

    a. Low incidence.

    b. Amelanotic 5%.

    c. Associated with perineural invasion.

10. Mucosal:

    a. 2%, poorer prognosis.

Pathology and Staging

1. Clark level—histological stages I–V:

    a. Level I: Epidermis only, not invasive (in situ).

    b. Level II: Papillary dermis only.

    c. Level III: Expands in papillary dermis but does not enter reticular dermis.

    d. Level IV: Extends to reticular dermis.

    e. Level V: Extends to subcutaneous tissue.

2. Breslow thickness:

    a. Based on maximum vertical dimension.

    b. Refer to AJCC staging. Note that there was a change in Breslow thickness staging between 6th and 7th AJCC editions.

3. Seventh AJCC edition incorporates Breslow thickness (rather than Clark level), mitotic rate, and ulceration in staging.

4. Clark level and Breslow thickness vary by site. For example, an ear melanoma and a scalp melanoma with the same Breslow thickness may have very different Clark levels.

5. Nodal staging dependent on number of lymph nodes and micro/macrometastasis status:
   a. *Micrometastasis*: Metastases only seen on microscopic evaluation of lymph nodes.
   b. *Macrometastasis*: Clinically detectable nodal metastases.
   c. *Satellite metastasis*: Intralymphatic metastasis within 2 cm of the primary lesion.
   d. *In-transit metastasis*: Intralymphatic metastasis outside 2 cm from the primary melanoma, but not in the first echelon lymph node.
6. M staging dependent on the site of metastasis.

Treatment

1. Surgery typically used for stage I–III disease.
2. Primary management:
   a. Wide local excision with negative margins.
   b. In an intergroup melanoma trial, 2-cm versus 4-cm margins showed no difference.
   c. *NCCN recommendation*: 1 mm for in situ, 1 cm for <2 mm depth, 2 cm for 2–4 mm depth, and >2 cm for >4 mm depth of invasion.
3. Nodal management:
   a. Sentinel lymph node biopsy (SLNBx) recommended for T2 or higher primary lesions or high-risk T1 lesions (ulceration, Clark level IV or greater, high mitotic rate) for N0 neck evaluation.
   b. Sentinel lymph node biopsy is a diagnostic procedure. It identifies high-risk patients for potentially further treatment but does not treat the patient.
   c. Lymphadenectomy is generally recommended following positive SLNBx, although this remains under investigation.
   d. Therapeutic lymphadenectomy is generally recommended for N+, M0 patients. Radiation may be considered as adjuvant treatment.

4. Metastatic melanoma:
    a. Currently under significant investigation due to new agents with clinical efficacy.
    b. Ipilimumab: Anti-CTLA4 antibody.
    c. Pembrolizumab: Anti-PD1 antibody.
    d. Vemurafenib: Small molecular inhibitor in V600E BRAF mutation positive tumors.

REFERENCES

1. Iwasaki JK, Srivastava D, Moy RL, et al. The molecular genetics underlying basal cell carcinoma pathogenesis and links to targeted therapeutics. J Am Acad Dermatol. 2012;66(5):e167-78.
2. Leibovitch I, Huilgol SC, Selva D, et al. Basal cell carcinoma treated with Mohs surgery in Australia I. Experience over 10 years. J Am Acad Dermatol. 2005;53(3):445-51.
3. Rowe DE, Carroll RJ, Day CL, Jr. Prognostic factors for local recurrence, metastasis, and survival rates in squamous cell carcinoma of the skin, ear, and lip. Implications for treatment modality selection. J Am Acad Dermatol. 1992;26(6):976-90.
4. Brantsch KD, Meisner C, Schönfisch B, et al. Analysis of risk factors determining prognosis of cutaneous squamous-cell carcinoma: a prospective study. Lancet Oncol. 2008;9(8):713-20.
5. Wu S, Han J, Laden F, et al. Long-term ultraviolet flux, other potential risk factors, and skin cancer risk: a cohort study. Cancer Epidemiol Biomarkers Prev. 2014;23(6):1080-9.

Chapter 24

Nasopharynx Cancer

Jeffrey C Liu

DEMOGRAPHICS
- Incidence of cancer varies widely with geography.
- United States/North America: <1/100,000.
- North Africa and Greenland: 3–8/100,000.
- Southeast China and Indonesia: 25–80/100,000.
- Highest incidence is among Eskimos and Southeast Asian Chinese.

HISTOLOGY
- World Health Organization's Classification of nasopharynx squamous cell carcinoma (SCC):
    - *Class I*: Well differentiated, keratinizing.
    - *Class II*: Nonkeratinizing.
    - *Class III*: Undifferentiated, also known as lymphoepithelioma.
    - *Class I/II*: Usually tobacco/alcohol abuse associated; Class III: Epstein-Barr virus (EBV) associated.

EBV-ASSOCIATED NASOPHARYNX CANCER
- Certain at-risk populations to nasopharynx cancer (NPC) are thought to be due to EBV association.
- Centered on endemic regions such as Southeast Asia and North Africa.

- No clear gene or cluster of genes that are specifically thought to predispose to NPC.
- Thought to be interaction between endemic EBV strains and human leukocyte antigen alleles (environment and host factors, respectively).
- EBV associated is usually Class III NPC, undifferentiated aka lymphoepithelioma.
- Surveillance, Epidemiology, and End Results (SEER) data show the place of birth and race matter in development of NPC. In the United States, most patients are keratinizing or nonkeratinizing due to tobacco and alcohol as causative agents.[1]

RELEVANT NASOPHARYNX ANATOMY (FIG. 24.1) AND PATTERNS OF SPREAD

- Nasopharynx boundaries:
  - *Superior*: Basisphenoid and clivus.
  - *Posteriorly*: Retropharyngeal and prevertebral space.

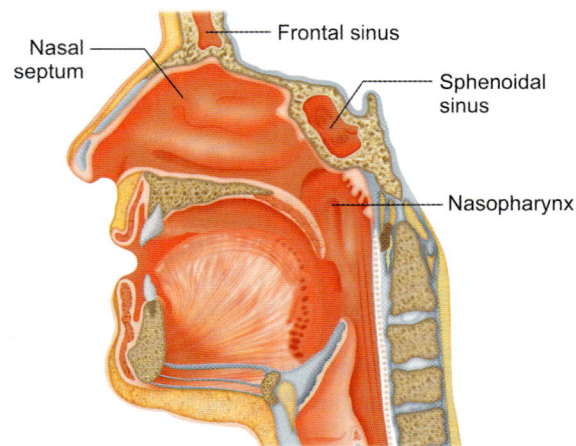

Fig. 24.1: Nasopharynx anatomy.

- – *Anteriorly*: Nasal choanae.
- – *Laterally*: Parapharyngeal space.
- Direct extension patterns of NPC:[2]
  - – *Anterior*: Into choanae; into pterygopalatine fossa via sphenopalatine foramen; from there into V2, inferior orbital fissure, vidian canal.
  - – *Lateral*: Through pharyngobasilar fascia (or via sinus of Morgagni) into parapharyngeal space; directly into V3 in infratemporal fossa.
  - – *Posterior*: Retropharyngeal space, prevertebral space.
  - – *Superior*: Into the clivus; through foramen lacerum or ovale into cranial cavity.
  - – *Inferior*: Into oropharynx.
- Nodal patterns of spread of NPC:
  - – Retropharyngeal nodes are often involved first, also known as nodes of Rouviere.
  - – 75% have cervical lymph node involvement at presentation.
  - – Jugulodigastric lymph nodes and level Vb are common metastatic sites.
- Distant metastasis:
  - – Slightly different pattern and frequency compared with other mucosal SCC.
  - – From 5–41% depending on the literature and treatment.
  - – Supraclavicular lymphadenopathy poses greater risk of metastasis.
  - – Metastases: Bone (20%), lung (13%), and liver (9%).

STAGING

- Staging for NPC is different from other head and neck subsites.
- Unlike other head and neck cancers, N1 and N2 diseases can be stage II.
- Primary staging (Table 24.1):
  - – *T1*: Tumor confined to the nasopharynx or tumor extends to oropharynx and/or nasal cavity without

Table 24.1: Staging of nasopharynx cancer.

Stage	T	N	M
0	Tis	N0	M0
I	T1	N0	M0
II	T1	N1	M0
	T2	N1	M0
	T2	N1	M0
III	T1	N2	M0
	T2	N2	M0
	T3	N0	M0
	T3	N1	M0
	T3	N2	M0
IVA	T4	N0	M0
	T4	N1	M0
	T4	N2	M0
IVB	T Any	N3	M0
IVC	T Any	N Any	M1

parapharyngeal extension (e.g. without posterolateral infiltration of tumor).

– *T2*: Tumor with parapharyngeal extension (posterolateral infiltration of tumor).

– *T3*: Tumor involving bony structures of skull base and/or paranasal sinuses.

– *T4*: Tumor with intracranial extension and/or involvement of cranial nerves, hypopharynx, or orbit, or with extension to the infratemporal fossa/masticator space.

– Nodal staging is also different from all other head and neck subsites.

– *NX*: Regional nodes cannot be assessed.

– *N0*: No regional lymph node metastasis.

– *N1*: Unilateral metastasis in cervical lymph nodes ≤6 cm in greatest dimension, above the supraclavicular fossa, and/or unilateral or bilateral retropharyngeal lymph nodes ≤6 cm in greatest dimension (midline nodes are considered ipsilateral nodes).

- *N2*: Bilateral metastasis in cervical lymph nodes ≤6 cm in greatest dimension, above the supraclavicular fossa (midline nodes are considered ipsilateral nodes).
- *N3*: Metastasis in a lymph node >6 cm and/or to the supraclavicular fossa (midline nodes are considered ipsilateral nodes).
- *N3a*: Metastasis in a lymph node >6 cm in dimension.
- *N3b*: Extension to the supraclavicular fossa.

Tumor stage for TNM is different than head and neck subsites.

TREATMENT

- Radiation alone is indicated for stage I tumors.
- Chemoradiation therapy is indicated for all stage II and higher diseases without distant metastasis.
- Chemotherapy, usually cisplatin, is given concomitantly with radiation. In addition, cisplatin and 5-fluorouracil (5FU) are often given following concomitant chemotherapy. This is commonly referred to as "adjuvant," "piggyback," or "outback" chemotherapy.

INTERGROUP 99 TRIAL[3]

- Major randomized trial in head and neck demonstrating benefit of chemotherapy with radiation therapy (RT) for NPC.
- Randomized trial of radiation alone versus cisplatin + RT and adjuvant cisplatin/5FU.
- Three-year actuarial progression-free survival rates were 24% versus 69% ($p < 0.001$).
- Three-year actuarial overall survival was 47% versus 78% ($p < 0.005$).
- The trial was terminated early due to significant benefit of chemotherapy arm over RT.
- Summary: The addition of chemotherapy to radiation therapy for NPC offers significant benefit.
- The role of adjuvant chemotherapy after chemo/RT remains a controversy.

REFERENCES

1. Marks JE, Phillips JL, Menck HR. The National Cancer Data Base report on the relationship of race and national origin to the histology of nasopharyngeal carcinoma. Cancer. 1998;83(3):582-8.

2. Dubrulle F, Souillard R, Hermans R. Extension patterns of nasopharyngeal carcinoma. Eur Radiol. 2007;17(10):2622-30.

3. Al-Sarraf M, LeBlanc M, Giri PG, et al. Chemoradiotherapy versus radiotherapy in patients with advanced nasopharyngeal cancer: phase III randomized Intergroup study 0099. J Clin Oncol. 1998; 16(4):1310-7.

Chapter 25

Neck Dissection and Patterns of Metastasis

Jeffrey C Liu

ANATOMY (FIG. 25.1)

- There are seven total levels.
- Levels I–V are for lateral cervical lymph nodes.
- Levels VI and VII are central compartment and mediastinum, respectively.
- Levels I, II, and V have both A and B parts.
- Levels II–IV = anterior triangle.
- Level V = posterior triangle.
- Boundary between levels II and III is the hyoid.
- Boundary between levels III and IV is the cricoid (radiographic) or omohyoid (surgical).
- Boundary between levels IA and IB is the digastric muscle.
- Boundary between levels IIA and IIB is the spinal accessory nerve (CN XI).
- Boundary between levels VA and VB is the cricoid (radiographic) or CN XI (surgical).

Other Lymph Node Basins

Parotid Gland

- It has multiple lymph nodes.
- Lymph node basin at risk for anterior cutaneous malignancies.

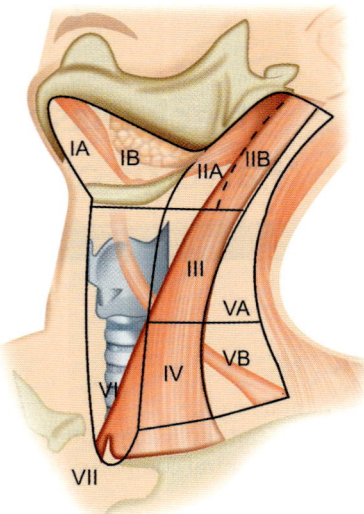

Fig. 25.1: Levels of the neck.

Suboccipital Basin

- Posterior cutaneous skin lesions.

PATTERNS OF NECK METASTASIS

Patterns of neck metastasis depend on lymphatic drainage of primary site.

Oral Cavity

- Supraomohyoid: Neck levels I–III.
- Ipsilateral, except midline structures where bilateral lymph nodes are at risk.

Oropharynx, Larynx, Hypopharynx

- Neck levels II–IV.
- Supraglottis and subglottis are bilateral risk.
- Base of tongue is bilateral risk. Tonsil is primarily unilateral risk.
- Medial piriform sinus has increased contralateral risk.[1]

Nasopharynx

- Bilateral levels II–V, supraclavicular.
- Posterior triangle is specifically at risk.

Cutaneous Squamous Cell Carcinoma (SCC)[2]

- Lymph node metastasis is rare—about 5%.
- Anterior to external auditory canal (EAC): Parotid, II–IV.
- Posterior to EAC: Occipital, II–IV (Va).
- External jugular node is at risk for cutaneous lesions.

Thyroid Cancer

- Level VI is usually primary drainage basin.
- May also drain to levels II–V, supraclavicular as first echelon.
- Very rarely to level I.

TYPES OF NECK DISSECTION

Supraomohyoid

- *Levels I–III*: Above omohyoid muscle.
- It is used for oral cavity.
- *Modified radical neck dissection*: Preservation of one or more of the three major structures.
- *Major structures*: Spinal accessory nerve, sternocleido-mastoid, and internal jugular vein.
- *Type I*: Only one structure is preserved.
- *Type II*: Two structures are preserved.
- *Type III*: All three structures are preserved.
- Levels II–V (and sometimes I).

Selective Neck Dissection

- Only specific neck levels are addressed.

Radical Neck Dissection

- Sacrifice of internal jugular vein, spinal accessory nerve, sternocleidomastoid muscle.
- Levels II–V (and sometimes I).

WHEN TO DO NECK DISSECTION

- Neck dissection may be performed as an isolated procedure, such as treatment for recurrent disease in the neck.
- It may be performed as part of a complex procedure, such as addressing regional lymphatics in glossectomy or laryngectomy.
- Elective (N0) versus staging (N0) versus therapeutic neck dissection (N+).
  - *Elective neck dissection*: Removal of lymph nodes performed when lymph nodes are considered to be at risk without evidence of metastasis. Elective implies it is performed at the discretion of the surgeon, e.g. neck dissection in a small parotid cancer.
  - *Staging neck dissection*: Removal of lymph nodes performed as part of pathological staging of lymph nodes where lymph nodes are considered to be high risk; usually a stronger indication than elective neck dissection, e.g. neck dissection in a high-risk oral cancer without evidence of neck disease.
  - *Therapeutic neck dissection*: Removal of lymph nodes performed as part of treatment of node positive disease. It is often followed by adjuvant radiation.
  - *Salvage neck dissection*: Removal of lymph nodes following initial treatment of a head and neck cancer now with suspected or proven persistent disease, e.g. when performing a neck dissection for an advanced tonsil

cancer initially treated with chemoradiation, and now with a persistent neck mass biopsy proven to be SCC.

- In the N0 neck, choice of observation versus elective neck dissection depends on tumor subsite and pathology. There is a need to weigh risks of metastasis versus morbidity. Addressed neck levels depend on drainage patterns.
- In the N+ neck, a therapeutic neck dissection is often performed, often followed by radiation.
- When patients are managed nonoperatively, e.g. chemo/radiation for an advanced larynx cancer, neck dissection may not be performed at all.

ROLE OF ADJUVANT RADIATION THERAPY IN NECK DISSECTION

- Generally advocated if positive nodes. The role of adjuvant radiation for pN1 neck disease remains somewhat controversial.
- Byers reviewed 967 neck dissection outcomes for clinically positive neck disease and noted significant benefit with adjuvant radiation therapy.[3]

NECK STAGING—ALL HEAD AND NECK SUBSITES EXCEPT NASOPHARYNX

- *N0*: No regional lymph node metastasis.
- *N1*: Metastasis in a single ipsilateral lymph node, ≤3 cm in greatest dimension.
- *N2a*: Metastasis in a single ipsilateral lymph node, >3 cm but ≤6 cm in greatest dimension.
- *N2b*: Metastasis in multiple ipsilateral lymph nodes, ≤6 cm in greatest dimension.
- *N2c*: Metastasis in bilateral or contralateral lymph nodes, ≤6 cm in greatest dimension.
- *N3*: Metastasis in a lymph node, >6 cm in greatest dimension.

REFERENCES

1. Johnson JT, Bacon GW, Myers EN, et al. Medial vs lateral wall pyriform sinus carcinoma: implications for management of regional lymphatics. Head Neck. 1994;16(5):401-5.

2. D'Souza J, Clark J. Management of the neck in metastatic cutaneous squamous cell carcinoma of the head and neck. Curr Opin Otolaryngol Head Neck Surg. 2011;19(2):99-105.

3. Byers RM. Modified neck dissection. A study of 967 cases from 1970 to 1980. Am J Surg. 1985;150 (4):414-21.

The Nose

Section Editor: Elina M Toskala

Chapter 26

Rhinitis

Samir Ketan Bhandutia, Elina M Toskala

> ***Chief Complaint***
> *"My nose is runny and I sneeze a lot".*

RHINITIS

Rhinitis is inflammation of the nasal lining. Symptoms can include nasal congestion, rhinorrhea, or sneezing. Rhinitis is diagnosed if the patient has two out of three symptoms that occur for over 2 weeks. This is divided, in general, into allergic (AR) and nonallergic (NAR) on the basis of skin testing for allergen-specific immunoglobulin E.

DEFINITIONS

Allergic rhinitis versus nonallergic rhinitis versus cerebrospinal fluid (CSF) rhinorrhea.

Allergic Rhinitis

Symptoms can include nasal congestion, rhinorrhea, nasal pruritus, postnasal drainage, anosmia, hyposmia, or ocular pruritus. Allergic rhinitis is very common in childhood in addition to being common in a positive family history. In the general population, AR prevalence varies between 10% and 30%. It is one of the most common complaints that patients have.

It can be due to seasonal allergens (grass, trees, pollen, and ragweed) or perennial allergies (insects, dust mites, and cats); see Figure 26.1.

Nonallergic Rhinitis

Symptoms can include nasal congestion, rhinorrhea, and posterior nasal drainage. Nonallergic rhinitis may be distinguished from AR by the consistent presence of symptoms and a lack of nasal or ocular pruritus. Possible triggers include

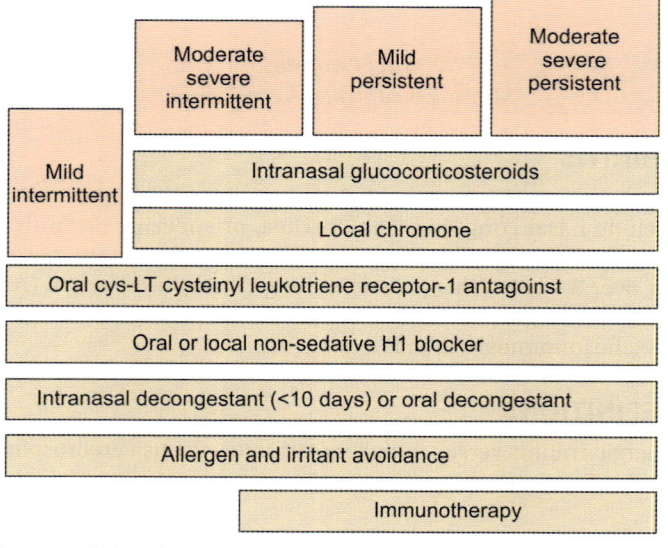

Fig. 26.1: Rhinorrhea. ARIA recommendations for treatment of allergic rhinitis.
Source: Reproduced with permission from Jurado-Palomo J, Bobolea ID, Belver Gonzalez MT, et al. Treatment of allergic rhinitis: anticholinergics, glucocorticotherapy, leukotriene antagonists, omalizumab and specific allergen immunotherapy. In: Gendeh BS (Ed). Otolaryngology. Rijeka, Croatia: Intech; 2012.

strong fragrances, cleaning products, cold air, or tobacco smoke. It can be divided in subgroups as discussed below.

Subclassifications

- *Infectious rhinitis*: Viral subtypes are most common and include rhinovirus, respiratory syncytial virus (RSV), parainfluenza virus, adenovirus, influenza virus, enterovirus; bacterial subtypes include diphtheria, pertussis, chlamydia, and syphilis.
- *Vasomotor rhinitis*: Parasympathetic system predominates, leading to vasodilation and mucosal edema. It occurs mainly in the elderly. Strong odors and cold air exacerbate symptoms, which include nasal obstruction and copious watery anterior rhinorrhea.
- *Hormonal rhinitis*: This is associated with hormonal imbalance (e.g. pregnancy and puberty).
- *Occupational rhinitis*: This is usually due to inhaled irritant such as cigarette smoke. Cessation from these stimuli results in control of symptoms. Occupational rhinitis can be allergic or nonallergic.
- *Drug-induced rhinitis*: Examples of this include angiotensin-converting enzyme inhibitors, beta-blockers, oral contraceptives, nonsteroidal anti-inflammatory drugs.
- *Rhinitis medicamentosa*: Tachyphylaxis associated with prolonged use of nasal sympathomimetic; rebound congestion can occur due to overuse of decongestants.
- *Gustatory rhinitis*: Rhinorrhea due to vasodilation after eating spicy or hot foods. Response is mediated by parasympathetic stimulation.
- *Nonallergic rhinitis of eosinophilia syndrome*: Rhinitis with approximately 10–20% eosinophils on nasal smears. Symptoms include nasal congestion, rhinorrhea, sneezing, pruritus, and hyposmia.
- *Atrophic rhinitis*: Mucosal colonization with *Klebsiella* and other organisms; patients often present with foul smell as well

as yellow or green nasal crusting with atrophy and fibrosis of mucosa.
- *Rhinitis of infancy*: Onset at birth or within first month of life; more common in fall and winter.

Cerebrospinal Fluid Rhinorrhea

Cerebrospinal fluid rhinorrhea may occur spontaneously or due to iatrogenic injury to the ethmoid roof during sinus surgery. Patients can present with watery rhinorrhea as well as a "halo sign," which is the fluid that is dropped onto gauze that separates into a clear outer ring with blood in the center. The drain can often be provoked by leaning the patient forward with the head lowered. Typically, the drainage has a salty or metallic taste. In order to test for CSF rhinorrhea, several modalities can be used such as computed tomography (CT), magnetic resonance imaging, radioactive pledget scan, or B-2 transferrin assay. For a known iatrogenic injury, CT with coronal view can verify the site of injury. Initial conservative management of CSF rhinorrhea includes bed rest, head elevation, and diuretic agents such as mannitol and furosemide. If drainage persists after 2–3 days, lumbar drain or surgical exploration may be considered. Surgical management is individualized as the skull base can be repaired with endoscopic instruments from below or via a neurosurgical approach from above.

ANATOMY AND PHYSIOLOGY OF OLFACTION

See Figure 26.2.

DIAGNOSTIC WORKUP

"My nose is runny and I sneeze a lot."

History

It is important to document the family and the personal history of atopy or allergies, medications, abnormal hormonal status, work environment, pregnancy, or use of smoking.

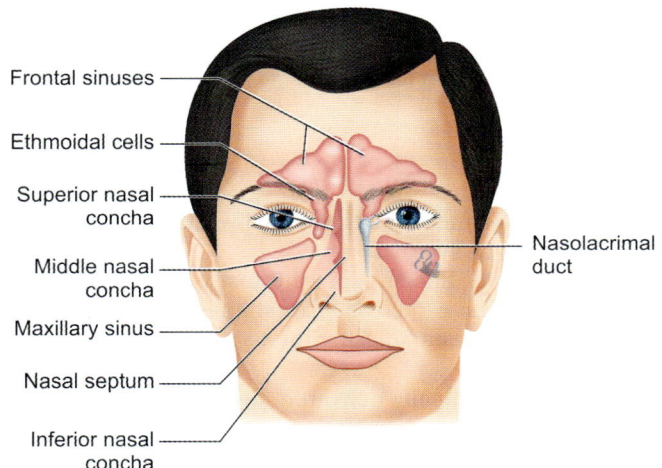

Frontal sinuses

Ethmoidal cells

Superior nasal concha

Middle nasal concha

Maxillary sinus

Nasal septum

Inferior nasal concha

Nasolacrimal duct

Fig. 26.2: Overview of sinuses and nasal cavity.
Source: Redrawn with permission from Chandra R, Patel Z. Sinus anatomy. American Rhinology Society. [online] Available from http://care.american-rhinologic.org/sinus_anatomy [Accessed March 2015].

Physical Examination

Diagnosis requires a full ear, nose, throat, head, and neck examination.

Ancillary Tools

- Skin prick allergy tests (tiny amounts of test substances are placed on the skin and a pin prick is made; a positive result leads to a small raised, red, itchy patch).
- Anterior rhinoscopy (examine for enlarged turbinates or nasal polyps).
- Nasal endoscopy (examine upper, middle, and lower meatus, for mucus or polyps).
- Radioallergosorbent (RAST) test (a blood test that indicates if patients are allergic to a range of test substances).

- Peak flow (many patients with rhinitis also have asthma and their peak flow may be reduced).
- Pulmonary function tests.

Management

Medical

- Irritating substances, allergens, cold weather, and offending foods should be avoided.
- *Anticholinergics*: Effective for watery vasomotor-type rhinitis.
- *Antihistamines*: Effective against sneezing, itching, and watery rhinorrhea in AR, not useful for symptoms of blockage.
- *Nasal steroids*: Ideally delivered topically to nasal mucosa using sprays or drops for AR.
- *Oral steroids*: These can be very effective but their systemic effects limit long-term use (ideal for important events such as examinations and weddings).
- *Nasal decongestants*: Only useful in short term at start of other therapy, since prolonged use can produce intractable rhinorrhea of rhinitis medicamentosa.
- *Sodium cromoglicate*: Mast cell stabilizer and useful for AR.

Surgical

- Surgery may be a useful adjunct to other treatments. It is worth obtaining a CT scan of paranasal sinuses if surgery is considered to review the need for sinus surgery.
- *Turbinate reduction*: Surgery may be effective in improving nasal obstruction, but additional medical therapy is needed to prevent recurrence of hypertrophied mucosa.
- *Septal surgery*: Deviated septum may need to be corrected to improve nasal function and help medication delivery.
- *Functional endoscopic sinus surgery*: This aims to remove blockage in critical area and restore the normal function and drainage of sinuses. It could benefit rhinitis patients with sinusitis who do not respond to medical treatments.

SUGGESTED READING

1. AAO HNSF (US)—American Academy of Otolaryngology—Head and Neck Surgery Foundation. Clinical Practice Guideline: Allergic Rhinitis. Alexandria, VA: The American Academy of Otolaryngology—Head and Neck Surgery Foundation; 2015. [online] Available from http://www.entnet.org/. Accessed May 22, 2015.
2. Bousquet J, Khaltaev N, Cruz AA, et al. Allergic Rhinitis and its Impact on Asthma (ARIA) 2008 Update (in collaboration with the World Health Organization, GA(2)LEN and AllerGen). Allergy. 2008;63(Suppl 86):8-160.
3. Hellings PW, Scadding G, Alobid I, et al. Executive summary of European Task Force document on diagnostic tools in rhinology. Rhinology. 2012;50(4):339-52.
4. Licari A, Ciprandi G, Marseglia A, et al. Current recommendations and emerging options for the treatment of allergic rhinitis. Expert Rev Clin Immunol. 2014;10(10):1337-47.

Chapter 27

Acute Sinusitis

Samir Ketan Bhandutia, Elina M Toskala

> ***Chief Complaint***
> *"I have postnasal drip and it is difficult to smell".*

ACUTE SINUSITIS

Sinusitis is a common inflammation of the nose and paranasal sinuses. It is caused by an acute bacterial infection that often develops after a preceding viral illness, such as a cold. Symptoms include nasal blockage, congestion, nasal discharge, facial pain, and hyposmia or anosmia. Acute sinusitis is diagnosed by the patient having two or more of the symptoms that last for <12 weeks with complete resolution.

Definitions

Acute viral rhinosinusitis versus acute bacterial rhinosinusitis versus acute fungal rhinosinusitis.

Acute Viral Rhinosinusitis

Rhinovirus and *Influenza* are the most common agents. Symptoms are self-limited and usually last for <14 days.

Acute Bacterial Rhinosinusitis

Haemophilus influenza, *Streptococcus pneumoniae*, and *Moraxella catarrhalis* are the most common agents.

Acute Fungal Rhinosinusitis

Bipolaris, *Curvularia*, *Exerohilium*, *Alternaria*, and *Aspergillus* are the most common agents.

Physiology/Pathophysiology of Olfaction

Effective sinus drainage occurs through the osteomeatal complex. Obstruction in this area due to anatomical or mucosal problems impairs sinus drainage and leads to obstructed air flow. Anatomic abnormalities may predispose one to acute sinusitis such as septal deviation and spur, turbinate hypertrophy, middle turbinate concha bullosa, prominent ethmoidal bulla, pneumatization, and inversion of uncinated process.

Diagnostic Workup

"I have postnasal drip and it is difficult to smell."

History

It is important to document nasal symptoms as well as any facial signs and symptoms.

Physical Examination

Diagnosis requires a full ear, nose, throat (ENT), head, and neck examination.

Ancillary Tools

- Anterior rhinoscopy.
- Nasal endoscopy shows the presence of pus in the middle meatus or edematous mucosa elsewhere in the nasal cavities.

Management

Medical

- Analgesics, decongestants, mucolytics, and saline irrigations are recommended.
- Empiric oral antibiotics (first line includes amoxicillin or amoxicillin/clavulanate for 10–14 days; penicillin-allergic

patients can receive macrolides or trimethoprim-sulfa-methoxazole [TMP-SFX].
- Switch to quinolones or high-dose amoxicillin/clavulanate if no improvement in 72 hours.
- Nasal corticosteroids have been shown to be effective.

Surgical
- Surgery is limited to patients with complications of sinusitis.

ORBITAL CELLULITIS AND ABSCESS

Orbital cellulitis can result as a complication of unresolved acute sinusitis and most commonly occurs in pediatric patients. Signs and symptoms can include orbital pain, edema, proptosis, difficulty with extraocular movements, and nasal discharge. Orbital abscess is a collection of pus in the orbital tissue. It may result in complete opthalmoplegia with severe visual impairment. Orbital cellulitis and abscess require immediate attention as both of these conditions can progress to blindness.

Chief Complaint

"My eye is swollen and it hurts to move."

Pathophysiology

Infection under pressure in the ethmoid sinus can traverse the thin bony plate of the medial orbital wall. This can lead to edema formation and abscess formation.

Definitions

Anatomically, the orbital is bounded by the paranasal sinuses and infection can spread to the orbit directly. Orbital cellulitis is classified according to the Chandler classification system.
- *Stage 1*: Preseptal cellulitis
- *Stage 2*: Orbital cellulitis

- *Stage 3*: Subperiosteal abscess
- *Stage 4*: Orbital abscess
- *Stage 5*: Cavernous sinus septic thrombosis

Diagnostic Workup

"My eye is swollen and it hurts to move."

History

It is important to document any nasal symptoms along with any facial signs or symptoms. Obtain a full history regarding the duration and location of eye pain.

Physical Examination

Diagnosis requires a full ENT, head, and neck examination.

Ancillary Tools

Contrast-enhanced computed tomographic (CT) scanning with coronal and axial views.

Management

- *Mild preseptal cellulitis*: Outpatient antibiotics (third-generation cephalosporins in children and older patients) are double covered with clindamycin for anaerobes; topical vasoconstrictors are useful (oxymetazoline); ensure that regular eye observations are performed.
- If symptoms persist, admit to hospital and obtain a coronal CT scan of the sinus and axial views through the orbits. Start intravenous (IV) antibiotics (e.g. Co-Amoxiclav) and topical decongestants.
- Obtain an ophthalmology consultation.
- Any compromise in visual acuity or intraorbital abscess requires urgent surgical intervention.
- Surgical exploration if no improvement with IV antibiotics.

SUGGESTED READING

1. AAO HNSF (US)—American Academy of Otolaryngology Head and Neck Surgery Foundation. Clinical Practice Guideline: Adult Sinusitis. Alexanfria, VA: American Academy of Otolaryngology Head and Neck Surgery Foundation; 2015. [online] Available from http://www.entnet.org/. Accessed May 22, 2015.
2. Fokkens WJ, Lund VJ, Mullol J, et al. European position paper on rhinosinusitis and nasal polyps 2012. Rhinol Suppl. 2012;50(23):3.

Chapter 28

Nasal Obstruction

Derrick Tint, Elina M Toskala

> ***Chief Complaint***
> *"My nose is blocked".*

OVERVIEW

Nasal obstruction is a nonspecific symptom that is caused by a mass, including various sinonasal tumors, both malignant and benign, and infectious/inflammatory processes that cause edema to the sinus mucosa and blockage of airflow through the nasal passages. This chapter will provide an overview of different benign sinonasal tumors and infectious processes that may cause a patient to experience nasal obstruction.

BENIGN SINONASAL TUMORS

Osteoma

Osteomas are the most common benign tumors of the sinonasal tract. They are usually slow-growing lesions that affect the frontal sinus most frequently and are found incidentally on radiographic imaging between the second and fifth decades of life. Osteomas can be associated with Gardner's syndrome (colon polyps, osteomas of the skull, and multiple soft tissue tumors).

Diagnosis

Osteomas are typically asymptomatic; however, they cause obstruction to sinus drainage pathways and can lead to acute sinusitis symptoms. Advanced lesions can cause compression to surround structures. They are rarely visualized on endoscopy because they are located in the sinus cavity. When visualized, they appear as a protrusion of bone in the nasal cavity with normal or thinned mucosal covering.

Imaging

Osteomas are usually found incidentally on computed tomographic (CT) imaging. Osteomasare well-circumscribed lesions. The density can be variable, from high density similar to that or cortical bone to low density with ground glass appearance.

Histology

Osteoma can be divided into three categories:
1. *Ivory or "eburnated" osteoma*: Lobulated, compact, dense bone, minimal fibrous tissue, no Haversian ducts.
2. *Mature osteoma/osteoma spongiosum*: Spongy, mature bone with bony trabeculae and copius fibrous tissue.
3. *Mixed osteoma*: It contains features of both ivory and mature osteomas.

Treatment

Treatment is based on symptoms. When asymptomatic and not close to any critical structures, these lesions are typically managed by observation with serial imaging. When the lesion is causing obstructive or compressive symptoms, surgical removal of the lesion is recommended.

Inverted Papilloma (Schneiderian Papilloma, Inverted Type)

Inverted papillomas are the second most common tumors of the sinonasal tract. They have a strong association with squamous cell carcinoma with a transformation rate between 4% and 10%. They are more commonly found in men and occur between the fifth and sixth decades of life.

Diagnosis

Symptoms of inverted papillomas are related to the size of the mass. Unilateral nasal obstruction and clear rhinorrhea are common for smaller lesions. Epiphora, proptosis, diplopia, and headache can signify more advanced lesions. On nasal endoscopy, they appear as pale, polypoid lesions protruding from the middle meatus. These lesions are most commonly located on the lateral nasal wall in the fontanelle area, followed by the maxillary sinus.

Imaging

- *Magnetic resonance imaging (MRI) with contrast*: Inverted papilloma has a characteristic cribriform/columnar pattern that reflects multilayered histology.
- *Computed tomography*: CT shows lesion with soft tissue density. Areas of focal hyperostosis and osteitic changes indicate the tumor origin.

Histology

Inverted papillomas are composed of hyperplastic ribbons of basement membrane and endophytic epithelium.

Treatment

Surgical removal is the treatment for this lesion. The goal is complete removal of the inverted papilloma and creation of a large marsupialized cavity for easy visualization due to high rate of residual tissue after surgery.

Endoscopic Techniques

1. *Type I resection*: Removal of the middle turbinate, superior turbinate ethmoids, and sphenoid sinus.

2. *Type II resection*: Medial maxillectomy, indicated for tumors extending into maxillary sinus and nasolacrimal duct.
3. *Type III resection (Sturman-Canfield operation)*: Removal of medial portion of anterior wall of maxillary sinus, for anterior involvement of maxillary sinus.

Juvenile Angiofibroma

Juvenile angiofibromas (JNAs) are benign sinonasal tumors that occur most frequently in young adolescent males and originate in the pterygopalatine fossa. They are thought to be a vascular anomaly that arises from a brachial artery with incomplete degeneration.

Diagnosis

Symptoms of JNA include unilateral nasal obstruction, epistaxis, and rhinorrhea. Advanced lesions may exhibit check swelling, proptosis, and headache. On endoscopy, they appear as smooth, hypervascularized lesions originating behind the middle turbinate. In-office biopsy is not recommended due to high risk of hemorrhage.

Imaging

Computed tomography or MRI characteristically shows tumor originating from the pterygopalatine fossa, hypervascular appearance on contrast enhancement, and anterior bowing of the posterior wall of the maxillary sinus (Holman-Miller sign).

Histology

Juvenile angiofibromas demonstrate vascular endothelium-lined spaces embedded in fibrous stroma.

Treatment

Surgical removal with either open or endoscopic approaches is the main treatment modality. Preoperative embolization has been used to reduce bleeding.

Lobular Capillary Hemangioma

Lobular capillary hemangiomas are another form of vascular anomaly that occur in the sinonasal tract. They occur in men and women equally and have a peak incidence in the fifth decade of life.

Diagnosis

Symptoms are usually unilateral nasal obstruction and epistaxis. On nasal endoscopy, these lesions appear as a red or purple mass that is usually < 1 cm in size.

Imaging

Computed tomographic scan shows a unilateral mass with soft tissue density. Magnetic resonance imaging shows a lesion that is hyperintense on T2 and hypointense on T1 with vivid contrast enhancement.

Histology

Definitive diagnosis is made on histologic examination. Histologic sectioning shows proliferation of capillaries arranged in lobules, separated by loose connective tissue stroma with inflammatory cell infiltration.

Treatment

Endoscopic surgical excision.

Fibro-osseous Lesions

Fibro-osseous lesions are a diverse group of lesions characterized by bone marrow that has been replaced by fibrous tissue and minerals. Ossifying fibroma and fibrous dysplasia are fibro-osseous lesions that occur within the sinonasal tract.

Ossifying Fibroma

Ossifying fibroma is a benign neoplasm that occurs during the third and fourth decades of life and more commonly affects

African American women. The psammomatoid variant affects men and is more locally aggressive. On histology, ossifying fibromas are characterized by islands of osteoid rimmed by osteoblast-forming lamellar bone. The stroma has parallel and whorled arrangements of collagen.

Imaging: Computed tomographic scan reveals a sharply circumscribed lesion with an eggshell rim and central radiolucency.

Treatment: Radical resection with either open or endoscopic approach.

Fibrous Dysplasia

Fibrous dysplasia is a developmental anomaly of bone-forming mesenchyme that leads to replacement of normal bone with immature bone. It occurs within the first two decades of life. There are three forms of fibrous dysplasia: monostotic, polyostotic, and disseminated (McCune-Albright syndrome).

Imaging: Computed tomographic scan shows a lesion in the paranasal sinus with hazy borders and homogeneous ground glass appearance.

Treatment: Surgical resection with intent to decompress and correct esthetic deformities rather than removal of the entire lesion.

INFECTIOUS/INFLAMMATORY CAUSES

Chronic Rhinosinusitis

Chronic rhinosinusitis (CRS): This is inflammation of the nasal and paranasal sinus mucosa for at least 12 weeks.

Acute Exacerbation of CRS (AECRS)

Intermittent flare-ups of symptoms in the context of chronic rhinosinusitis. It is characterized by increased mucus, purulence, congestion, and anosmia.

Pathophysiology

The pathophysiology of chronic rhinosinusitis is multifactorial, with any factor, not just limited to bacterial infections, that causes inflammation to the nose and sinuses as a possible inciting factor for CRS. A combination of host, microbial, and environmental factors all contributes to the pathophysiology of CRS (Flowchart 28.1).

Microorganisms

The organisms identified in patients with CRS differ significantly from patients with acute bacterial rhinosinusitis.

- *Chronic rhinosinusitis*: *Aureus*, coagulase-negative staphylococci, anaerobic, gram-negative bacteria, *Streptococcus pneumoniae,* and *Haemophilus influenzae* are the organisms that are commonly identified.
- *AECRS*: It increases in both aerobic organisms seen in ABRS and gram-negative and anaerobic organisms seen in CRS.

Flowchart 28.1: A combination of host, microbial, and environmental factors leading to inflammation.

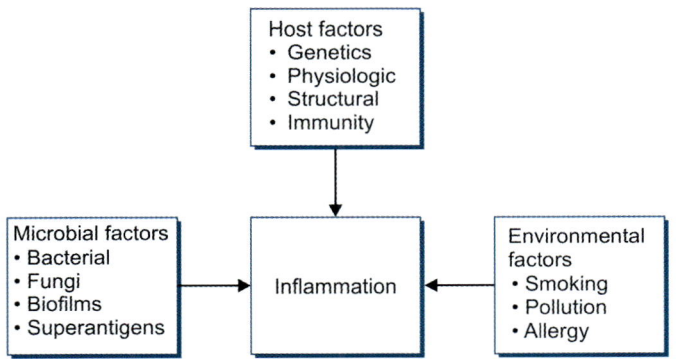

Source: Rosenfeld RM, Andes D, Bhattacharyya N, et al. Clinical practice guideline: adult sinusitis. Otolaryngol Head Neck Surg. 2007;137(3 Suppl):S1-31.

Diagnosis

The diagnosis of CRS according to the Clinical Practice Guidelines requires the presence of symptoms for at least 12 weeks as well as inflammation (Table 28.1).

Physical Examination

- *Anterior rhinoscopy*: Examination of mucosa for edema and inflammation, turbinates for hypertrophy, and the presence of purulence or polyps.
- *Nasal endoscopy*: Examination of the entire nasal cavity, under the inferior turbinate, medial and lateral to the middle turbinate; look for anatomic abnormalities, signs of inflammation, and purulence.

Table 28.1: Chronic and recurrent rhinosinusitis definitions.

Term	Definition
Chronic rhinosinusitis (CRS)	Twelve (12) weeks or longer of two or more of the following signs and symptoms: • Mucopurulent drainage (anterior, posterior, or both) • Nasal obstruction (congestion) • Facial pain-pressure-fullness, or • Decreased sense of smell AND inflammation is documented by one or more of the following findings: • Purulent (not clear) mucus or edema in the middle meatus of ethmoid region, • Polyps is nasal cavity or the middle meatus, and/or • Radiographic imaging showing inflammation of the paranasal sinuses
Recurrent acute rhinosinusitis	Four (4) or more episodes per year of ABRS without signs or symptoms of rhinosinusitis between episodes: • Each episode of ABRS should meet diagnostic criteria

Source: From Rosenfeld RM, Andes D, Bhattacharyya N, et al. Clinical practice guideline: adult sinusitis. Otolaryngol Head Neck Surg. 2007;137(3 Suppl):S1-31.

Imaging

- *Computed tomographic scan*: CT provides objective evidence for the diagnosis of CRS. It also provides excellent bony detail.
- *Magnetic resonance imaging*: A good adjunct to CT scan for soft tissue and fluid delineation, but inferior to CT for bony detail.

Culture

- *Endoscopic*: Cultures of purulent secretions can be obtained using either sterile suction traps or small wire swabs.
- *Maxillary sinus puncture and aspiration*: The nose is decongested and anesthetized topically. An antral tap trocar or needle is inserted through the thin bone of the lateral inferior meatus into the maxillary sinus. The contents are then aspirated with a syringe and sent for culture.

Treatment

- *Medical*: Therapy includes addressing and reversing immunocompromised state, aggressive antifungal drugs and repeat endoscopic examination with debridement.
- *Surgical*: Functional endoscopic sinus surgery is the main surgical treatment for patients with CRS that is refractory to medical therapy.

FUNGAL SINUSITIS

Overview

There are several different manifestations of fungal sinusitis that are related to the immunologic status of the patient. Patients who are immunocompromised tend to have invasive forms of fungal sinusitis, while patients with normal or hyper-reactive immune systems have noninvasive forms.

Invasive

Invasive fungal sinusitis tends to occur in patients who are immunocompromised. Diagnosis is based on culture specimens and biopsy with histopathologic findings of hyphae within tissue.

Subtypes

Acute invasive fungal sinusitis:

- *Symptoms*: Rapid development of symptoms over days of fever, nasal congestion, facial pain, and orbital swelling.
- *Examination*: Edema and erythema of nasal mucosa, occasional necrosis of nasal mucosa, or fungal sporulation.
- *Immune status*: Immunocompromised, diabetics.

Chronic invasive fungal sinusitis:

- *Symptoms*: Slow development of symptoms over weeks to months.
- *Immune status*: Immunocompetent or limited immunocompromised.

Microbiology

- *Aspergillus* (*A. fumigatus* and *A. flavus*): It is usually associated with chronic invasive subtype and demonstrates narrow hyphae with narrow, regular septations and 45° branches.
- *Mucormycosis* (*Rhizopus oryzae*): Rapid onset, acutely fatal infection in humans. Broad, irregular hyphae with rare septations.

Imaging

Computed tomographic scan is often similar to patients with bacterial rhinosinusitis with heterogeneous opacification of sinuses, focal or diffuse areas of hyperintensity, and erosion of bony septations.

Treatment

Multimodality therapy to address and reverse immunocompromised state, aggressive antifungal therapy (amphotericin B) and endoscopic debridement.

Noninvasive

Noninvasive fungal sinusitis tends to occur in patients who are immunocompetent or have limited immunocompromise (i.e. systemic steroids).

Subtype

Fungus ball:
- *Symptoms*: Indistinguishable from patients with chronic rhinosinusitis. Sometimes asymptomatic.
- *Examination*: Darkened, crumbly mass with visible sporulation.
- *Microbiology*: Usually *Aspergillus* species.
- *Imaging*: Computed tomographic scan shows metallic or calcified densities. High-negative predictive value.
- *Treatment:* Surgical debridement.

Allergic Fungal Rhinosinusitis

This is the sinonasal form of allergic bronchopulmonary asthma. Patients with allergy to fungal spores are exposed by inhalation of spores, leading to allergic mucin production.

Signs and Symptoms

These are similar to CRS. Patients present with atopic symptoms and recurrent nasal polyposis. It has a strong association with asthma.

Imaging

Computed tomographic scan commonly shows heterogeneous soft tissue density and nasal polyposis, and there is often bony erosion.

Diagnosis

Histologically, allergic fungal rhinosinusitis shows allergic mucin with necrotic inflammatory cells, eosinophils, and Charcot-

Leyden crystals with no evidence of fungal invasion. Elevated immunoglobulin E antibodies to fungi found on histology.

Microbiology

Bipolaris, *Exserohilum robustum*, *Curvularia lunata*, *Alternaria*, and *Aspergillus* species.

Treatment

This entity requires multimodality treatment:
- Surgical debridement of nasal polyps
- Systemic or topical steroids
- Nasal lavage

Other treatment modalities such as immunotherapies, antifungals, antibiotics, and anti-inflammatory agents have been tried, but efficacy is unclear.

ODONTOGENIC SINUSITIS

Odontogenic sinusitis accounts for 10–12% of cases of maxillary sinusitis. Risk factors include a history of odontogenic infection, dentoalveolar surgery, periodontal surgery, and patients with resistant sinusitis.

Diagnosis

Symptoms include dental pain, headache, maxillary tenderness, nasal obstruction, and purulent rhinorrhea. Examination requires thorough inspection of the maxillary teeth, gums, and alveolus and nasal endoscopy for evidence of sinusitis.

Imaging

Panorex should be obtained to evaluate for maxillary tooth disease and CT scan to evaluate sinus disease.

Microbiology

1. *Aerobic*: α-Hemolytic *Streptococcus*, microaerophilic *Streptococcus, S. aureus.*

2. *Anaerobes*: *Peptostreptococcus* species, *Fusobacterium* species.

Treatment

1. Thorough dental devaluation with removal of infected source.
2. Closure of any oroantral communication.
3. Antibiotics with oral and anaerobic coverages for 3–4 weeks.
4. Treatment of nasal symptoms with nasal decongestants, steroid nasal sprays, and nasal saline.

OROANTRAL FISTULA

Oroantral fistulas are fistulous tracts between the maxillary sinus and oral cavity. They occur most commonly after extraction of posterior maxillary teeth, in patients with pre-existing periapical abnormalities, and in maxillary sinus perforation > 5 mm.

Diagnosis

Symptoms include nasal congestion, fluids entering nose when eating or drinking, sanguineous discharge, dental discomfort, and acute sinusitis symptoms. Examination reveals odontogenic drainage from a tooth socket.

Treatment

Initially, any maxillary sinusitis should be treated with antibiotics and saline lavage through the oral cavity. Cultures and sensitivities should be obtained for purulent discharge. A Caldwell-Luc procedure can be performed to remove sinus polyps and disease.

Closure

Locoregional soft tissue flaps, such as a buccal sliding flap or a palatal rotational flap, are most commonly employed. Other techniques such as fat plugs and bone grafts have also been used to successfully close oroantral fistulas.

SUGGESTED READING

1. Brook I. Sinusitis of odontogenic origin. Otolaryngol Head Neck Surg. 2006;135(3):349-55.
2. Dym H, Wolf JC. Oroantral communication. Oral Naxillofac Surg Clin North Am. 2012;24(2):239-247, viii-ix.
3. Eller R, Sillers M. Common fibro-osseous lesions of the paranasal sinuses. Otolaryngol Clin North Am. 2006;39(3):585-600, x.
4. Rosenfeld RM, Andes D, Bhattacharyya N, et al. Clinical practice guideline: adult sinusitis. Otolaryngol Head Neck Surg. 2007;137(3 Suppl):S1-31.

Chapter 29

Anosmia

Jennifer R Cracchiolo, Elina M Toskala

Chief Complaint
" I cannot smell".

DEFINITIONS

Anosmia: Complete inability to smell or detect odors.

Hyposmia: Reduced ability to smell and to detect odors.

Parosmia: Distorted perception of odorants.

Phantosmia: Constant perception of an odor usually foul in character.

ANATOMY AND PHYSIOLOGY OF OLFACTION

Experiencing normal olfaction requires the following:
1. *Nasal airflow*: Odorant molecules reaching the olfactory mucosa at the top of the nasal cavity.
2. *Olfactory mucus*: In order for odorant molecules to reach the olfactory region, they are solubilized in mucus produced by (1) Bowman's glands and (2) goblet cells.
3. *Olfactory epithelium*:
   a. Pseudostratified columnar cells' neuroepithelium.
   b. It is located in the superior cleft between the middle and superior turbinates and the septum.

Four cell types: (1) ciliated olfactory receptors, (2) microvillar cells, (3) supporting (sustentacular) cells, and (4) basal cells.

4. *Cranial nerves (CNs)*:
   a. CN I (olfactory): Axons extending from the receptor neurons coalesce into bundles (CN I) that travel through the cribriform plate to make primary synapses with the olfactory bulb.
   b. CN V, VIII, X (trigeminal, glossopharyngeal, and vagus nerves): They provide added chemoreceptivity in the mucosa of the respiratory tract. Example: They are sensitive to the burn of ammonia and the bite of hot pepper.

5. *Olfactory bulb*: It lies at the base of the frontal cortex in the anterior fossa and serves as the first relay station in the olfactory pathway, where the primary olfactory neurons synapse with secondary neurons.

6. *Central olfactory connections*: Olfactory tubercle, the prepiriform cortex, part of the amygdaloid nuclei, and the nucleus of the terminal stria, the hypothalamus.

Review: Olfaction Pathway

Nasal airflow carries odorant molecules to olfactory mucosa at the cranial aspect of the nasal cavity → odorant is loosely captured by mucus (produced by goblet cells and Bowman's glands) → solubilized odorant lands on olfactory epithelium → axons extending from olfactory epithelium coalesce, form CN I, travel through cribriform plate and synapse with olfactory bulb → primary olfactory neurons from olfactory bulb synapse with secondary neurons and travel to their central olfactory destination.

Disruption in this pathway can result in both physiologic and pathologic olfactory functions. Additionally, congenital loss of the sense of smell should also be considered in patients who present with the chief complaint "I cannot smell," and often, "I have lost my sense of taste."

HUMAN OLFACTORY DYSFUNCTIONS

Physiologic

Aging: Olfactory thresholds have been found to decline with age; this effect is slightly less dramatic in women.

Pathologic

- *Obstructive nasal*: Total obstruction by polyps or simple nasal occlusion can result in anosmia. Obstruction of the olfactory cleft can occur with mucosal edema or tumor. Enlargement or medialization of the middle turbinate, of the superior turbinate, or of both can be seen on nasal endoscopy and computed tomography (CT) and also have contributed to olfactory dysfunction.
- *Treatment*: When the obstruction is released, olfactory ability should return, although the minimal nasal opening at which the return occurs is not known.

Chronic Rhinosinusitis

1. *Obstruction*: Edematous mucosa and polyps in chronic rhinosinusitis may play a role in the olfactory dysfunction.
2. *Damage to olfactory epithelium*: Olfactory mucosa biopsy specimens from patients with chronic rhinosinusitis show inflammatory changes within olfactory epithelium. Active apoptosis of olfactory epithelium has also been observed.
3. *Treatment*: Treat chronic rhinosinusitis with topical and systemic medications.

Post Upper Respiratory Infection

In a small number of patients, olfactory complaints persist after the acute symptoms of an upper respiratory infection have resolved. It occurs more often in women; patients tend to be otherwise healthy individuals in the fourth, fifth, or sixth decade of life. Biopsy specimens of the olfactory cleft in these patients show decreased numbers of olfactory receptors. Magnetic resonance imaging measurements of olfactory bulb volume in these patients reveal a decrease in size that correlates with severity of loss. Prognosis is often poor, with one third of the patients recovering their olfactory ability.

Head Trauma

Olfactory loss occurs in 5–10% patients after head trauma. It is more likely with frontal trauma than occipital; however, total anosmia is five times more likely with an occipital trauma. The mechanism is thought to be due either to shearing of the olfactory nerves as they exit the top of the cribriform plate or to contusion of the olfactory bulbs. Compromise of central processing areas is another potential mechanism. It has a poor prognosis.

Treatment

No current treatment; hypothesized therapy would include re-establishing contact between the olfactory axons and the olfactory bulb if viable.

Toxic Exposure

A long list of agents, mostly gases or aerosols, have been reported to be associated with olfactory dysfunction. History of exposure with resultant olfactory dysfunction is a key for diagnosis.

Neoplasm

Tumors originating from the olfactory cleft or extending into the olfactory cleft can result in olfactory dysfunction. Associated signs of obstruction, epistaxis, and visual lesions should be included in the history.

Differential diagnosis of tumors includes inverting papillomas, adenomas, squamous cell carcinomas, and esthesioneuroblastomas.

CONGENITAL DYSFUNCTION

Kallmann's Syndrome (Hypogonadotropic Hypogonadism)

- It is often present in elementary school when social interactions reveal that the patient does not appreciate a smell noted by the group.
- Males > females (1 in 8,000 vs 1 in 40,000).
- *Genetics*: X chromosome and autosomal-dominant cases reported. KAL1 gene (encodes the protein anosmin-1) and KAL2 gene (fibroblast growth factor receptor-1).
- *Pathophysiology*: Agenesis of the olfactory bulbs and stalks and incomplete development of the hypothalamus. Absence of olfactory epithelium in the olfactory cleft has also been observed.
- *Associated defects*: Renal abnormalities, cryptorchidism, deafness, midline facial deformities, and diabetes.

Central Pathologies

- These are often characterized by parosmia and phantosmia; however, hyposmia and anosmia are also observed in dementia-related diseases, including Alzheimer's disease and Parkinson's disease.
- *Epilepsy*: It is associated with olfactory auras.
- *Depression and schizophrenia*: Olfactory hallucinations.
- *Temporal lobe tumors*: Up to 25% may cause olfactory disturbance.
- *Alzheimer's disease and Parkinson's disease*: They can be the early sign of dementia-related diseases.

Iatrogenic

Olfactory disturbance can be a complaint following septoplasty, sinus surgery (less so with functional endoscopic techniques), rhinoplasty, total laryngectomy, and skull base surgery in the region of the olfactory bulbs. Pathophysiology is related to alterations in airflow dynamics, olfactory epithelium, or damage to olfactory bulbs.

DIAGNOSTIC WORKUP: "I CANNOT SMELL" (FLOWCHART. 29.1)

History

- "Is your smell decreased, absent, or distorted?"
- "Was your change in smell always absent, was lost suddenly, changed over days, weeks, months, or years?"
- "Did you have an upper respiratory infection, head trauma, toxin exposure, change in medication, surgery around the time you noticed a change in smell?"
- "Do you have associated nasal symptoms of unilateral nasal congestion, epistaxis, nasal crusting, or dry nasal passages?"
- "Do you have associated symptoms including headache, visual disturbance, seizures, memory loss, and tremor?"

Physical Examination

- Anterior rhinoscopy (septal deviations and mucosal changes).
- Endoscopic nasal examination (look for nasal mass, polyps, signs of chronic sinusitis, enlarged turbinates); specifically, look into olfactory cleft (superior cleft between the middle and superior turbinates and the septum).

Ancillary Tools

Smell Identification Test

University of Pennsylvania Smell Identification Test (UPSIT): Chance identification performance is 25% correct. If one does

Flowchart. 29.1: Physical examination including nasal endoscopy is essential in evaluating patients with distorted olfaction. Imaging of brain and nasal cavity including olfactory bulbs (CT/MRI) augments clinical findings. (URI: Upper respiratory infection).

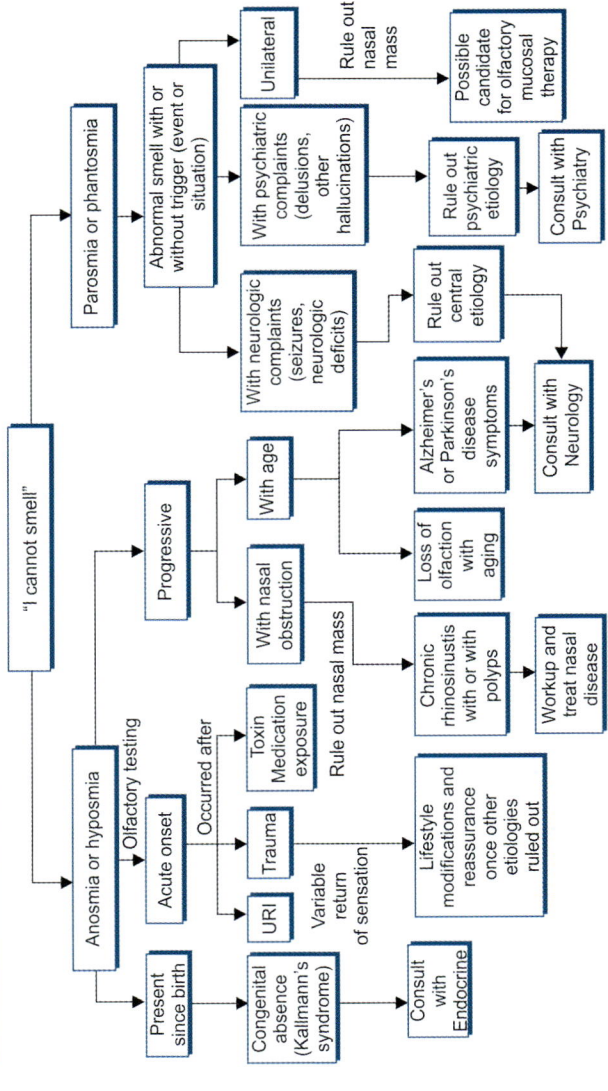

significantly worse than that, one is classified as probably malingering.

SUGGESTED READING

1. Barresi M, Ciurleo R, Giacoppo S, et al. Evaluation of olfactory dysfunction in neurodegenerative diseases. J Neurol Sci. 2012;323(1-2):16-24.
2. Gaines A. Olfactory disorders. Am J Rhinol Allergy. 2013;27(Suppl 1):S45-7.
3. Higgins TS, Lane AP. What is the best imaging modality to investigate olfactory dysfunction in the setting of normal endoscopy? Laryngoscope. 2014;124(1):4-5.
4. Leopold DA, Holbrook EH. Physiology of olfaction. In: Flint PW, Haughey BH, Lund VJ, et al. (Eds). Cummings Otolaryngology: Head and Neck Surgery, 5th edition. St Louis, MO: Mosby; 2010. pp. 597-623.

Chapter 30

Epistaxis

Derrick Tint, Elina M Toskala

Chief Complaint
"My nose is bleeding".

DEFINITIONS

- *Epistaxis*: Bleeding from the nose.
- *Anterior epistaxis*: Bleeding from the nose originating anterior to the maxillary sinus ostium.
- *Posterior epistaxis*: Bleeding from the nose originating posterior to the maxillary sinus ostium.

EPIDEMIOLOGY

- *Prevalence*: Approximately 60% of population have epistaxis in their lifetime. Approximately 6% require medical attention.
- *Age*: Epistaxis has a bimodal distribution that peaks between 5 and 15 years and again between 65 and 85 years.
- *Gender*: Between 20 and 50 years of age, there is a male predominance of 2:1. However, above 50 years of age, the male-to-female ratio is closer to 1:1.

ANATOMY

- *Anterior and posterior epistaxis*: The dividing line is the maxillary sinus ostium.

- *Blood supply*: The nasal cavity receives blood from both the external carotid (ECA) and internal carotid artery (ICA) systems. The ECA provides blood supply from branches of the facial artery and internal maxillary artery.

1. *Facial artery*: This supplies the anterior septum from the superior labial branch.

2. *Internal maxillary artery*: This supplies the sphenopalatine artery and the greater palatine artery. The sphenopalatine artery exits the pterygopalatine fossa through the sphenopalatine foramen, giving off lateral and medial branches to supply the lateral nasal wall and septum, respectively. The greater palatine artery descends along the pterygopalatine fossa, travels along the hard palatine, and enters the floor of the nasal cavity anteriorly through the incisive foramen.

The ICA provides blood supply from its first branch, the ophthalmic artery. The ophthalmic artery first gives off the posterior ethmoid artery, which travels through the posterior ethmoid canal and provides blood supply to the posterior superior nasal septum. It then gives off the anterior ethmoid artery, which travels through the anterior ethmoid canal and provides blood supply to the posterior superior nasal septum.

Kiesselbach's plexus (Little's area): This is a plexus of blood vessels located in the anterior nasal septum. It receives blood supply from both the ECA and ICA via the superior labial, greater palatine, anterior ethmoid, and posterior ethmoid arteries (Fig. 30.1).

ETIOLOGY

In general, epistaxis can be categorized as primary (idiopathic) or secondary. Secondary epistaxis refers to bleeding when the cause is known and can be further divided into local versus systemic factors (Table 30.1). Although there are many different causes of secondary epistaxis, the majority are post-traumatic.

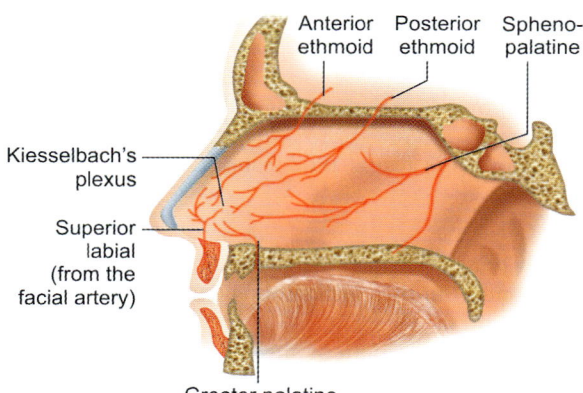

Fig. 30.1: Sagittal view of the nasal septum highlighting anterior vessel contribution to Kiesselbach's plexus.

Table 30.1: Secondary epistaxis.	
Local	*Systemic*
Trauma (digital, nasogastric tube)	Drugs (blood thinners, NSAIDs)
Surgery (sinus, skull base)	Bleeding diatheses
Anatomic (septal spur, perforation)	Hypertension
Sinonasal tumors (JNA, vascular tumors)	Liver disease
Foreign bodies	Alcoholism
Inflammatory disease (Wegener's)	Connective tissue disorder
Topical medication (topical steroids)	Malnutrition
Low humidity (winter, nasal cannula)	

(NSAIDs: Nonsteroidal anti-inflammatory drugs; JNA: Juvenile nasopharyngeal angiofibroma).

HISTORY AND PHYSICAL EXAMINATION

Initial Assessment

- Estimate blood loss (soaked through tissue, handkerchief, facecloth, and towel?).

- General assessment (pale, sweating, or cool)—look for signs of significant hypovolemia.
- Vital signs.
- Initial laboratory results (CBC, PT, INR, aPTT), type, and screen/cross.
- Intravenous (IV) access, fluid resuscitation.

Conservative Measures

- *Holding pressure*: Apply firm pressure to the ala (not over the nasal bones, but the cartilaginous anterior part of the nose) for 20 minutes.
- *Lean forward*: The patient should be leaning forward over a bowl. It allows for further estimation of blood loss and prevents patients from swallowing and possibly later vomiting or aspirating blood.

Examination

- *Gather supplies*: Headlamp, suction, nasal speculum, bayonet forceps, scissors, protective gear including facemask and eye protection, flexible fiberoptic endoscope.
- Perform anterior rhinoscopy. Suction all blood clots out of the nose. Identify the bleeding source. If the source cannot be identified, then perform nasal endoscopy.

TREATMENT

Treatment methods are presented in Table 30.2.

Conservative Treatment

Topical Therapy

- *Moisturizers*: Nasal saline, bacitracin, and vaseline can be applied regularly to keep the nasal cavity moist and as a preventative measure against nosebleeds.
- *Vasoconstrictors*: Oxymetazoline, phenylephrine, cocaine, and epinephrine have been shown to be effective as a single measure to stopping nosebleeds.

Table 30.2: Treatment for epistaxis.	
Treatment	*Types*
Conservative	Hold pressure, lean forward
	Saline, vaseline, bacitracin
Topical	Vasoconstrictors (oxymetazoline)
	Chemical cautery (silver nitrate)
	Hemostatic agents (topical thrombin)
Packing	Anterior pack (ribbon gauze, Merocel)
	Posterior pack (foley, Epistat)
Surgical	Electrocautery
	Sphenopalatine artery ligation
	Anterior ethmoid ligation
Embolization	Sphenopalatine artery embolization
	Facial artery embolization

- *Chemical cautery, silver nitrate*: Silver nitrate can be applied to the site of bleeding, working peripherally toward the center.
- *Hemostatic agents*: Bovine-derived thrombin (Floseal), oxidized cellulose polymer (Surgicel), and microfibrillar collagen (Avitene) are better tolerated and can sometimes be used instead of nasal packing.

Nasal Packing

If bleeding continues despite the application of topical vasoconstrictions, cautery, and adequate placement of pressure, nasal packing should be considered. A myriad of nasal packs are available. Selection of the appropriate nasal packing is dependent upon a number of factors, including location, availability, provider's preference, and patient's comfort. Once packing has been placed and bleeding has been adequately controlled, it is left in the nares for 48–72 hours and then removed. The patient should be started on an oral or IV antibiotic to cover for *Staphylococcus aureus* (controversial). If bleeding continues, packing in the contralateral nares or placement of a posterior pack should be considered.

Anterior Pack

- *Balloon (i.e. Rapid Rhino)*: This is a balloon catheter with carboxymethylated cellulose mesh. Placement of an anterior balloon catheter is a quick, simple, and effective method to stop nosebleeds and is well tolerated by patients. It requires a headlight, nasal speculum, and bayonet forceps. First, it must be soaked in sterile water for 30 seconds to allow for appropriate lubrication. Then the catheter is placed along the nasal floor and inflated with air or saline.

- *Nasal tampon (i.e. Merocel)*: This is made of synthetic open-cell foam polymer. It requires a headlight, nasal speculum, bayonet forceps, and lubrication. Before placing the Merocel, one should check for the presence of a string for easy removal. If one is not present, it can be easily fashioned by the placement of a 2.0 silk suture at one end. The Merocel is coated in lubrication (surgical lubricant or bacitracin) and inserted parallel to the nasal floor. It is then expanded with 10 mL of saline or oxymetazoline solution.

- *Ribbon gauze*: This is a strip of woven cotton that is impregnated with bacitracin or petroleum jelly. It requires a headlight, nasal speculum, and bayonet forceps. Once the nasal cavity is visualized with a speculum, a single strip of this ribbon gauze is layered parallel to the nasal floor to the roof of the nose. If more than one piece of the gauze is used, each piece should be tied together to create a single continuous strip. The total number of pieces used should be accurately recorded.

Posterior Pack

- Patients who have posterior packs placed should be admitted with telemetry and continuous pulse-oximetry monitoring due to nasopulmonary reflex and other respiratory problems.

- *Epistat nasal catheter (Medtronic)*: This is a balloon catheter with two independently inflatable cuffs. The anterior cuff can be inflated with up to 30 cc of air. The posterior cuff is designed to stop sphenopalatine artery bleeds and can be filled with up to 10 cc of air.

- *Foley*: The catheter is advanced along the floor of the nose until it is visualized in the oropharynx. The tip of the catheter is then secured with a string and inflated with 10 mL of sterile water. The catheter is retracted and guided into the nasopharynx using a finger, while the string remains outside the oral cavity. The ribbon gauze is placed into the nasal cavity. The pack is then secured using an umbilical clip or chest tube clamp. The device should be checked daily. Severe complications include alar necrosis and palate necrosis.

Invasive Treatment

- *Indications*: Bleeding refractory to conservative measures, chronic recurrent episodes, single life-threatening bleeding.
- *Goal*: Isolate and ligate the bleeding vessel.
- *Sphenopalatine artery ligation*: The artery is identified endoscopically in the posterolateral mucosa within the orbital process of the palatine bone. The sphenopalatine foramen can be identified after locating the crista ethmoidalis. The artery is identified and ligated using clips or bipolar cautery.

Ethmoid Artery Ligation

- *Open*: Medial canthal incision. The anterior ethmoid is identified at the frontoethmoidal suture line and ligated using clips, suture, or bipolar cautery.
- *Endoscopic*: The artery is identified within the ethmoid roof and ligated with bipolar diathermy.
- *Endovascular embolization*: Embolization can be considered for selected patients who are poor surgical candidates for bleeding arising from the internal maxillary system. Bleeding from the anterior or posterior ethmoid system should be addressed surgically, due to the risk of ophthalmoplegia.

HEREDITARY HEMORRHAGIC TELANGIECTASIA (OSLER–WEBER–RENDU)

Hereditary hemorrhagic telangiectasia (HHT) is a hereditary condition (autosomal dominant) characterized by arteriovenous (AV) malformations in the sinonasal tract, lungs, brain, skin, and gastrointestinal (GI) tract.

Epidemiology: Its prevalence is 1 in every 5000–8000 people, with a higher prevalence in the Afro-Caribbean population. Clinical features include frequent epistaxis, telangiectasias of mucosa of the aerodigestive tract, GI bleeding, and AV malformations of the lungs, liver, and heart.

Diagnosis

Refer to Table 30.3.

Management

- *Conservative measures*: Prevention of epistaxis using the techniques described above can be applied to patients with HHT. However, often these patients are refractory to conservative measures and require surgical procedures to achieve long-term benefit.
- *Endoscopic laser excision*: The use of endoscopic techniques and Nd:YAG laser has been described to excise telangiectasias and AV malformations of the nasal mucosa.

Table 30.3: Curacao criteria for clinical diagnosis of hereditary hemorrhagic telangiectasia.

Criteria	Epistaxis Telangiectasia Visceral lesions Family history
Diagnosis	*Definite*: Three or more criteria present *Possible/suspected*: Two criteria present *Unlikely*: Fewer than two criteria present

- *Septodermoplasty*: This consists of resection of mucosa on the septum, the floor of the nasal cavity, and inferior turbinate using a microdebrider and suction cautery, followed by placement of a split thickness skin graft overlying the resected tissue.
- *Young's procedure*: The nostrils are sewn to the septum. Patients are obligate mouth breathers. It is effective for the treatment of HHT; however, patients lose the ability to smell and taste.

SUGGESTED READING

1. Koh E, Frazzini VI, Kagetsu NJ. Epistaxis: vascular anatomy, origins, and endovascular treatment. AJR Am J Roentgenol. 2000;174:845-51.
2. Krempl GA, Noorily AD. Use of oxymetazoline in the management of epistaxis. Ann Otol Rhinol Laryngol. 1995;104:704-6.
3. Nikoyan L, Matthews S. Epistaxis and hemostatic devices. Oral Maxillofac Surg Clin North Am. 2012;24:219-28, viii.
4. Small M, Murray JA, Maran AG. A study of patients with epistaxis requiring admission to hospital. Health Bull. 1982;40:20-9.
5. Taylor MT. Avitene—its value in the control of anterior epistaxis. J Otolaryngol. 1980;9:468-71.
6. Tomkinson A, Roblin DG, Flanagan P, et al. Patterns of hospital attendance with epistaxis. Rhinology. 1997;35:129-31.

Chapter 31

Endoscopic Sinus Surgery

Lori A Lemonnier

> **Chief Complaint**
> *"I have had problems with my sinuses as long as I can remember".*

DEFINITIONS

- *Rhinorrhea*: Nasal discharge.
- *Nasal obstruction*: The absence of airflow through the nasal cavity.
- *Paranasal sinuses*: Because there are other anatomic sinuses located in the human body, the sinuses surrounding the nasal cavity are clearly identified by the term paranasal sinuses.
- *Ostium*: The hole that is the natural drainage pathway of the sinus.
- *Rhinosinusitis*: The symptomatic inflammation of the nasal cavity and paranasal sinuses. As put forth in the Clinical Practice Guidelines on adult sinusitis,[1] diagnostic symptoms are defined as purulent rhinorrhea accompanied by nasal obstruction, facial pain/pressure/fullness, or both. Additional symptoms may include fever, malaise, cough, halitosis, dental pain, hyposmia, and anosmia (*see* Chapter 29). Classification of rhinosinusitis is determined on the basis of the duration of symptoms.
  - *Acute*: < 4 weeks

- – *Subacute*: 4–12 weeks
- – *Chronic*: >12 weeks.

- *Recurrent acute sinusitis*: Four or more episodes of acute rhinosinusitis per year, with complete resolution of symptoms between episodes.
- *Nasal endoscopy*: Examination of the nasal cavity performed with a nasal endoscope.
- *Functional endoscopic sinus surgery*: Sinus surgery, performed with a nasal endoscope, in a manner that preserves the mucosal lining of the sinuses.

ANATOMY AND PHYSIOLOGY OF THE PARANASAL SINUSES

The average adult has four paired paranasal sinuses, eight in total, including the maxillary, ethmoid, sphenoid, and frontal sinuses. The sinus cavities are lined with respiratory mucosa, a pseudostratified ciliated columnar epithelium with goblet cells. The cilia are preprogrammed to beat toward the natural drainage pathway of each sinus, resulting in clearance of the mucus that it produces, a process termed mucociliary clearance. Only the maxillary and ethmoid sinuses are present at birth. These sinuses continue to enlarge, or pneumatize, and are followed by the development of the sphenoid and frontal sinuses. Sinuses that fail to develop or are underdeveloped are called aplastic or hypoplastic, respectively.

1. *Maxillary sinus*: Housed in the maxilla, the maxillary sinus is the most inferiorly located sinus, bordering the floor of the orbit and the lateral nasal wall (Fig. 31.1).
2. *Ethmoid sinuses*: Composed of multiple small air cells, the ethmoid sinuses are located between the eyes, bordering the medial orbital wall and anterior skull base. The ethmoid cavity is divided into anterior and posterior portions by a structure called the basal lamella, which is the horizontal attachment of the middle turbinate to the lateral nasal wall (Fig. 31.1).

3. *Sphenoid sinus*: The most posterior of the paranasal sinuses, the sphenoid sinus borders the anterior skull base, as well as multiple important neurovascular structures including the optic nerve, carotid artery, and cavernous sinus (Fig. 31.2).

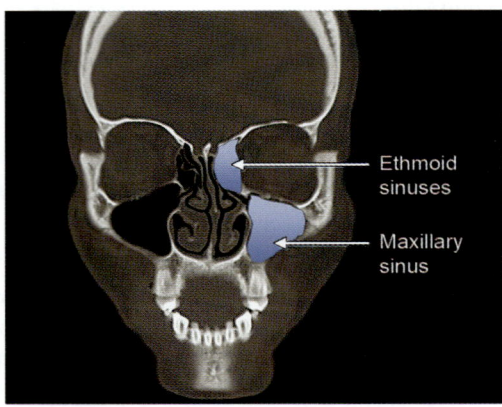

Ethmoid sinuses

Maxillary sinus

Fig. 31.1: Maxillary and ethmoid sinuses.

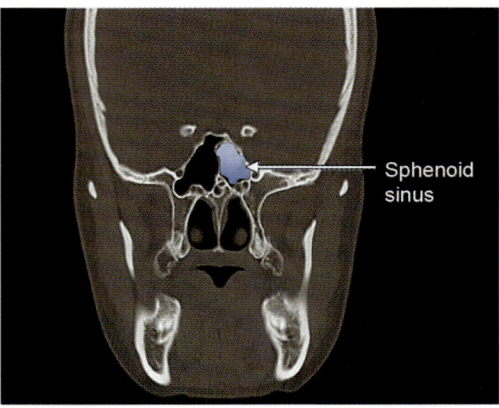

Sphenoid sinus

Fig. 31.2: Sphenoid sinus.

4. *Frontal sinus*: Housed in the frontal bone, the frontal sinus is the most superiorly located sinus, bordering the roof of the orbit and the anterior skull base (Fig. 31.3).

5. *Anterior osteomeatal complex (OMC)*: The anterior OMC is the collective drainage pathway of the anterior sinuses, which include the maxillary, anterior ethmoid, and frontal sinuses.

6. *Posterior osteomeatal complex*: The posterior OMC, or sphenoethmoidal recess, is the common drainage pathway of the sphenoid and posterior ethmoid sinuses.

7. *Turbinates*: There are three sets of turbinates in each nasal cavity—the inferior, middle, and superior turbinates. A fourth set of turbinates, the supreme turbinates, is also present in some individuals. The turbinates are mucosal-covered bony structures that play a role in airflow, filtration, and humidification of inspired air (Fig. 31.4).

INDICATIONS FOR ENDOSCOPIC SINUS SURGERY

1. *Chronic rhinosinusitis (CRS)*: This condition, with persistent symptoms despite medical therapy, is the most common indication for endoscopic sinus surgery.

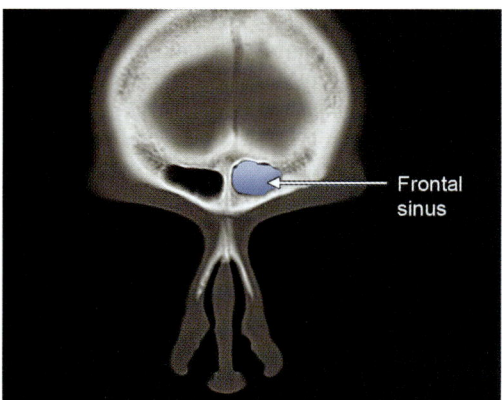

Fig. 31.3: Frontal sinus.

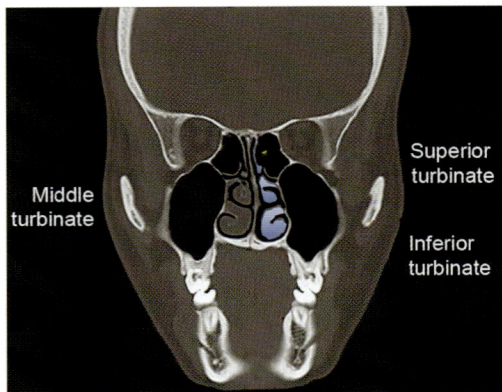

Middle turbinate

Superior turbinate

Inferior turbinate

Fig. 31.4: Inferior, middle, and superior turbinates.

2. *Recurrent acute sinusitis*: Patients with recurrent acute sinusitis who have an anatomic variant contributing to the problem may be candidates for endoscopic sinus surgery. An example is the patient who has an extra cell in the maxillary sinus, called a Haller cell, which results in narrowing of the osteomeatal complex.

3. *Complications of acute sinusitis*: Orbital and intracranial complications of acute sinusitis that require surgical drainage also call for surgical management of the responsible sinus. For example, a subperiosteal abscess of the orbit is commonly treated by endoscopic sinus surgery with ethmoidectomy and medical orbital wall decompression.

4. *Sinus neoplasm*: It is widely accepted that the standard of care for the treatment of the benign sinonasal neoplasms is endoscopic resection. Many malignant sinonasal lesions can also be resected endoscopically. However, in order to be able to achieve an oncologic resection, the importance of careful patient selection cannot be overemphasized.

5. *Mucocele*: A mucocele is a pseudocyst of the sinuses, which typically forms as a result of scar tissue formation secondary

to facial trauma or prior surgery and secondary obstruction of the sinus. As the pseudocyst produces mucus, it enlarges and exerts pressure on the surrounding bone, in time resulting in bony erosion. Erosion of the orbit and skull base then leaves the eye and brain vulnerable to the pressure exerted by mucocele. Mucoceles are treated by marsupialization, which entails surgically draining and widely opening the pseudocyst cavity. Mucoceles should be differentiated from mucosal cysts, which form within the patent sinus and rarely cause symptoms.

6. *Facial trauma*: Facial trauma can result in fractures of the paranasal sinuses. If the frontal sinus outflow tract is involved, endoscopic sinus surgery may be required to restore its patency, in order to prevent scarring and long-term complications such as mucocele formation.

7. *Cerebrospinal fluid (CSF) leak*: Leakage of CSF into the sinuses and nasal cavity may occur due to a number of etiologies: traumatic, iatrogenic, congenital, tumor-related, and spontaneous. Spontaneous leaks are typically associated with raised intracranial pressure. The majority of CSF leaks can be repaired endoscopically, from within the affected sinus cavity.

PROCEDURE

Sinus surgery was initially performed through external incisions of the skin with the use of a headlight, with or without surgical loops or an operating microscope. However, since its introduction to the United States in 1985 by Dr David Kennedy, endoscopic sinus surgery has become the gold standard for surgical management of CRS. The nasal endoscope provides dynamic visualization, illumination, and magnification. Because the endoscope is placed through the nasal cavity, skin incisions are avoided. The goal of endoscopic sinus surgery is to identify and enlarge the nature sinus ostia in order to restore ventilation and drainage, thereby improving the patient's symptoms.

The following are the key steps involved in endoscopic sinus surgery:

1. *Decongestion*: Topical decongestion of the nasal mucosa is typically performed with oxymetazoline, neosynephrine, or cocaine.

2. *Injection*: To aid in hemostasis, the nasal mucosa and region of the sphenopalatine artery can be injected with a local anesthetic and vasoconstrictive agent, such as 1% lidocaine with 1:100,000 epinephrine.

3. *Nasal endoscopy*: The nasal endoscope is first used to systematically examine the anatomy of the nasal cavity. Straight and angled endoscopes can be used for visualization throughout the procedure.

4. *Maxillary antrostomy*: A small bone called the uncinate process must first be removed in order to identify the opening of the maxillary sinus, or the ostium. Once identified, the ostium is then enlarged, revealing the maxillary sinus cavity.

5. *Ethmoidectomy*: Because the ethmoid sinuses are composed of multiple small cells, each cell must be entered and its bony walls removed.

6. *Sphenoidotomy*: The sphenoid ostium is identified between the nasal septum and the superior turbinate. As with a maxillary antrostomy, the ostium is then enlarged, revealing the underlying sphenoid sinus.

7. *Frontal sinusotomy*: The frontal sinus recess is the space that leads to the frontal sinus ostium located above. Because the recess is part of the anterior ethmoid sinuses, it often involves multiple small cells that must be opened in order to clear the pathway to the ostium. If indicated, the ostium can then be further enlarged.

8. *Implants*: A number of implantable materials are available for use in the sinuses, many of which are dissolvable and do not require removal. Examples include stents to help prevent postoperative scar tissue formation, as well as powders, foams, and packing that aid in hemostasis.

9. *Dressing*: A moustache, or drip dressing, may be placed under the nose to contain postoperative bleeding if needed.
   Image guidance is a system that can be used to allow the surgeon to correlate intraoperative anatomy with that seen on computed tomographic (CT) imaging. Image guidance can be a valuable tool during procedures that involve areas of complex anatomy or lack endoscopic landmarks secondary to prior surgery or polypoid disease.

COMPLICATIONS OF ENDOSCOPIC SINUS SURGERY

When counseling a patient on the option of endoscopic sinus surgery, the following potential complications should be discussed preoperatively:

1. *Synechiae*: The most common complication of endonasal surgery is synechiae or scar band formation. Although potentially asymptomatic, synechiae can result in nasal obstruction and compromise access to the sinonasal cavities during postoperative endoscopy and debridement. They are treated by lysis, typically in the office setting.

2. *Bleeding*: Both major and minor bleeding complications can occur during or after endoscopic sinus surgery. Major bleeding may result from injury to the anterior ethmoid, posterior ethmoid, sphenopalatine, or internal carotid artery.

3. *Infection*: As with any surgical procedure, infection of the operating field and surrounding structures is a potential complication of endoscopic sinus surgery. Current evidence, however, does not support the use of routine antibiotic prophylaxis.

4. *Hypoesthesia*: Decreased facial sensation may occur as a result of damage to branches of the fifth cranial nerve (CN). The maxillary branch, CNV2, runs along the floor of the orbit, making it susceptible to injury during endoscopic sinus surgery.

5. *Epiphora*: Increased tearing may result from damage to the nasolacrimal system during endonasal procedures.

The nasolacrimal duct runs directly anterior to the natural maxillary ostium, making it vulnerable to injury.

6. *Intracranial injury*: Penetration of the anterior skull base during endoscopic sinus surgery may result in complications such as CSF leak, meningitis, abscess, bleeding, and parenchymal injury. Although the diagnosis of intracranial complications may be delayed, if identified intraoperatively immediate repair of a CSF leak is indicated.

7. *Orbital complications*: Inadvertent injury to the orbital contents may result in complications such as diplopia and vision loss. Such injury may occur directly or via transection of the anterior ethmoid artery, which can result in retraction of the proximal portion into the orbit, leading to orbital hematoma, a surgical emergency. Early recognition of the signs of orbital hematoma, such as proptosis and pain, and swift orbital decompression are keys in preventing permanent loss of vision.

8. *Persistent or recurrent symptoms*: It is important to educate patients undergoing endoscopic sinus surgery that medical therapy is a necessary adjunct to the procedure. Surgery alone, without treatment of the underlying etiology, often results in persistent or recurrent symptoms. Ongoing medical therapy and endoscopic surveillance of the mucosa are essential until such time as the mucosa re-stabilizes.

9. *Complications of general anesthesia*: Major morbidity, including myocardial infarction and cerebrovascular accident, as well as mortality may result from the administration of general anesthesia. Patients must be thoroughly screened preoperatively and sent for medical or cardiac clearance, if indicated.

REFERENCE

1. Kennedy DW, Hwang PH (Eds). Rhinology: Diseases of the Nose, Sinuses, and Skull Base. New York: Thieme; 2012.

Chapter 32

Septoplasty

Lori A Lemonnier

> **Chief Complaint**
> *"I cannot breathe through my nose".*

DEFINITIONS

- *Nasal obstruction*: The absence of airflow through the nasal cavity.
- *Septal deformity*: Abnormality of the nasal septum, i.e. septal deviation or spur, that is congenital, traumatic, or iatrogenic in nature.
- *Septoplasty*: Surgical procedure for the correction of a septal deformity.
- *Scoring*: Superficial incisions made to weaken and improve the contour of the septal cartilage.

ANATOMY OF THE NASAL SEPTUM

The nasal septum is a vertical midline structure that divides the nasal cavity into right and left sides and consists of cartilage and bone covered by respiratory mucosa. The cartilage is lined by a thin fibrous layer of connective tissue called perichondrium. The bone is lined by a similar thin fibrous connective tissue layer termed periosteum. Respiratory mucosa, a pseudostratified ciliated columnar epithelium, composes the most superficial layer of the nasal septum.

1. *Cartilage (Fig. 32.1)*: Quadrangular cartilage—forms the most anterior portion of the septum.
2. *Bone (Fig. 32.1)*:
   a. Perpendicular plate of the ethmoid bone—forms the superior septum.
   b. Vomer—the posterior septum.
   c. Sphenoid rostrum—the posterior superior septum.
   d. Palatine crest—the posterior inferior septum.
   e. Maxillary crest—the anterior inferior septum.
3. Blood supply:
   a. *Superior labial artery (a.)*: External a. → Facial a. → Superior labial a. → Anterior nasal septum.
   b. *Greater palatine artery*: Maxillary a. → Descending palatine a. → Greater palatine a. → Anterior inferior septum.

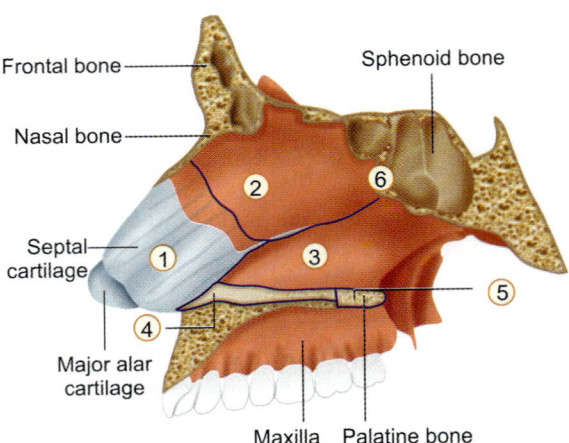

Fig. 32.1: The cartilaginous and bony anatomy of the nasal septum. 1, quadrangular cartilage; 2, perpendicular plate of the ethmoid bone; 3, vomer; 4, maxillary crest; 5, palatine crest; 6, sphenoid rostrum.

   c. *Sphenopalatine artery, septal branch*: Maxillary a. →
      Sphenopalatine a. → Septal (posterior medial) branch of
      the sphenopalatine a. → Posterior septum.
   d. *Anterior ethmoid artery*: Internal a. → Ophthalmic a.
      → Anterior ethmoid a. → Nasal branch of the anterior
      ethmoid a. → Anterior superior septum.
   e. *Posterior ethmoid artery*: Internal a. → Ophthalmic a. →
      Posterior ethmoid a. → Medial branch of the posterior
      ethmoid a. → Posterior superior septum.

INDICATIONS FOR SEPTOPLASTY

Septal Deformity

Septal deformity, diagnosed on anterior rhinoscopy or nasal
endoscopy, resulting in nasal obstruction is the most common
indication for septoplasty. For the patient with a septal deviation
or spur that does *not* compromise nasal breathing, septoplasty is
generally not indicated, with the following possible exceptions:

1. Recurrent epistaxis due to septal deformity.
2. Limited visualization during endoscopic sinus surgery as a
   result of septal deformity.
3. Decreased nasal continuous positive airway pressure
   tolerance in a patient with obstructive sleep apnea and septal
   deformity.
4. Septal deformity that contributes to the obstruction of the
   osteomeatal complex (drainage pathway of the anterior
   sinuses) in a patient with recurrent acute or chronic sinusitis.

    The last and most controversial indication for septoplasty
is headache that is felt to be the result of an intranasal contact
point, in which a deviated nasal septum or septal spur touches
one of the lateral nasal wall structures.

PROCEDURE

Septoplasty is most commonly performed under general
anesthesia. In a traditional septoplasty, the procedure is
performed by looking directly into the nasal cavity with the use

of a headlight for illumination. Alternatively, a nasal endoscope can be used and provides visualization, illumination, and magnification.[1]

The following are the key steps necessary to perform septoplasty, regardless of whether the traditional or endoscopic technique is utilized:

1. *Decongestion*: Topical decongestion of the nasal mucosa is typically performed with oxymetazoline, neosynephrine, or cocaine.

2. *Injection*: The septum is injected with a local anesthetic and vasoconstrictive agent such as 1% lidocaine with 1:100,000 epinephrine. Note that care is taken to inject between the layers of the septal cartilage and the perichondrium. This allows the injection to elevate the perichondrium off of the underlying cartilage, easing the dissection that follows.

3. *Incision*: An incision is made through the mucosa of the septum. When performed endoscopically, the incision is placed just anterior to the septal deformity and may be vertical or L shaped. When a traditional septoplasty technique is used, the following incisions are most commonly utilized:
   a. *Hemitransfixion*: At the most caudal edge of the septal cartilage, through one side of the mucosa only.
   b. *Kilian*: 1–2 cm posterior to the caudal edge of the septal cartilage.

4. *Dissection*: The following steps are included in the dissection of the nasal septum:
   a. *Elevation of a submucoperichondrial flap*: The plane between the cartilage and the perichondrium is identified and the overlying perichondrium and mucosa are raised off from the cartilage.
   b. *Incision of the septal cartilage*: The cartilage is incised anterior to the deformity, taking care to avoid incising the mucosa on the opposite side.
   c. *Elevation of the submucoperichondrial flap on the contralateral side*: As described above, it is performed on the opposite side.

d. *Correction of the septal deformity*: The deviated septal cartilage is commonly resected, but may also be released from the adjacent bone and repositioned, crushed, or scored (see definitions) in order to address the deformity.

e. *Removal of septal bone (if indicated)*: Removal of portions of the maxillary crest may be required to correct the deformity.

5. *Closure*: The right and left mucoperichondrial flaps are laid back together and the nasal cavities are inspected to ensure adequate correction of the septal deformity. A variety of techniques can be used to close the incision and secure the flaps in place, including the following:

a. *Simple sutures*: The mucosal incision may be sutured closed.

b. *Quilting sutures*: A quilting stitch can be performed by suturing the opposing mucoperichondrial flaps together.

c. *Nasal stents*: A nasal stent may be placed in each nasal cavity to approximate the mucoperichondrial flaps. Stents are typically removed within 7 days of surgery.

d. *Nasal packing*: May similarly be used to stent the nasal cavities, approximate the mucoperichondrial flaps and aid in hemostasis.

6. *Dressing*: A moustache, or drip dressing, is commonly placed under the nose to contain postoperative bleeding.

COMPLICATIONS OF SEPTOPLASTY

When counseling a patient on the option of septoplasty, the following potential complications should be discussed preoperatively:[2]

1. *Nasal obstruction*: The most common complication of endonasal surgery is synechiae or scar band formation. Although potentially asymptomatic, synechiae can result in nasal obstruction, compromising symptomatic improvement following septoplasty. Synechiae are treated by lysis, typically in the office setting. It is important to note that postoperative

nasal obstruction is not always the result of scar tissue formation. Although the vast majority of patients note significant symptomatic improvement following septoplasty, due to the resiliency of the septal cartilage, septal deviation may persist or recur following the procedure.

2. *Bleeding*: Both epistaxis and septal hematoma formation are potential complications of septoplasty. Intraoperative hemostasis, quilting sutures, nasal stents, nasal packing, and postoperative epistaxis precautions are measures employed to prevent bleeding complications. Septal hematoma formation should be suspected in patients who present with significant nasal pain accompanied by septal fullness on anterior rhinoscopy. Although most cases of epistaxis can be managed with nasal packing, septal hematoma requires evacuation of the blood clot in addition to obtaining hemostasis. When left untreated, septal hematoma may lead to avascular necrosis of the septal cartilage with resultant septal abscess and/or saddle-nose deformity (*see* Rhinoplasty in Chapter 9).

3. *Septal perforation*: A septal perforation, or hole, may form if opposing tears occur in the mucoperichondrial flaps during septoplasty. Perforations can often be prevented in this situation by suturing the tears closed and placing a piece of cartilage between the two sites. While perforations of the posterior septum are typically asymptomatic, anterior perforations may cause whistling, bleeding, and crusting. If symptomatic, septal perforation may necessitate surgical repair or, alternatively, placement of a septal button, a prosthetic device placed to occlude the perforation.

4. *Hypoesthesia*: Hypoesthesia, or numbness, of the anterior hard palate, maxillary incisors, upper lip, and nasal septum my occur postoperatively due to stretching of or damage to the nasopalatine nerve, a branch of the maxillary division of the trigeminal nerve, CNV2, which traverses the nasal septum. Hypoesthesia is typically transient, but may be permanent in nature.

5. *Cosmetic deformity*: The quadrangular cartilage is an integral component of the structural support of the external nose. If care is not taken during septoplasty to preserve superior and caudal cartilaginous struts of 1–1.5 cm, cosmetic deformities such as tip ptosis or saddle-nose deformity may result (*see* the discussion of rhinoplasty in Chapter 9).

6. *Infection*: As noted earlier, septal abscess is a potential complication of septoplasty. Another rare but potentially life-threatening infectious complication is toxic shock syndrome (TSS). This syndrome is caused by a toxin, most commonly associated with *Staphylococcus aureus* infection, and leads to multiorgan system failure. Because TSS can occur secondary to nasal packing, patients must always be placed on an antibiotic with staphylococcal coverage while nasal packing is in place.

7. *Cribriform plate injury*: Because the perpendicular plate of the ethmoid bone is contiguous with the cribriform plate, torque placed on the nasal septum during septoplasty can result in injury to the cribriform plate with the following serious sequelae. By taking care to sharply separate the superior nasal septum from the area of dissection, such complications are drastically reduced.

   a. *Anosmia*: Lack of sense of smell (*see* Chapter 29).

   b. *Cerebrospinal fluid (CSF) rhinorrhea*: Cerebrospinal fluid may leak into the nasal cavity through a fracture of the cribriform plate. Cerebrospinal fluid rhinorrhea is associated with an increased risk of meningitis and requires immediate repair if noted intraoperatively. When CSF leaks occur postoperatively, conservative measures such as bed rest and lumbar drain placement can be considered prior to surgical repair.

   c. *Tension pneumocephalus*: Tension pneumocephalus occurs when air enters the intracranial cavity via a cribriform plate fracture. The air is unable to escape through the fracture site, expanding pneumocephalus leads to compression of the brain parenchyma, resulting in mental status changes. Tension pneumocephalus is a surgical emergency requiring neurosurgical evacuation.

8. Although exceedingly rare, unilateral blindness and death have also been reported to occur as complications of septoplasty.

REFERENCES

1. Lemonnier LA. Endoscopic septoplasty. Oper Tech Otolaryngol. 2014;25(2):156-9.
2. Bloom JD, Kaplan SE, Bleier BS, et al. Septoplasty complications: avoidance and management. Otolaryngol Clin North Am. 2009;42(3):463-81.

Section

7

Pediatric ENT

Section Editor: *Donald Solomon*

Chapter 33

Embryology of Head and Neck Congenital Malformations

Glenn Isaacson

EMBRYOLOGY OF EAR ANOMALIES

Outer Ear

The auricle or pinna is formed from the fusion of six raised soft tissue swellings (hillocks) on the surface of the embryo. Three of these hillocks are derived from the first branchial arch (Meckel) and three from the second branchial arch (Reichert) during the 5th and 6th weeks of intrauterine life. Growth of the fused tissues, guided by the pull of the intrinsic muscles of the ear, creates the folds of the helix, antihelix, and tragus.

The ear canal is formed from an invagination of surface epithelium in the 5th week of intrauterine life. This solid core of cells meets a similar evagination from the pharynx, trapping a layer of mesothelium in between. Fusion of these cells at the juncture results in the formation of the three layers of the tympanic membrane. Recanalization of the external ear canal occurs in the second trimester and is complete at ~28 weeks' gestation; vernix-like material is left behind. The external auditory meatus is formed from an invagination of squamous epithelium from the first branchial cleft. This solid core of tissue recanalizes at the beginning of the third trimester.

Microtia: Incomplete development and growth of the pinna can lead to a small, deformed, or absent pinna. Microtia and anotia occur in1–3 per 10,000 births. They occur more frequently in boys, at increased altitude, with increasing birth order, in infants of diabetic mothers, and infants with prenatal exposure to isotretinoin, thalidomide, or alcohol.

Preauricular pits: Preauricular pits, which are small indentations located anterior to the helix and superior to the tragus of the ear (bilateral in 25–50% of cases), represent the most common fusion abnormality of the auricular hillocks. They are present in 1% of White, 5% of Black, and 10% of Asian children and occur with increased frequency in some families. Associated congenital anomalies occur in approximately one third of the sporadic cases and none of the familial ones. Children with preauricular pits or tags are at five times the risk of the general population for permanent hearing impairment.

Infants with preauricular pits should have formal audiologic evaluation. Preauricular pits may be the first indication of branchio-oto-renal syndrome (BOR), the most common inherited syndrome causing hearing loss. Branchio-oto-renal syndrome is an autosomal dominant syndrome characterized by sensorineural hearing loss, preauricular pits, branchial cysts, malformed ears, and renal anomalies, including renal dysplasia and bifid renal pelvises. Patients with BOR have a variety of mutations that range from single nucleotide changes to complex genomic rearrangements. Approximately 70% of cases are due to mutations in the EYA1 gene.

Aural atresia: Failure of complete invagination of the external auditory canal results in an absent or stenotic ear canal and improper formation of the eardrum. Failure of recanalization results in membranous stenosis or atresia.

Formation of the ossicles occurs at the same time as the invagination of the first branchial cleft. Associated abnormalities of the ossicles, particularly fusion of the ossicles to each other or to atretic bone in the auditory canal, occur commonly in children with aural atresia.

Children who have unilateral aural atresia seldom require surgery if the pinna is well formed and the contralateral ear has normal hearing. Such children receive limited benefit from a bone-conduction hearing aid, since they have normal hearing perception and bone-conduction hearing aids do not help localize sound. Amplification is important if the child has hearing loss in the contralateral ear. There may be benefit to the use of a bone-anchored aid.[1]

Children with unrepaired aural atresia also have a risk of developing middle ear cholesteatoma. Persistent ear pain or fever may be the only clues to this condition, which is diagnosed with computed tomography (CT).[2,3]

Bilateral aural atresia is associated with a maximal conductive hearing loss (~ 60 dB) and requires early intervention. Children with bilateral aural atresia should be fitted with a bone-conduction hearing aid within weeks of birth to assist with early language acquisition. Bone-anchored hearing aids have gained greater acceptance as an alternative for hearing habilitation in children with bilateral aural atresia.[4]

Surgery to correct aural atresia usually is performed toward the end of the first decade of life, when substantial mastoid development has occurred. Surgery entails the creation of a new ear canal and ear drum, providing a skin lining for the canal and drum, and mobilizing or repositioning the ossicles to allow transmission of sound. Surgery is more likely to be successful if extensive pneumatization of the mastoid air cells is present and the stapes is mobile. One of the major risks of this surgery is injury to the facial nerve or the dura of the middle cranial fossa. Thus, the procedure should be performed by an experienced otologist and with electrophysiologic facial nerve monitoring. The new ear canal often requires cleaning and care for life.[5]

Middle Ear

The ossicles are formed by condensation of mesenchyme derived from the first and second branchial arches. Cartilage develops and gradually is replaced by bone in the second and third trimesters. The ossicles are near adult size and adult ossification at the time of birth. Cartilage remains only at the articulations.

The cavity of the middle ear forms when endoderm evaginating from the first pharyngeal pouch invades the mesoderm of the middle ear. This pouch narrows to form the lining of the eustachian tube near the nasopharynx and spawns finger-like projections that surround the developing ossicles. The lateral-most projection of endoderm creates the inner layer of the tympanic membrane.

At birth, the middle ear is narrow and contains residual mesenchyme and amniotic fluid. Within minutes of birth and spontaneous breathing, air enters the eustachian tube, displacing amniotic fluid to create a pneumatized cavity.

Middle ear malformations: Congenital malformations of the ossicles may cause conductive hearing loss. Ossicular and other middle ear malformations occur as part of syndromes (e.g. Treacher Collins, branchio-oto-renal, Stickler, Shprintzen, or Beckwith–Wiedemann), and occasionally as isolated events. The most common abnormalities of the ossicles are fixation of the malleus and/or incus, incudostapedial discontinuity, and stapes fixation. Each of these abnormalities is surgically correctable; correction of stapes fixation is most likely to fail because of the delicate attachment of the stapes to the inner ear.[6]

Inner Ear

The cochlea and vestibular system is derived from epithelium that migrates deep from within the embryonic surface early in development. This epithelium forms a fluid-filled cyst called the otic vesicle. The otic vesicle folds, spirals, and elongates to form the membranous labyrinth. Neural cells arising in the eighth cranial nerve invade the labyrinth. By the end of the second trimester, the inner ear is developed sufficiently to transduce vibratory energy into neural impulses that are transmitted to the brain.

Inner ear malformations: The cochlea arises from a cystic invagination of surface epithelium (the otocyst) that pulls away from the vestibular portion of the inner ear during the first trimester and forms an elongating spiral. Failure of development along this pathway results in the Michel and Mondini anomalies, which can be detected with high-resolution CT. The Michel malformation occurs when the labyrinth is absent or reduced to a single cystic cavity. The Mondini malformation is present when cochlear growth is arrested at < 1 complete turn (2.75 turns are normal). It is associated with complete deafness and vestibular malformations.[7]

Minor abnormalities in the labyrinthine structure can also result in partial or progressive hearing loss. The large vestibular aqueduct syndrome is one of the better known syndromes; it may affect one or both ears. The hearing loss in children with large vestibular aqueduct syndrome may be sensorineural or mixed. Some patients have normal hearing at birth, followed by progressive or fluctuating hearing loss. Sudden hearing loss may occur spontaneously or after minor head trauma.[7]

EMBRYOLOGY OF THE NOSE

The nose arises from the nasal placodes during the 3rd and 4th weeks of intrauterine life. Each nasal placode is a local thickening of the surface ectoderm on the lateral surface of the head of the embryo, just above the oral stoma. The nasal placodes sink into the mesenchyme to form the depressions that will become the nostrils. Hypertrophy of the tissue surrounding the nasal placodes creates the medial and lateral nasal prominences.

The nostrils migrate medially, and their soft tissues fuse as the orbits begin their medial migration. The medial nasal processes form the anterior nasal septum, mid-upper lip, and a portion of the anterior hard palate.[8] The nasofrontal process originates from the floor of the anterior cranial fossa as a division of the prosencephalon. The nasofrontal process forms the posterior nasal septum and the ethmoid, nasal, and premaxillary bones. The posterior nasal and oral cavities are separated by the oronasal membrane until the 6th or 7th week of intrauterine life, when the oronasal membrane is resorbed to form the primitive choanae.

The prenasal space is located between the nasal and frontal bones during embryogenesis. It extends from the nasal skin to the foramen cecum, an area of the anterior cranial fossa where some prolapse of the dura may occur. The foramen cecum fuses with the fonticulus frontalis to form the cribriform plate.[9]

Holoprosencephaly

Improper segmentation and growth of the prosencephalon affects the brain and the face; the series of midface and central nervous system (CNS) malformations that result are collectively known as the holoprosencephalies. The etiology of holoprosencephaly is heterogeneous, with both genetic and environmental causes. Holoprosencephalies are characterized by varying degrees of hypotelorism, facial clefts, nasal malformations, and incomplete separation of the two halves of the brain. These abnormalities may be detected prenatally through ultrasound examination.[10]

The clinical manifestations of holoprosencephaly range from an isolated single maxillary incisor to cebocephaly (e.g. small mouth, single nostril, and close-set eyes) or cyclopia. The brain may be normal, but incomplete separation of the hemispheres (semilobar holoprosencephaly), single common ventricle, and absence of the corpus callosum (alobar holoprosencephaly) are frequent occurrences. As a general rule, the more severe the facial malformations, the worse the abnormalities of the CNS.[11] The more severe forms of holoprosencephaly often are lethal. Mental retardation and seizures are common occurrences in survivors. Children with semilobar holoprosencephaly may be asymptomatic and have normal mentation.[12]

Nasal Encephaloceles

Nasal encephaloceles result from congenital fusion abnormalities at the nasal root. These are herniations of brain, meninges, and/or cerebrospinal fluid through a defect in the skull. They communicate freely with the subarachnoid space and intracranial ventricular system. They occur in ~ 1 in 4,000 live births and are thought to be caused by the defective closure of the anterior neuropore during the 4th week of embryogenesis.

Nasal encephaloceles may be frontoethmoidal (60%), basal (30%), or both (10%). Frontoethmoidal cephaloceles usually are evident at birth, presenting as a skin-covered mass at the root of the nose. Lesions that retain a connection with the subarachnoid space enlarge when the infant cries or strains. Basal cephaloceles are not apparent externally; they may cause nasal obstruction or symptoms related to the herniation of basal structures.[13]

Surgical correction of nasal cephaloceles improves appearance and decreases the risk of developing meningitis. Cephaloceles typically are treated through a frontal craniotomy. The soft tissue and nose are approached only after dysplastic brain tissue is transected and a watertight closure of the dural defect is achieved. Neurologic outcome depends upon the extent of excision that is necessary. Normal mentation is possible after correction of pure meningoceles or small encephaloceles. In contrast, persistent neurologic deficits are common occurrences after excision of large portions of brain parenchyma.[14]

THYROGLOSSAL DUCT ANOMALIES

The thyroid gland forms from a diverticulum (median thyroid anlage) located between the anterior and posterior muscle complexes of the tongue at week 3 of gestation. As the embryo grows, the diverticulum is displaced caudally into the neck and fuses with components from the fourth and fifth branchial pouches (lateral thyroid anlage). The descent continues anterior to or through the hyoid bone with the median anlage elongating into the thyroglossal duct. By weeks 5–8 of gestation, the thyroglossal duct obliterates, leaving a proximal remnant, the foramen cecum, at the base of the tongue and a distal remnant, the pyramidal lobe of the thyroid. If the duct fails to obliterate before the formation of the mesodermal anlage of the hyoid bone, it will persist as a cyst.[15]

Thyroglossal duct anomalies are the second most common neck mass behind adenopathy, and the most common congenital anomaly of the neck. Two thirds of thyroglossal duct anomalies will be diagnosed within the first three decades of life, with over half being identified before 10 years of age. The most common presentation is that of a painless cystic neck mass near the hyoid bone in the midline. Although they will most commonly be found immediately adjacent to the hyoid (66%), they can also be located between the tongue and hyoid, between the hyoid and pyramidal lobe, within the tongue, or within the thyroid. The mass will usually move with swallowing or protrusion of the tongue. Approximately one third will present with a concurrent or prior infection, which is the more common presentation in adults.[16] One fourth of patients will present with a draining sinus, which results from spontaneous drainage or surgical drainage of an abscess.

Elective surgical excision is the treatment of choice for uncomplicated thyroglossal duct cysts in order to prevent infection of the cyst. The Sistrunk procedure rather than simple excision is performed to reduce recurrence risk. In this operation, the central portion of the hyoid bone is excised in continuity with the cyst, and the tract is dissected with a core of tissue from the muscle at the base of the tongue to the foramen cecum. No attempt is made to locate the thyroglossal duct tract above the hyoid as it is fragile and often branches within the tongue musculature.[17] Recurrent thyroglossal duct cysts are best treated by en bloc central neck dissection rather than re-excision.[18]

BRANCHIAL CLEFT ANOMALIES

Branchial anomalies compose ~30% of congenital neck masses and can present as cysts, sinuses, or fistulae. They are equally common in men and women, and usually present in childhood or early adulthood. By the end of the 4th week of gestation, there are four well-defined pairs of arches and two rudimentary arches. These are lined externally by ectoderm and internally by endoderm, with mesoderm in between. The mesoderm contains the dominant artery, nerve, cartilage rod, and muscle for each arch. Each arch is separated by clefts externally and pouches internally. In humans, the clefts and pouches are gradually obliterated by mesenchyme to form the mature head and neck structures. Branchial anomalies result from incomplete obliteration of the clefts and pouches.

Branchial anomalies are classified by the cleft or pouch of origin, which is determined by the internal opening of the sinus and its relationship to nerves, arteries, and muscles.

First cleft anomalies account for only 1% of branchial cleft malformations. The first arch, or mandibular arch, forms the mandible, part of the maxillary process of the upper jaw, and portions of the inner ear. The first cleft and pouch form the external auditory canal, eustachian tube, middle ear cavity, and mastoid air cells. Therefore, first cleft anomalies enter either the external auditory canal or occasionally the middle ear. First cleft anomalies course close to the parotid gland, especially the superficial lobe, traveling above, between, or below the facial nerve branches. First cleft anomalies are classified as type I or type II. Type I lesions are duplications of the membranous external auditory canal, are composed of ectoderm only, course lateral to the facial nerve, and present as swellings near the ear. Type II lesions have ectoderm and mesoderm, can contain cartilage, pass medial to the facial nerve, and present as preauricular, infra-auricular, or postauricular swellings inferior to the angle of the mandible or anterior to the sternocleidomastoid (SCM) muscle.[19]

The surgical resection of first arch anomalies often requires at least partial facial nerve dissection and superficial parotidectomy. It is also necessary to excise any involved skin or cartilage of the external auditory canal. If the tract extends medial to the tympanic membrane, it may be necessary to transect the tract and remove the medial portion during a second procedure. Compared to tracts that go to the external auditory canal, tracts going to the middle ear tend to lie deep to the facial nerve. However, tracts can split around the nerve.

Second branchial cleft anomalies are the most common. The second arch, or hyoid arch, forms the hyoid bone and adjacent areas of the neck. The second pouch develops into the palatine tonsil and tonsillar fossa. Thus, second cleft anomalies enter the tonsillar fossa pass close to the glossopharyngeal and hypoglossal nerves on their course to the fossa.[20]

Second brachial cleft anomalies present as a fistula or cyst in the lower, anterolateral neck. Cysts are most commonly diagnosed in adults during the third and fifth decades as a nontender mass, which can acutely increase in size after an upper respiratory infection.[21] The enlargement can lead to respiratory compromise, torticollis, or dysphagia. Fistulae, however, are usually diagnosed in infancy or childhood and present as chronic drainage from an opening along the anterior border of the SCM in the lower third of the neck.

Surgical resection of second cleft anomalies can be approached via a transverse cervical incision placed within a natural skin fold. Cysts can be located either superficially or deep to the cervical fascia. A careful exploration of an associated fistula tract must be performed with a complete excision of the entire tract if one is found. Fistulas are dissected from cervical opening to the tonsillar fossa. This sometimes requires stairstep incisions. Tonsillectomy or cauterization of the proximal tract is occasionally required for recurrent lesions.

Third and fourth branchial anomalies are rare. The third and fourth pouches form the pharynx below the hyoid bone; thus these sinuses and fistulae will enter into the pyriform sinus. Third and fourth branchial anomalies normally contain thymic tissue, as will cysts and sinuses that result from thymic or parathyroid rests, but only branchial anomalies will have the connection to the pyriform sinus. Third arch anomalies present as cystic structures located at the lower, anterior border of the SCM at the level of the superior pole of the thyroid. In childhood, they may present as "thyroid abscess" that recur after surgical drainage.[22] Endoscopic cauterization of the tract or open excision prevents recurrence.[23] Resection of a portion of the thyroid ala may be necessary to expose the proximal end of the tract at the pyriform sinus.[24]

EMBRYOLOGY OF LARYNGEAL ATRESIA, STENOSIS, AND CLEFT

The formation of a median pharyngeal groove presages the appearance of the respiratory tract. At ~25 days of intrauterine life, the anlagen of the larynx, trachea, bronchi, and lungs arise from a ventromedial diverticulum of the foregut called the tracheobronchial groove. The cartilage of the trachea and connective tissue and the muscle of the trachea and esophagus are derived from splanchnic mesenchyme. Lateral furrows develop on each side of the ventromedial diverticulum, deepen, and join to form the tracheoesophageal septum.

During the 5th and 6th weeks, the tracheoesophageal septum extends to the first tracheal ring. By the time the embryo is 13–17 mm in length, laryngeal cartilage and muscle development are clearly identifiable, and lateral cricoid condensation is underway. By the 7th week of development, the cricoid ring is complete, and the cartilaginous hyoid is visible below the epiglottis. Definitive tracheal cartilage appears at this stage, and the esophagus has four discrete layers. The larynx, trachea, and esophagus are well formed by the end of the embryologic period.[25]

Atresia and Stenosis

Laryngeal atresia is thought to be caused by the failure of epithelial growth and recanalization in the vestibule and subglottic regions.[26] The three types of laryngeal atresia are as follows:

- *Type 1*: Supraglottic obstruction, absent vestibule, and stenotic subglottis.
- *Type 2*: Supraglottic obstruction separates the primitive vestibule from the normal subglottis.
- *Type 3*: Perforated membrane partly obstructs the glottis (laryngeal web).

Most infants with laryngeal atresia present with asphyxia at the time of birth. Performing an emergent tracheotomy soon after delivery is necessary for survival because the imperforate larynx cannot be intubated.

Laryngeal Clefts

Posterior laryngeal clefts are thought to result from failed fusion of the two lateral growth centers of the posterior cricoid cartilage at 6–7 weeks of intrauterine life. Further aborted development of the tracheoesophageal septum may result in a laryngotracheoesophageal cleft that extends to the carina. Laryngeal clefts occur in ~ 1 in 10,000 to 1 in 20,000 live births. They are more common in boys than girls, with a male to female ratio of 5:3.

Posterior laryngeal clefts and laryngotracheoesophageal clefts may be classified according to anatomic or clinical criteria. The Benjamin classification describes five types:

- Occult clefts can be appreciated only by palpation and measurement of the interarytenoid height.
- Type 1 clefts are limited to the supraglottic, interarytenoid area.
- Type 2 clefts show partial clefting of the posterior cricoid cartilage, sometimes with a mucosal bridge across the cartilaginous gap.
- Type 3 clefts involve the entire cricoid and the cervical portion of the tracheoesophageal membrane, stopping above the thoracic inlet.
- Type 4 clefts involve a major portion of the intrathoracic tracheoesophageal wall.[27]

The treatment for these disorders depends upon the type of cleft and severity of associated symptoms. Alternatives to surgery for type 1 clefts may include endoscopic injection augmentation of the posterior glottis and medical therapy to control gastroesophageal reflux and aspiration.[28]

REFERENCES

1. Danhaeur JL, Johnson CE, Mixon M. Does the evidence support use of the Baha implant system (Baha) in patients with congenital unilateral aural atresia? J Am Acad Audiol. 2010;21:274-86.

2. Casale G, Nicholas BD, Kesser BW. Acquired ear canal cholesteatoma in congenital aural atresia/stenosis. Otol Neurotol. 2014;35(8):1474-9.

3. Sone M, Naganawa S, Yoshida T, et al. Imaging findings in a case with cholesteatoma in complete aural atresia. Am J Otolaryngol. 2010;31(4):297-9.

4. Ricci G, Volpe AD, Faralli M, et al. Bone-anchored hearing aids (Baha) in congenital aural atresia: personal experience. Int J Pediatr Otorhinolaryngol. 2011;75(3):342-6.

5. Rosen EJ. Congenital aural atresia. Grand Rounds Presentation, Department of Otolaryngology, University of Texas Medical Branch, January 8, 2003. Available from http://www.utmb.edu/otoref/Grnds/Congenital-Aural-Atresia-2003-01/Congenital-Aural-Atresia-slides-030108.pdf. Accessed on May 26, 2016.

6. Swartz JD, Faerber EN. Congenital malformations of the external and middle ear: high-resolution CT findings of surgical import. AJR Am J Roentgenol. 1985;144:501-6.

7. Niknejad MT. Mondini malformation. [online] Available from http://radiopaedia.org/cases/mondini-malformation.

8. Som PM, Naidich TP. Illustrated review of the embryology and development of the facial region, part 1: early face and lateral nasal cavities. AJNR Am J Neuroradiol. 2013;34:2233-40.

9. Balasubramanian T. Embryology nose and paranasal sinuses. [online] Available from www.slideshare.net/drtbalu/embryology-nose-and-paranasal-sinuses.

10. Department of Pediatrics, Division of Genetics and Metabolism, University of Florida. Teaching resources: holoprosencephaly. [online] Available from www.peds.ufl.edu/divisions/genetics/teaching/brain_malformations/holoprosencephaly.htm. Accessed on May 26, 2016.

11. Rabou AA. Holoprosencephaly-semilobar type. [online] Available from http://radiopaedia.org/cases/holoprosencephaly-semilobar-type.

12. Winter TC, Kennedy AM, Woodward PJ. Holoprosencephaly: a survey of the entity, with embryology and fetal imaging. Radiographics. 2015;35(1):275-90.

13. Knipe H, Hosn SS, et al. Nasal encephalocele. [online] Available from http://radiopaedia.org/articles/nasal-encephalocoele.

14. Gun R, Tosun F, Durmaz A, et al. Predictors of surgical approaches for the repair of anterior cranial base encephaloceles. Eur Arch Otorhinolaryngol. 2013;270(4):1299-305.

15. Gaillard F. Thyroglossal duct: diagram. [online] Available from http://radiopaedia.org/cases/thyroglossal-duct-diagram.

16. Gaillard F. Thyroglossal duct cyst. [online] Available from http://radiopaedia.org/cases/thyroglossal-duct-cyst-2.

17. Christiansen LL. Iowa Head and Neck Protocols: Thyroglossal duct cyst excision. [online] Available from https://wiki.uiowa.edu/display/protocols/Thyroglossal+Duct+Cyst+Excision.

18. Kim MK, Pawel BR, Isaacson G. Central neck dissection for the treatment of recurrent thyoglossal duct cysts in childhood. Otolaryngol Head Neck Surg. 1999;121(5):543-7.

19. Cagley JR. Iowa Head and Neck Protocols: First branchial cleft cyst. [online] Available from https://wiki.uiowa.edu/display/protocols/First+Branchial+Cleft+Cyst+-+Rads.

20. Ghorayeb BY. Pictures and imaging of branchial cleft cysts. [online] Available from www.ghorayeb.com/branchialcleft.html.

21. Hsu CCT. Infection 2nd branchial cleft cyst and fistula tract from tonsillitis. [online] Available from http://radiopaedia.org/cases/infected-2nd-branchial-cleft-cyst-and-fistula-tract-from-tonsilits.

22. Kruiff S, Sywak MS, Sidhu SB, et al. Thyroidal abscesses in third and fourth branchial anomalies: not only a paediatric diagnosis. ANZ J Surg. 2015;85(7-8):578-81.

23. Sun JY, Berg EE, McClay JE. Endoscopic cauterization of congenital pyriform fossa sinus tracts: an 18-year experience. JAMA Otolaryngol Head Neck Surg. 2014;140(2):112-7.

24. Rosenfeld RM, Biller HF. Fourth branchial pouch sinus: diagnosis and treatment. Otolaryngol Head Neck Surg. 1991;105(1):44-50.

25. Valcamonico A, Goncalves LF, Jeanty P. Larynx, atresia. [online] Available from www.sonoworld.com/fetus/page.aspx?id=401.

26. Embryology of the respiratory system: clinical correlations. [online] Available from http://embryology4genius.weebly.com/clinial-correlations.html. Accessed on May 26, 2016.

27. McCulloch TM, Jaffe D. Head and neck disorders affecting swallowing. [online] Available from www.nature.com/gimo/contents/pt1/fig_tab/gimo36_F1.html.

28. Rahbar R, Rouillon I, Roger G, et al. The presentation and management of laryngeal cleft: a 10-year experience. Arch Otolaryngol Head Neck Surg. 2006;132(12):1335-41.

Chapter 34

Congenital Hearing Loss

Gillian R Diercks, Michael S Cohen

Chief Complaint
"Failed newborn hearing screen".

DEFINITIONS

Pars superior: Utricle and semicircular canals.

Pars inferior: Saccule and cochlea.

Michel's aplasia: Failure of inner ear development (no cochlea or labyrinth) during the 3rd week of development. Contraindication to cochlear implantation.

Mondini's aplasia: Fewer than 2.5 cochlear turns due to incomplete partitioning during the 7th week of development (Figs. 34.1A to C). It may be associated with enlarged vestibular aqueduct (EVA) and abnormal labyrinth. Often autosomal-dominant inheritance pattern, associated with Pendred, Waardenburg, Treacher Collins, CHARGE (coloboma, heart defects, choanal atresia, retarded growth and development, genital abnormalities, and ear anomalies), and branchio-oto-renal (BOR) syndromes.

Bing–Siebenmann aplasia: Complete absence of the membranous labyrinth.

Scheibe dysplasia: Malformation of the cochlea and saccule (pars inferior). The most common cochlear deformity, associated with Jervell and Lange-Nielsen, Usher, and Waardenburg syndromes.

Alexander aplasia: Partial aplasia of the cochlear duct. It is associated with high-frequency hearing loss.

Enlarged vestibular aqueduct: Width is >1.5 mm or greater than the width of the posterior semicircular canal on computed tomography (CT) scan (Figs. 34.1A to C). It results in progressive or sudden hearing loss after minor head trauma or barometric pressure changes. It is the most common inner ear anomaly, associated with Mondini aplasia, Pendred syndrome, and BOR.

EMBRYOLOGY AND DEVELOPMENT

The external, middle, and inner ear structures form from different precursors and at different times during development. Errors that occur early in development are associated with more severe anomalies. External and middle ear deformities are often concurrent.

External Ear

The auricle forms during the 6th week of development from mesoderm of the first and second branchial arches, which form six hillocks of His. The hillocks fuse during the 12th week. Failure of appropriate formation results in microtia and failure of fusion results in branchial sinus formation. The external ear canal begins to form from the ectodermally derived first groove at 8th week, core hollows from 21–28 weeks.

Middle Ear

Ossicles form from branchial arch mesoderm during weeks 6–16 of development. First arch: malleus head and neck, incus short process. Second arch: manubrium, stapes, incus long, and lenticular processes.

Inner Ear

Otic placode is composed of neural tissue and ectoderm surrounded by mesoderm forms during 3rd and 4th weeks of

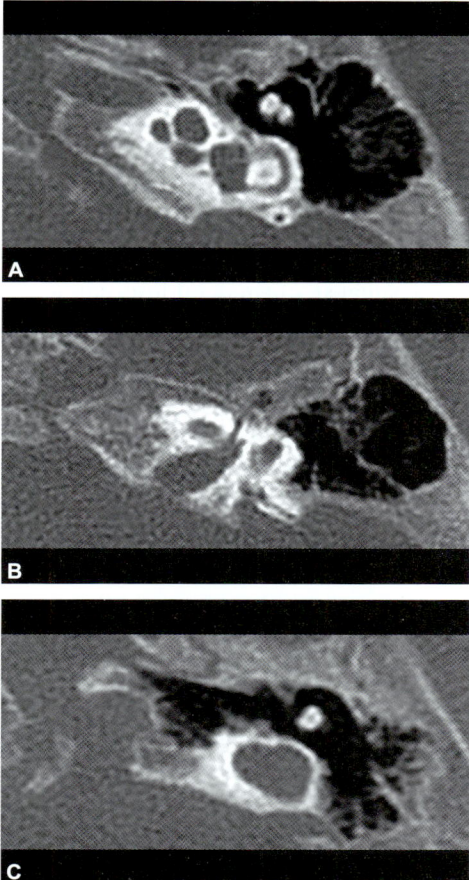

Figs. 34.1A to C: Congenital inner ear deformities and their appearance on computed tomography imaging (all left ears and axial plane). (A) Mondini aplasia with abnormal labyrinth—incomplete partition between turns of cochlea, dilated vestibule. (B) Enlarged vestibular aqueduct—vestibular aqueduct larger than diameter of posterior semicircular canal. (C) Common cavity deformity—absence of cochlea and semicircular canals, dilated vestibular organ.

gestation. The pars superior forms by the 6th week and pars inferior by the 12th week. The organ of Corti, including the stria vascularis, tectorial membrane, and inner and outer hair cells, does not form even after the 20th week of development.

AUDIOLOGIC EVALUATION OF THE NEWBORN AND CHILD (FLOWCHART 34.1)

- *Otoacoustic emissions*: Produced by outer hair cells spontaneously (50% of individuals) or in response to "click" stimuli, and suggest normal middle ear and cochlear function, used in newborn hearing screening. They are absent if middle ear pathology or sensorineural hearing loss (SNHL) > 30 dB are present.
- *Auditory brainstem response (ABR):* Evoked responses by the auditory (eighth) nerve, brainstem, and brain to sound. Response is not affected by sedation; used after failed newborn hearing screen. Thresholds are typically 10–20 dB above behavioral thresholds. Absent if SNHL > 60 dB; response is impaired by lidocaine, phenytoin, diazepam.
- *Behavior observation audiometry*: Age 0–6 months. Observation of reflexive and unconditioned responses to a sound stimulus. Problems: unable to test ears separately and early habituation.
- *Visual reinforcement audiometry:* Age 6 months–2 years. Operant conditioning in which lights, motion, or a toy are used to positively reinforce a response to sound stimulus.
- *Conditioned play audiometry:* Age 2–5 years. Use of a game or task to reinforce a response to sound stimulus.

ETIOLOGY

Causes of congenital hearing loss are 50% environmental or idiopathic and 50% genetic (Flowchart 34.2).

Flowchart 34.1: Newborn hearing screen algorithm.

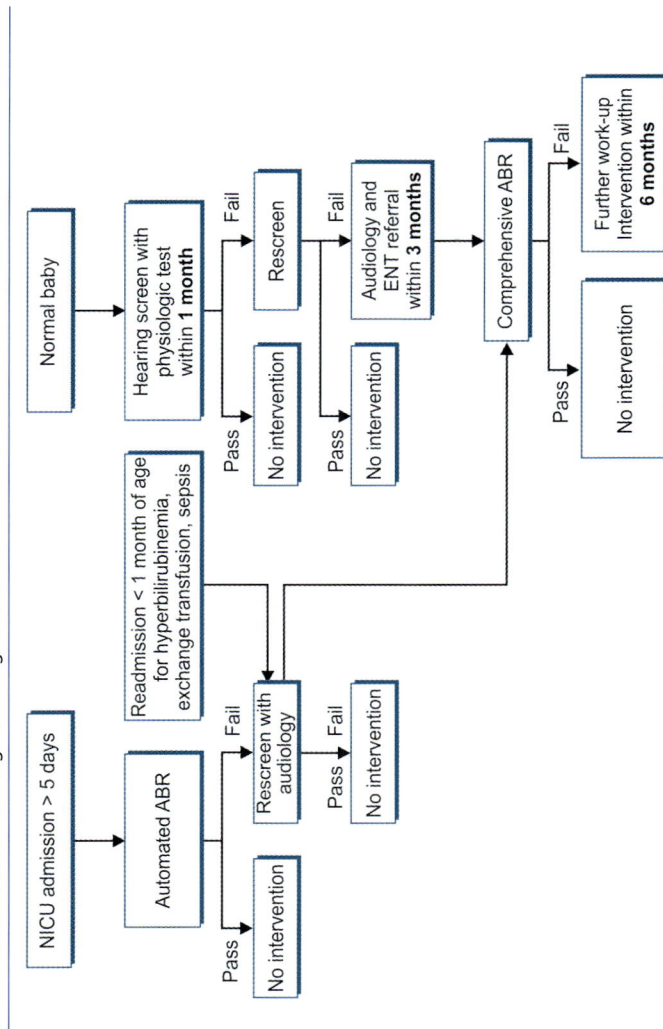

(NICU: Neonatal intensive care unit; ABR: Auditory brainstem response; ENT: Ear, nose and throat).

Flowchart 34.2: Hearing loss etiology.

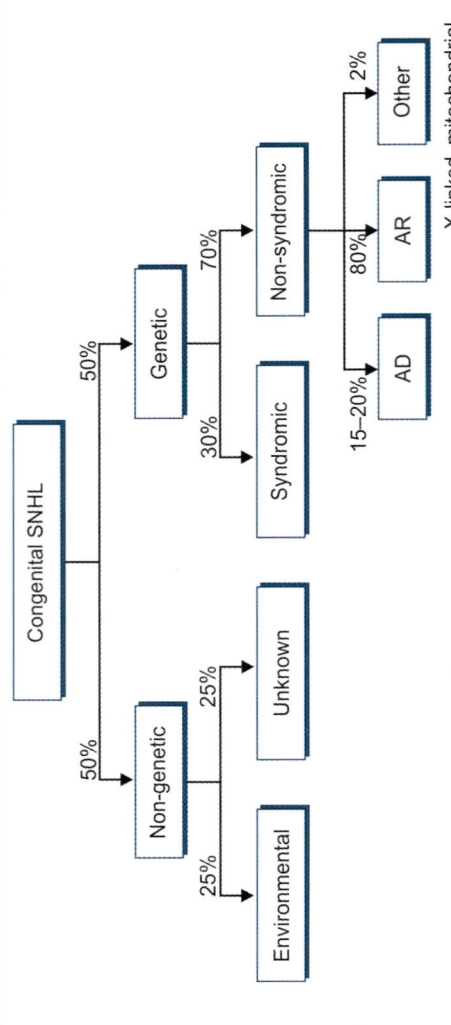

(SNHL: Sensorineural hearing loss; AD: Autosomal dominant; AR: Autosomal recessive).

Environmental Causes

Environmental causes of congenital hearing loss are presented in Table 34.1.

Genetic Causes

Genetic causes of congenital hearing loss are 30% syndromic and 70% nonsyndromic; 80% of nonsyndromic are autosomal recessive (Table 34.2).

DIAGNOSTIC WORKUP

Careful history and physical examination are required as they may provide important clues about etiology.

History

- *Prenatal history:* Maternal infections and exposures.
- *Birth history:* Weight, Apgar score, prematurity, exposure to ototoxic medications, history of jaundice, perinatal infection, history of intubation, neonatal intensive care unit admission, hypoxia, and extracorporeal membrane oxygenation (ECMO).
- *Developmental history:* Speech and motor milestones.
- *Medical/surgical history:* Disease or abnormalities involving other organ systems.
- Medications.
- *Family history:* Family history of vestibular or hearing disorders (go back three generations), family history of sudden death or cardiac abnormalities, and history of consanguinity.

Physical Examination

- *General appearance*: Tone.
- *HEENT (head, eye, ear, nose, and throat examination):* Presence/absence of nystagmus, appearance of external ear, presence of pitting in preauricular or cervical regions,

Table 34.1: Environmental causes of congenital hearing loss.

Etiology	Type of hearing loss	Defining characteristics
Exposure to ototoxic medications		
Perinatal factors		
Birth weight <1,500 g		
Apgar 0–4 at 1 min; 0–6 at 5 min		
Mechanical ventilation >5 days		
History of ECMO		
Hyperbilirubinemia	SNHL	Deposition and injury to dorsal and ventral cochlear nuclei
Infectious		
Rubella	Bilateral SNHL "Cookie bite" pattern audiogram Hearing loss may be delayed	Strial atrophy, injury to organ of Corti Deafness, congenital cataracts, mental retardation, cardiac defects
Cytomegalovirus	Unilateral or bilateral SNHL Hearing loss may be delayed	Most common cause of nongenetic deafness Associated with hepatosplenomegaly, petechiae, jaundice, intracerebral calcifications

Contd...

Contd...

Etiology	Type of hearing loss	Defining characteristics
Syphilis	SNHL, often bilateral May be progressive	Osteitis, endolymphatic hydrops Saddle nose, cranial bossing, saber shin, Hutchinson's teeth, short stature, interstitial keratitis Hennebert sign (+ fistula test) Tullio phenomenon
Meningitis (neonate: *Escherichia coli*, Group B β-hemolytic streptococcus; older children: *Haemophilus influenza, Neisseria meningitis, Streptococcus pneumoniae*)	Bilateral SNHL	Associated with early development of labyrinthitis ossificans

(ECMO: Extracorporeal membrane oxygenation; SNHL: Sensorineural hearing loss)

Table 34.2: Genetic causes of congenital hearing loss.

Etiology	Gene	Type of hearing loss	Defining characteristics
Syndromic			
Autosomal recessive (mnemonic PUJ)			
Usher syndrome	Three types	Varying degrees of SNHL and vestibular dysfunction	Retinitis pigmentosa (RP) *Type 1: profound SNHL, absent vestibular function, early RP* *Type 2: moderate SNHL, normal vestibular function, RP at puberty* *Type 3: progressive SNHL, variable vestibular function, RP at puberty*
Pendred syndrome	SLC26A4 Chromosome 7	Variable SNHL, can be progressive	Mondini deformity EVA Euthyroid goiter after puberty (tyrosine iodination impaired)
Jervell and Lange-Nielsen	KVLQT1 mutation Chromosome 11	Profound SNHL	Potassium channel mutation QT interval prolongation Family history of sudden death or syncope
Autosomal dominant (mnemonic WANT CBS)			
Waardenburg syndrome	Pax 3 mutation Chromosome 2 Four types	SNHL	**Most common AD syndrome** White forelock Iris heterochromia Confluent brow Dystrophia canthorum (types 1 and 3) Limb abnormalities (type 3) Hirschsprung's disease (type 4)

Contd...

Contd...

Contd...

Etiology	Gene	Type of hearing loss	Defining characteristics
Goldenhar syndrome	Multifactorial	CHL SNHL	Hemifacial microsomia Microtia and aural atresia Abnormal course of CN VII Oculoauriculovertebral spectrum
Treacher Collins syndrome	TCOF1 mutation Chromosome 5	CHL	Antimongoloid slant Coloboma Malar hypoplasia Microtia and aural atresia
Stickler syndrome	COL11A2 mutation Chromosome 12	Progressive SNHL Mixed HL	Type 2 collagen disorder Myopia, vitreoretinal detachment Midface hypoplasia Cleft palate Hyperextension of joints
Branchio-oto-renal syndrome (BOR)	EYA1 mutation Chromosome 8	Mixed > CHL > SNHL	External ear malformation Inner ear malformations (60%) Branchial anomalies Renal abnormalities
Apert syndrome	FGFR2 mutation Chromosome 10	CHL	Craniofacial dysostosis with maxillary hypoplasia, frontal prominence Exophthalmos Syndactyly Stapes fixation

Contd...

Etiology	Gene	Type of hearing loss	Defining characteristics
Crouzon syndrome	FGFR2 mutation Chromosome 10	Mixed hearing loss	Cranial synostosis Hypertelorism Exophthalmos Parrot-beak shaped nose Small maxilla
CHARGE syndrome	CHD7 mutation Chromosome 8	Mixed or SNHL	Coloboma Cardiac defects Choanal atresia Retarded development Genital hypoplasia Ear anomalies (external and inner ear), including Mondini and absence of semicircular canals
Neurofibromatosis type 1	NF1 mutation Chromosome 17	SNHL	Central nervous system tumors 5% acoustic neuromas, usually unilateral Café-au-lait spots Iris Lisch nodules, optic gliomas Multiple neurofibromas

Contd...

Contd...

Etiology	Gene	Type of hearing loss	Defining characteristics
Neurofibromatosis type 2	NF2 mutation Chromosome 22	SNHL	95% acoustic neuromas, usually bilateral Subcapsular cataracts Café-au-lait spots
X-linked			
Alport syndrome	COL4A5 mutation	Progressive SNHL (starts after the age 10)	Type-IV collagen disorder Spiral ganglia and stria vascularis affected Renal dysplasia or agenesis
Perilymph gusher	POU3F4 mutation DFN3 locus chromosome X		
Nonsyndromic			
Autosomal recessive			
GJB2 (Connexin 26)	DFNB1 locus Chromosome 13 35delG mutation	Prelingual Profound SNHL (usually bilateral)	Most common nonsyndromic genetic cause of HL Gap junction protein mutation

(SNHL: Sensorineural hearing loss; EVA: Enlarged vestibular aqueduct; AD: Autosomal dominant; CHL: Conductive hearing loss; HL: Hearing loss; GJB2: Gap junction protein beta 2; CHARGE: Coloboma, heart defects, choanal atresia, retarded growth and development, genital abnormalities, and ear anomalies).

maxillary and mandibular development, cranial nerve (CN) examination including facial symmetry, palate examination; ear canal, tympanic membrane, and ossicles.

Audiology

- Auditory brainstem response if newborn hearing screen is abnormal.
- Audiometry, if age appropriate (can usually obtain behavioral audiometry in children > 9 months of age).

Imaging

- *Renal ultrasound:* Obtain in cases of progressive SNHL or if BOR is suspected.
- *Computed tomography versus magnetic resonance imaging (MRI) of the temporal bones:* Temporal bone imaging is recommended for all children with SNHL. Noncontrast CT is appropriate in many cases. Consider MRI in children with sudden or progressive hearing loss, unilateral hearing loss, concern for retrocochlear lesion, history of meningitis (evaluate for labyrinthitis ossificans), or preoperatively prior to cochlear implantation. Evaluate for bony and membranous inner ear malformations, size of internal auditory canal (IAC) (<3 mm with normal CN VII suggests the absence of CN VIII; >10 mm associated with perilymph gusher), and course of CN VII. Sagittal oblique reconstructions or direct imaging through IAC allow visualization of CN VII and cochlear, inferior vestibular, and superior vestibular divisions of VIII.

Ancillary Testing

- *Cytomegalovirus (CMV) testing:* Urine or salivary polymerase chain reaction or urine shell vial culture should be performed for all newborns with SNHL, ideally within 21 days of birth. Blood serology is not accurate in infants due to the presence of maternal antibodies as well as relatively poor immune response in infants. Cytomegalovirus does not cause hearing loss when acquired postnatally, and treatment for CMV-related hearing loss is both available and time sensitive. Cytomegalovirus may cause isolated hearing loss without microcephaly or other neurologic findings.

- Electrocardiography for all congenital hearing loss cases (rule out QT prolongation).
- Ophthalmology evaluation at 1 year of age.

Genetic Testing

- *Connexin 26/30 testing:* Consider if no obvious syndrome. Seventy percent of genetic hearing loss is nonsyndromic; 50% of nonsyndromic genetic loss is due to connexin 26/30 mutations.
- GeneChip analysis is continually evolving.
- Whole genome/whole exome sequencing is in development.

TREATMENT

- *Hearing preservation:* Protect residual hearing by avoidance of loud sounds, use of noise-reducing ear plugs and personal listening device volume controls. For children with EVA, recommend avoidance of head trauma or sudden pressure changes (scuba diving, air travel).
- *Amplification:* Preferential seating, frequency modulation system in school, and hearing aids.
- *Osseointegrated bone conduction devices (Baha Connect, Baha Attract, Ponto, Sophono):* Indicated in cases of aural atresia, chronic otitis externa unable to accommodate hearing aids, and bone conduction <45 dB. Often recommended for single-sided deafness; however, the benefit is likely less than for conductive losses. Complications include skin overgrowth, wound infection, and implant extrusion. Baha Attract and Sophono use magnet rather than percutaneous abutment and reduce skin complications, while losing some gain in amplification.

- *Cochlear implant:* Indicated for severe to profound bilateral SNHL (>75–90 dB). Better results if implanted early in prelingually deaf children and in children with history of meningitis. Contraindications include Michel's aplasia, absence of cochlear nerve or narrow IAC (<3 mm width with normal CN VII function). Complications include device failure, perilymphatic gusher or cerebrospinal fluid leak, wound infection, and increased risk for meningitis (pneumococcal vaccination needed for prophylaxis).

- *Auditory brainstem implant*: Approved in adults with neurofibromatosis type 2. US Food and Drug Administration-approved clinical trials are underway to evaluate use in congenitally deaf children who are not anatomic candidates for cochlear implantation.

SUGGESTED READING

1. Diercks GR, Mankarious L. Congenital hearing loss. In: Benninger CJ (Ed.). Sataloff's Comprehensive Textbook of Otolaryngology—Head and Neck Surgery: Pediatric Otolaryngology. Philadelphia: Jaypee Brothers; 2016. pp. 55-68.
2. Lee KJ. Essential Otolaryngology: Head and Neck Surgery, 11th Edition. New York: McGraw Hill Professional Publishing; 2015.
3. US Preventive Services Task Force. Universal screening for hearing loss in newborns: US Preventive Task Force recommendation statement. Pediatrics. 2008;122(1):143-8.

Chapter 35

Cleft Lip and Palate

Scott R Owen, Deborah S F Kacmarynski

EPIDEMIOLOGY

More than 300 syndromes are associated with facial clefting. This is the most common congenital malformation in the face, and the second most common congenital malformation behind clubfoot deformity.

Incidence

- Twenty five percent lip alone
- Thirty percent palate alone
- Forty five percent cleft lip and palate
- Eighty percent unilateral, 20% bilateral
- Two-thirds of:
    - Cleft lips are left sided
    - Cleft lips are men
    - Cleft palates are women
- Right-sided clefts are more commonly associated with syndromes

Cleft lip with or without palate (CL±P) is epidemiologically a distinct entity from cleft palate only (CPO):

- CL±P:
    - 0.2–2.3/1,000 births
    - Thirty percent associated with syndromes
    - Male-to-female ratio: 1.5–2.0:1

- CPO:
- 0.1–1.1/1,000 births
- Fifty percent associated with syndromes/sequences
- Male-to-female ratio: 0.5-0.7:1

ANATOMY

An understanding of cleft anatomy is crucial for a viable and functional repair.

Upper Lip

- Orbicularis oris muscle creates a sphincter around the mouth.
    - *Blood supply*: Deep from superior labial artery.
    - *Innervation*: Cranial nerve VII, buccal branch.
- *Cleft lip:* Orbicularis oris muscle interrupted, with muscle remnants flowing superiorly toward the columella medially and nasal alar base laterally (Fig. 35.1).
- Incomplete clefts have a variable amount of muscle intact across cleft portion of lip.
- Bilateral complete clefts have no orbicularis oris in the central prolabium.

Palate

- *Primary palate*: Anterior to incisive foramen.
- *Secondary palate*: Posterior to the incisive foramen.
- *Muscles*:
    - *Tensor veli palatini*: Opens eustachian canal, tenses soft palate (V3).
    - *Levator veli palatini*: Elevates palate (pharyngeal plexus).
- In the noncleft setting, the levator palatini muscle forms a horizontal sling that elevates the soft palate and closes the nasopharynx from the oropharynx during speech and swallowing.
    - *Uvularis*: Moves uvula superior and anterior.

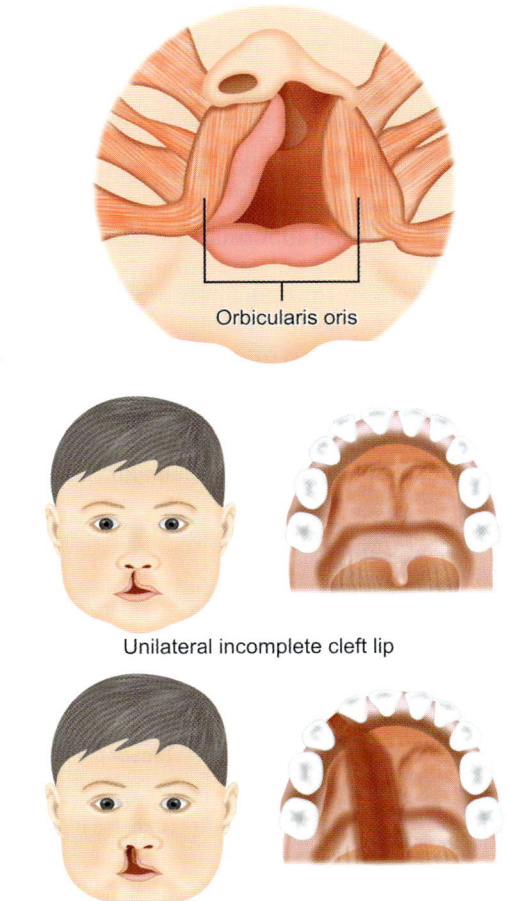

Orbicularis oris

Unilateral incomplete cleft lip

Unilateral complete cleft lip

Fig. 35.1: Aberrant oral musculature in the setting of cleft palate. In unilateral and bilateral cleft lips, the orbicularis oris is disrupted, maintaining only attachments to the inferior pyriform aperture.

- – *Palatopharyngeus*: Draws palate inferiorly (pharyngeal plexus).
- *Arterial supply*:
  - – *Hard palate*: Greater palatine artery.
  - – *Soft palate*: Descending palatine branch of the internal maxillary artery, ascending palatine branch of the facial artery, palatine branch of the ascending pharyngeal artery, lesser palatine artery.
- *Cleft palate*: Involves the abnormal orientation of the levator veli palatini, with aberrant attachments to the posterior hard palate anteriorly. Muscle fibers are oriented anterior-posterior, parallel to the cleft (Fig. 35.2).
  - – Submucous cleft involves an anterior–posterior orientation of musculature with intact mucosa.
  - – Tensor palatini muscle is also abnormally oriented in an anterior–posterior direction paralleling the cleft, resulting in inadequate opening of the eustachian canal.

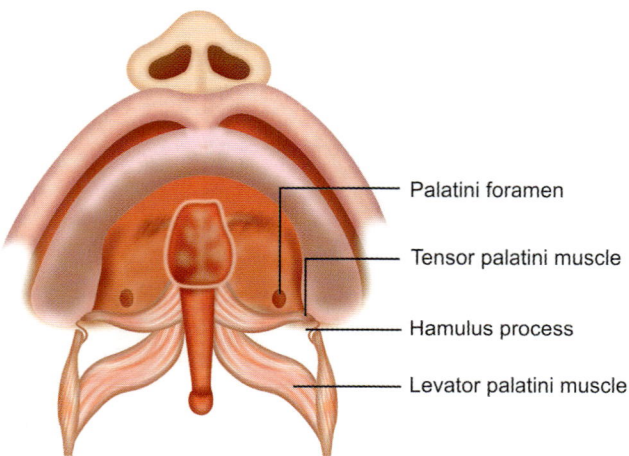

Palatini foramen

Tensor palatini muscle

Hamulus process

Levator palatini muscle

Fig. 35.2: Aberrant palate musculature in the setting of cleft palate. In palatal clefting, the muscular sling is disrupted. Instead, the intrinsic palate muscles insert on the posterior bony palate.

EMBRYOLOGY

It involves the creation of two distinct anatomic areas (Figs. 35.3A to F):

- *Primary palate*: Anterior to incisive foramen, includes lip, anterior alveolus, and premaxilla.
- *Secondary palate*: Incisive foramen and posterior.

The face develops in the first 12 weeks of gestation.

- *Critical lip development window*: 4–6 weeks
- *Critical palate development window*: 8–12 weeks

Five facial prominences form around the primordial mouth (stomodeum) during the fourth week of gestation.

- Frontonasal prominence
- Maxillary prominences (paired)
- Mandibular prominences (paired)

Bilateral nasal pits form inferior to the frontonasal prominence and the surrounding tissue develop into medial and lateral nasal prominences. The central portion of the maxilla is

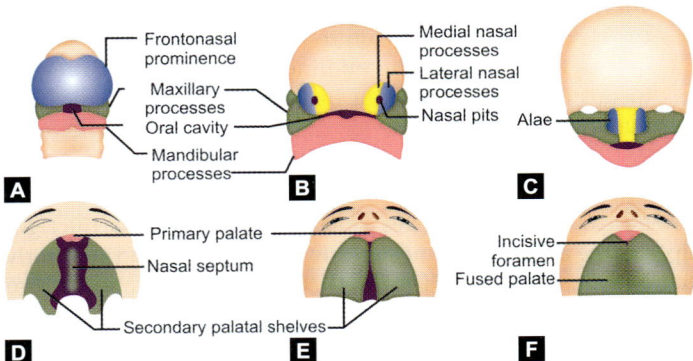

Figs. 35.3A to F: Embryology of the face. The midface is formed by the fusion of lateral maxillary prominences with the medial nasal prominence. Likewise, the palate is formed by the fusion of the premaxilla (a caudal extension of the medial nasal prominence) anteriorly, and the palatal shelves posteriorly. These form the primary and secondary palates.

formed by fusion of the medial nasal prominences. This leads to development of the philtrum, the columella, and the primary palate. The lateral lip is formed by fusion of the maxillary prominences with the prolabium. The secondary palate is formed by fusion of the maxillary prominences. These create the lateral palatine processes that fuse in an anterior-to-posterior direction to create the secondary palate. This fusion is reinforced by the migration of mesenchymal tissue derived from neuroectoderm; folic acid plays a prominent role in this process.

Cleft Embryology

- *Cleft lip*: Failure of the maxillary prominence to fuse with the medial nasal prominence, resulting in a defect between the lateral lip and the philtrum.
- *Cleft primary palate*: Failure of the maxillary prominence to fuse with the intermaxillary segment, resulting in a defect between the primary palate (anterior to the incisive foramen) and the secondary palate (posterior to the incisive foramen). This includes the cleft alveolus.
- *Cleft secondary palate*: Failure of the palatine processes to fuse to each other in the midline. It occurs in an anterior-to-posterior fashion when the tongue descends into the mandible.

CLASSIFICATION

LAHSHAL classification: Describes clefts beginning at the right lip, moving anatomically posteriorly to the palate, then anteriorly to describe the left lip (Fig. 35.4). The mnemonic moves from right to left (in descending order):

- L—Right lip
- A—Right alveolus
- H—Right hard palate
- S—Soft palate
- H—Left hard palate
- A—Left alveolus
- L—Left lip

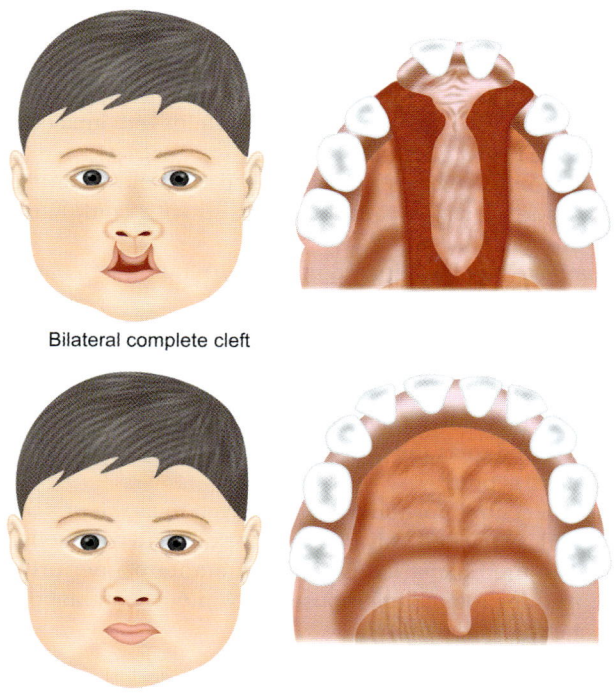

Bilateral complete cleft

Submucous cleft

Fig. 35.4: The LAHSHAL classification system.

Capital letter for complete clefting, lower-case letter for incomplete clefting, asterisk for microform, and a dash if uninvolved:

- Soft palate only: ---S---
- Left sided incomplete cleft lip: ------l
- Complete soft palate cleft, incomplete hard palate cleft: --hSh--
- Complete cleft lip and palate: LAHSHAL
- Submucous cleft palate: ---*---

Cleft Lip

- *Microform cleft lip*: *Forme fruste*; minimal clefting, may be as small as a notch in the vermilion.
- *Incomplete cleft lip*: Variable width cleft lip with intact bridge of tissue below nasal sill.
  - *Simonart's band* is often described as a band of connective tissue <1 cm in complete cleft lip with complete cleft alveolus.
- *Complete cleft lip*: Separation of lip extending into nasal sill, can involve alveolus into the palate.
- Unilateral versus bilateral
  - Bilateral cleft lips may also be complete or incomplete, and may be different on each side.
  - Complete bilateral cleft, central portion of the alveolus is referred to as the *premaxilla*, and is only attached to the nasal septum.
  - The central portion of lip is referred to as the *prolabium*, and is attached only to the premaxilla and columella.
  - The premaxilla tends to migrate anterosuperiorly and must be rotated inferoposteriorly into its natural position before lip repair.

Cleft Palate

- *Submucous cleft palate*: Intact mucosa, but aberrant anterior or posterior orientation of palatal musculature. Associated findings:
  - *Zona pellucida*: Hyperlucent gray line in the midline of the soft palate.
  - Bifid uvula.
  - Notch in the midline posterior palate.
- *Incomplete cleft palate*: Cleft of part of the soft palate or soft and part of the secondary palate. This can have a variable presentation from a wide cleft of the palate extending to the incisive foramen, to a narrow cleft of the posterior soft palate.

- *Complete cleft palate*: Complete dehiscence of mucosa and palatal musculature, and fully extends through the entire secondary palate.
- *Cleft alveolus*: Accompanies a cleft lip rather than a cleft palate, and can be bilateral and complete without causing any effect on secondary palate.

ETIOLOGY

Environmental Causes

- Anticonvulsant medication
- Retinoic acid derivatives (Accutane)
- Folic acid antagonists or deficiency (methotrexate)
- Tobacco use
- Fetal alcohol exposure
- Gestational maternal diabetes

Associations have been seen in animal models that have suggested cleft association with early gestational hypoxia and folic acid deficiency.[1] These are currently under investigation.

Genetics

There are hundreds of syndromes that can include cleft lip and palate. Overall, syndromic clefts make up <20% of total clefts.

DIAGNOSIS

Most cleft lips are identified in utero via ultrasound by the absence of muscle fibers across the upper lip. Cleft palates may be found by ultrasound, but most are not identified until birth. There are initiatives to improve prenatal ultrasound diagnosis of cleft palate.

MANAGEMENT

As recommended by the American Cleft Palate Association, the care of a child with a cleft requires a multidisciplinary approach with a team that may include a cleft surgeon, speech therapist, audiologist, pediatrician, dentist, orthodontist, otolaryngologist, oral maxillofacial surgeon, specialized nurse, and others. The goal is to provide the best results with the fewest number of procedures for the child. Most require multiple procedures in the first two decades of life.

Preoperative Considerations

- *Feeding*: A child should be evaluated initially for oral intake, as oral clefting may compromise the infant's ability to latch and feed to a nipple or a bottle. A custom nipple may improve feeding. Adequate oral intake is assessed by weight gain. Minimal acceptable weight gain is 1/2 oz per day.
- *Airway*: If the child's cleft is associated with *Pierre Robin sequence*, airway management may be necessary.
    - Diagnosing Pierre Robin sequence requires some airway or feeding difficulties and diagnostic criteria are not firmly established.
- *Genetics*: Genetic testing may be appropriate to identify any syndrome associated with the cleft.

Preoperative Orthopedic Manipulation

- May be considered in complete cleft lip and palate to reduce the width of the cleft and facilitate a tension-free repair.
- For incomplete cleft lip and alveolus, preoperative manipulation can facilitate inferior rotation of the premaxilla.
- Should be started in the first to second week of life and be continued until lip repair, after which the intact orbicularis oris provides tension to mold the position of the alveolar shelves.
- *Options*:
    - *Nasoalveolar molding*: Molding plates created and modified weekly by an orthodontist, pediatric dentist, or prosthodontist to allow narrowing of the cleft and stretching of the nasal ala.

– *Lip taping*: A less expensive and less labor-intensive option to narrow cleft width, this involves daily placement of tape over the cleft. Results can be less predictable, and involves extensive participation of the parents.
– *Lip adhesion*: Surgical procedure performed around 2 months of age involving elevation of flaps that unite the cleft segments, creating essentially an incomplete cleft. This allows for molding of the alveolar shelves without taping or appliance placement, but requires an additional definitive procedure to repair the lip, and creates scar tissue, which may impede final repair.

PROCEDURES

Cleft Lip

Goals of lip repair: Creation of symmetrical cupid's bow and lip fullness, maintain normal lip and philtrum contour, restore complete and competent orbicularis oris musculature, and create length on the side of the cleft.

Timing of repair in some protocols is based on the rule of 10s:
- 10 weeks old
- 10 lb
- Hemoglobin of 10
  This may be adjusted for prematurity or comorbidity.

Unilateral Cleft Lip

Challenges

- Releasing orbicularis oris from aberrant attachment, with recreation of sphincter
- Lengthening of cleft side lip
- Symmetric alignment of alar base
- Closure of nasal floor and sill
- Meticulous alignment at the vermillion–cutaneous junction at the cleft repair site, establishment of cutaneous roll
- Camouflage of incisional scars
- Establishment of normal relationships of nasal cartilage

Techniques

- *Rotation advancement cleft lip repair*: The Millard repair (Figs. 35.5A to H)
  - Involves back-cuts along superior lip of noncleft side
  - Z-plasty across philtrum
  - Restores lip length but leaves scars violating subunits
  - May flatten lip by losing anterior "pout" projection

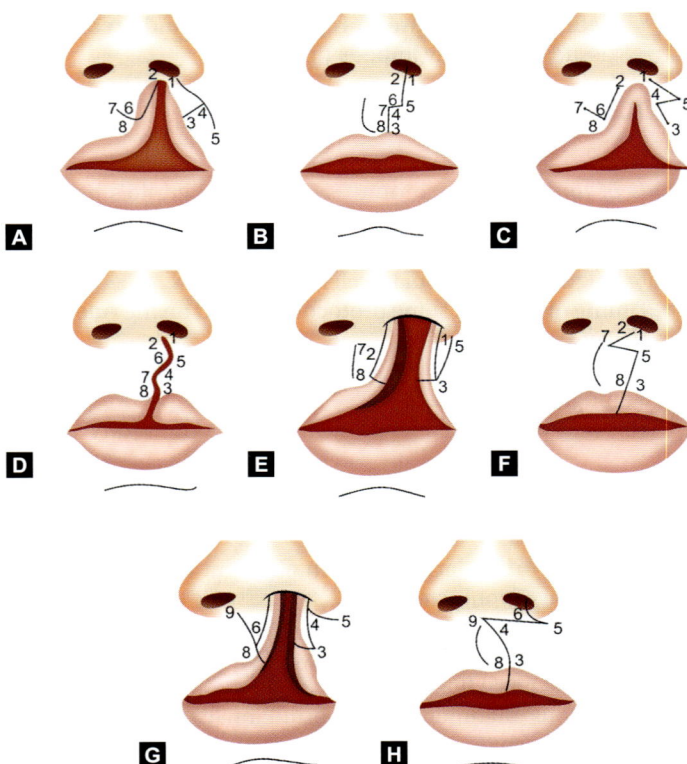

Figs. 35.5A to H: Millard rotational advancement flap technique.

- Modified rotation advancement
- *Triangle cleft lip repair*: Tennison–Randall cleft lip repair
  - Hides incisions along lip subunits
  - "Donation" of tissue from noncleft side via triangle tissue inset into cleft side
  - Improved anterior projection, conceals incisions
  - Less lip length
  - *Modification example*: Fisher cleft repair

Bilateral Cleft Lip Repair

Challenges

- Muscle fibers are absent in the prolabial segment.
- Vermillion is absent in prolabial segment.
- There is limited blood supply of prolabial segment.
- Prolabium tends to be too short and too wide.
- In complete bilateral cleft lips, nasal floor and sill are absent.
- Premaxilla is displaced anteriorly and superiorly.
- Premaxilla is mobile.
- Nasal tip is widened and there is hooding of the nostrils.

Techniques

- Challenge to re-establish the orbicularis oris sphincter within the prolabium.
- Bilateral cleft repair is typically performed as a single stage, but can be delayed with repair of the widest cleft first.
- Prolabium becomes neocolumella, red vermillion, and cutaneous roll donated from lateral lips that are advanced to meet midline inferior to neocolumella.

Cleft Palate

Goals

The main objective is to separate the oral and nasal cavities and to restore dynamic function to the palate.

Timing

Typically performed at 8–18 months of age.

The balance of palate repair is choosing a schedule early enough that normal speech development is not affected, but late enough to minimize complications from the procedure, or maxillary hypoplasia from stripping of periosteum from the palate. Consideration is also given to the size of the child's mouth, and the ability of a surgeon's fingers to work inside of the oral cavity. Most data suggest that in an otherwise healthy child, repair before 18 months of age is advantageous for normal speech development. This may be delayed for premature children or those with syndromes and developmental delay to 18–24 months of age.

Cleft Palate Repair

Challenges

- Separation of the oral and nasal cavities
- Prevention of postoperative fistula formation
- Restoration of orientation of levator veli palatini to re-establish velopharyngeal function
- Maintain nasal airway

Techniques

- *Two-stage repairs*: Akin to a lip adhesion, involves first repair of the soft palate cleft, then a second stage repair of the hard palate. Associated with worse speech outcomes, but improved facial growth.
- V-Y pushback—Veau-Wardill-Kilner repair
  - Elevation of mucoperiosteal flaps bilaterally pedicled off of greater palatine arteries
  - Used for wide clefts
  - Improves palatal length, but leaves significant exposed bone anteriorly, challenging facial growth
  - Greater risk of anterior fistulas

- Two-flap palatoplasty—Bardach repair
    - Elevation of extensive bilateral mucoperiosteal flaps pedicled off of greater palatine arteries
    - Muscle freed from the posterior maxilla and sling re-established for normal levator anatomy
    - Shortens palatal length
    - Used for wide clefts
- Bipedicled-flap palatoplasty—von Langenbeck repair
    - Bucket-handle mucoperiosteal flaps attached anteriorly and posteriorly
    - Blood supply from both mucosal attachments and blind dissection around greater palatine artery
    - Shortens palate length
    - Used for narrow clefts
- Double-opposing Z-plasty—Furlow repair (Figs. 35.6A to D)
    - Use of an opposing Z-plasty on oral and nasal sides of the soft palate
    - Allows for additional palatal length, and re-aligns levator palatini muscles in an overlapping fashion
    - Used for narrower clefts and submucous clefts

SECONDARY SURGICAL PROCEDURES

Bone Grafting

Alveolar bone grafting may be necessary before eruption of the permanent teeth occurs. This most commonly utilizes iliac crest bone, but may also come from rib or calvarium. In older individuals, oral donor sites may be used. Reasons for bone grafting include:

- Stabilization of the maxilla
- Support for the roots of adjacent teeth
- Closure of any residual anterior fistula
- Support for the alar base on the cleft side
- Support dental implant for missing incisors or canines

Otologic Disease

Chronic otitis media with effusion is present in 95% of children with clefts.

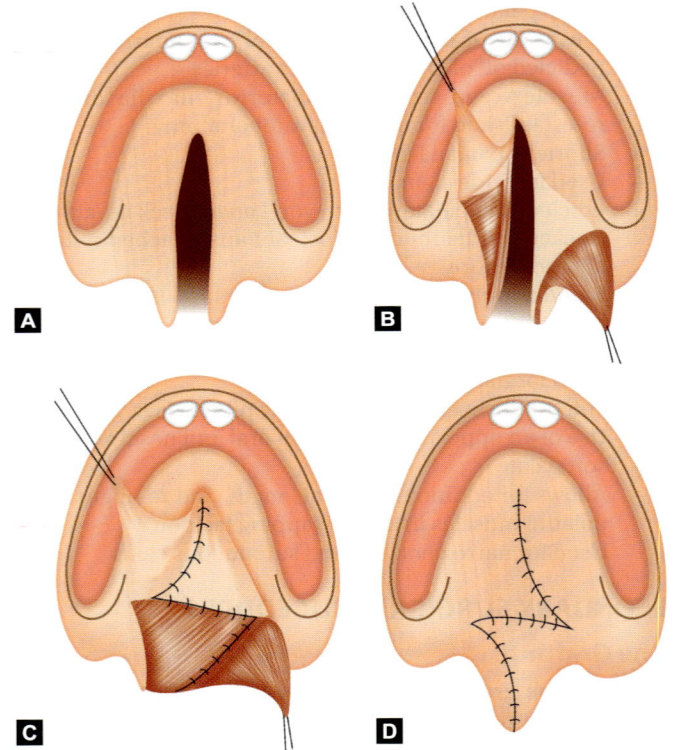

Figs. 35.6A to D: Furlow double-opposing Z-plasty palatoplasty technique.

- Longitudinal displacement of tensor veli palatini prevents proper opening of eustachian canal.
- Velopharyngeal reflux may exacerbate middle ear inflammation.
- Most require placement of ventilation tubes.
- Improves with growth and hardening of eustachian canal cartilage.

Velopharyngeal Insufficiency (VPI)

It can be seen postoperatively due to difficult patient anatomy, shortening of palatal repair with scar contracture, fistula, or wound dehiscence.

Speech evaluation by a speech pathologist to identify cause of VPI:

- Lateral cephalogram
- Nasal manometry
- Video fluoroscopy
- Nasal endoscopy

Need to differentiate phoneme-specific VPI, which would require speech therapy, from global VPI, which would suggest an anatomic cause.

Procedures

- *Pharyngeal flap*: Mucosa and muscular tissue taken from the posterior pharyngeal wall with a superior base near the adenoid tissue. The flap is insert into the posterior soft palate.
  - About 80–90% have improvement in VPI.
  - Up to 40% develop obstructive sleep apnea (OSA).
- *Sphincter pharyngoplasty*: Flaps made from posterior tonsillar pillars create a theoretically innervated flap. These flaps are sutured around an area of denuded mucosa on the posterior pharyngeal wall, creating a small central port.
  - About 90% success rate.
  - Best in patients with good velar motion and poor lateral wall motion.
  - Lower incidence of OSA than pharyngeal flap.
- *Furlow double-opposing Z-plasty*: Elevation of opposing oral and nasal mucosal/muscular flaps and interposition forming a double-opposing Z-plasty. This improves velar position with palatal tissue rearranged to add palatal length and rearranges palatal musculature, recreating levator sling, improving velar movement.

- Often combined with sphincter pharyngoplasty for similar results as a pharyngeal flap alone, but a lower incidence of OSA.
- *Injection veloplasty or pharyngoplasty*: Involves injectable fillers into the retropharyngeal space to create a "neo-Passavant's ridge."
  - Good for small defects or for "touch-up" after other intervention.
  - Can be fat transfer.
  - Many other injectable products have been tried with mixed long-term success.[2]
- *Nonsurgical measures*: For poor surgical candidates with high risk for general anesthesia or with extensive scarring of oral cavity/oropharynx.
  - *Speech bulb prosthesis*: Retainer with palatal lift appliance.
  - *Obturator*: Additional arm that obstructs the gap between palate and posterior oropharynx.

Lip revision: Revision surgeries are avoided if possible by adequately addressing anatomic issues with the initial procedure. These may become necessary as the lip heals and grows. Hypertrophic scarring may be addressed with steroid injections in early healing phase.

Rhinoplasty: Cleft anatomy results in distortion of the nasal cartilages. A rhinoplasty is frequently required in the teenage years.

Distinctive cleft nose deformities:
- Wide nasal base, short columella
- Flared nostrils, asymmetric or buckled lower lateral cartilages
- Oblique tip-defining points, or bifid nasal tip
- Asymmetric columellar–alar angles
- Poor tip projection
- Displaced caudal septum

Secondary cleft rhinoplasty is widely considered the most challenging nasal surgery, and care must be taken to correctly assess the nose, with careful consideration for nasal function and aesthetics. Advanced rhinoplasty techniques may be necessary to correct nasal deformity.

Orthognathic surgery: Maxillary hypoplasia is common in children with cleft. Around 10–15% of patients require orthognathic surgery, usually a maxillary advancement, sometimes maxillary distraction osteogenesis; sometimes mandibular jaw surgery is also needed.[3-9]

REFERENCES

1. Brooklyin S, Jana R, Aravinthan S, et al. Assessment of folic acid and DNA damage in cleft lip and cleft palate. Clin Pract. 2014;4(608):4-6.
2. Wise JB, Cabiling D, Yan D, et al. Submucosal injection of micronized acellular dermal matrix: analysis of biocompatibility and durability. Plast Reconstr Surg. 2007;120(5):1156-60.
3. Hoffman WY. Cleft Lip & Palate. CURRENT Diagnosis & Treatment in Otolaryngology—Head & Neck Surgery, 3e Lalwani AK. New York, NY: McGraw-Hill, 2012, http://accessmedicine.mhmedical.com/content.aspx?bookid=386&sectionid=39944056.
4. Fisher DM. Unilateral cleft lip repair: an anatomical subunit approximation technique. Plast Reconstruct Surg. 2005;116(61):61-71.
5. Moller KT, Glaze LE. Cleft Lip and Palate: Interdisciplinary Issues and Treatment, 2nd edn. Austin, TX: Pro-Ed; 2009:415-452.
6. Patel K, Senders C. Cleft lip and palate. In: Lee KJ (Ed). Essential Otolaryngology, New York, NY: McGraw Hill; 2012. pp. 285-99.
7. Furlow LT Jr. Cleft palate repair by double opposing Z-plasty. Plast Reconstr Surg. 1986;78(6): 724-38.
8. Van Beek AL, Hatfield AS, Schnepf E. Cleft rhinoplasty. Plast Reconstr Surg. 2004;114(4): 57e-69e.
9. Cantarella G, Mazzola RF, Mantovani M, et al. Treatment of velopharyngeal insufficiency by pharyngeal and velar fat injection. Otolaryngol Head Neck Surg. 2011;145:401-3.

Chapter **36**

Pediatric Tonsil and Adenoid Disorders

Sidrah M Ahmad, Gabriela Timoney, Donald Solomon

> ***Chief Complaint***
> *"Recurrent sore throat and snoring".*

DEFINITIONS

Apnea: Any pause in respiration.

Hypopnea: Reduction of airflow by 50% for two respiratory cycles accompanied by reduction of saturation by 3% or arousal from sleep.

Apnea–hypopnea index (AHI): Sum of apneas and hypopneas per hour of sleep.

Respiratory disturbance index: Sum of apneas, hypopneas, and respiratory-related arousals per hour of sleep.

ANATOMY AND PHYSIOLOGY

Adenoids

- *Blood supply*: Pharyngeal branch of internal maxillary artery, ascending palatine branch of facial artery, ascending cervical branch of thyrocervical trunk, and ascending pharyngeal artery.
- *Innervation:* Cranial nerves (CNs) IX and X.
- *Histology:* Ciliated pseudostratified columnar and stratified squamous.

Tonsils

- *Blood supply*: Tonsillar branch of facial artery, ascending palatine branch of facial artery, dorsal lingual branch of lingual artery, descending palatine artery, greater palatine artery, and ascending pharyngeal artery (Fig. 36.1).
- *Innervation*: General somatic afferent fibers from V2 and general visceral afferent fibers from CN IX.
- *Histology*: Stratified epithelium lining (including crypts) and lymphoid tissue.

TONSIL AND ADENOID DISORDERS

- Adenotonsillar hypertrophy
  - Obstructive sleep apnea (OSA)
    - Often diagnosed by history (witnessed apnea, enuresis, difficult morning arousal, poor school performance, behavioral problems/hyperactivity, poor weight gain) and physical findings (mouth breathing, stertor, pectus excavatum, tonsillar hypertrophy). If a polysomnogram (PSG) is obtained, OSA can be further classified based on AHI as follows:
      - Mild: AHI = 1–5
      - Moderate: AHI = 5–10
      - Severe: AHI >10

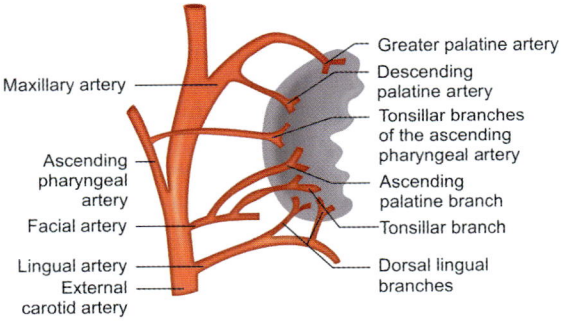

Fig. 36.1: Arterial supply of the tonsils.

- Often subdivided based on etiology:[1]
  - Type 1: Adenotonsillar hypertrophy
    - Collapse at level of tonsils
  - Type 2: Obesity related
    - Increasing prevalence
    - Upper airway narrowing results from fatty infiltration of upper airway structures and subcutaneous fat deposits in the anterior neck, which exert collapsing forces promoting increased pharyngeal collapse.
- Effects of OSA:
  - Neurocognitive dysfunction, pulmonary hypertension, cardiovascular disease, and hypertension[2]
- American Academy of Otolaryngology—Head and Neck Surgery Guidelines for PSG in children:[3]
  - Obtain PSG in children with complex medical conditions such as obesity, Down syndrome, craniofacial abnormalities, sickle cell disease, or mucopolysaccharidoses.
  - Obtain PSG if there is a discordance between history and physical examination or if need for intervention is uncertain.
- American Academy of Otolaryngology—Head and Neck Surgery Guidelines for tonsillectomy:[4]
  - Assess children with sleep-disordered breathing for comorbid conditions such as growth retardation, poor school performance, enuresis, and behavioral problems, which may improve after adenotonsillectomy.
  - Apnea–hypopnea index > 5 may require tonsillectomy. Recommended to base decision for surgical intervention on clinical history, examination, and likelihood of improvement in sleep-disordered breathing.
- Intraoperative/postoperative care:

- One dose of intravenous dexamethasone should be given intraoperatively.
- Preoperative antibiotics should not be given routinely.
- Children under the age of 3 undergoing tonsillectomy for OSA and those with severe OSA on PSG should be admitted overnight for observation.
- Caregivers should be counseled on the importance of pain management and good hydration.

- Recurrent tonsillitis
  - Pathophysiology
    - Common pathogens for pseudomembranous tonsillitis are Epstein–Barr virus (most common), Candidiasis, *Neisseria gonorrhoeae*, syphilis, *Corynebacterium diphtheriae*, and Group A beta-hemolytic *Streptococcus* (GABHS).
    - Bacterial tonsillitis accounts for 15–30% of pharyngotonsillitis cases, with GABHS being the most common pathogen.
    - Crypts may serve as reservoir for bacteria. More recently, biofilm formation in crypts has been proposed, although more research is necessary.[5]
  - American Academy of Otolaryngology—Head and Neck Surgery Guidelines for tonsillectomy:
    - Watchful waiting for < 7 episodes of tonsillitis in 1 year, < 5 episodes per year for 2 years, or < 3 episodes per year for 3 years. It is recommended that each episode be documented in the medical record and associated with one of the following in addition to complaint of sore throat: temperature > 38.3°C, cervical adenopathy, tonsillar exudate, or positive GABHS.
    - Clinicians may offer tonsillectomy for patients with recurrent tonsillitis who do not meet the above criteria but have modifying factors such as multiple drug allergies, PFAPA (periodic fever, aphthous stomatitis, pharyngitis, adenitis occurring every 3–5 weeks for at least 6 months), or history of a peritonsillar abscess.

- Pediatric autoimmune neuropsychiatric disorders associated with streptococcal infections (PANDAS)
  - Diagnosis criteria:
    - Presence of a tic disorder and/or obsessive–compulsive disorder (OCD).
    - Prepubertal onset.
    - Abrupt onset of symptoms or episodic with periods of mild or no symptoms.
    - Prior streptococcal infection with subsequent development of symptoms.
  - Pathophysiology
    - Not well understood.
    - *Molecular mimicry hypothesis:* Antibodies against streptococcus cross-react with neuronal tissue. The basal ganglia may be one target, which results in tics and OCD.[6]
  - Treatment
    - Selective serotonin reuptake inhibitor.
    - Antibiotic therapy may help with symptoms but is not well supported.
    - The role for tonsillectomy is not well defined but may improve symptoms.[7]
- Adenoiditis
  - Pathophysiology:
    - Viruses and bacteria chronically infect adenoid tissue.
      - Biofilm formation
        - Common pathogens: *Staphylococcus aureus, Streptococcus pneumonia*, and *Moraxella catharralis*[8]
  - Treatment:
    - Antibiotics
    - Adenoidectomy
      - Effective in children under the age of 6[9]
- Other indications for adenoidectomy
  - Chronic otitis media with/without effusion in children >4 years

- Adenoid hypertrophy with nasal obstruction and orofacial abnormalities (adenoid facies)
- Failure to thrive (not attributed to other causes)
- Additional consideration:
  - About 15% of lymphomas involve Waldeyer's ring.
    - Tonsillar asymmetry is the most common finding.[10]
    - Burkitt's lymphoma is the most common type involving Waldeyer's ring.

DIAGNOSTIC WORKUP (FLOWCHARTS 36.1 AND 36.2)
History: "Sore Throat"

- "How long have you had a sore throat?"
- "How many episodes of tonsillitis have you had in the past year? What about last year?"
- "Have you ever had a peritonsillar abscess?"
- "Have you ever been hospitalized for tonsillitis?"

Physical Examination

- General facial appearance (Craniofacial abnormalities? Adenoid facies?)
- Respiration (Mouth breathing? Stertor?)

Flowchart 36.1: Workup for sore throat.

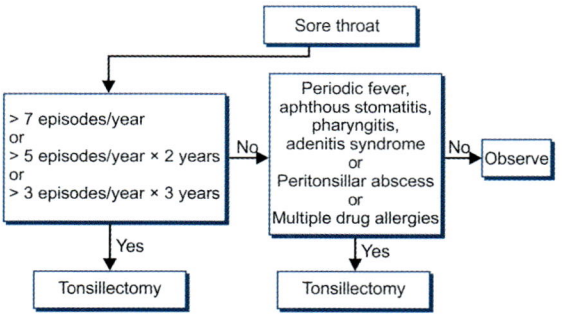

Flowchart 36.2: Workup for snoring.

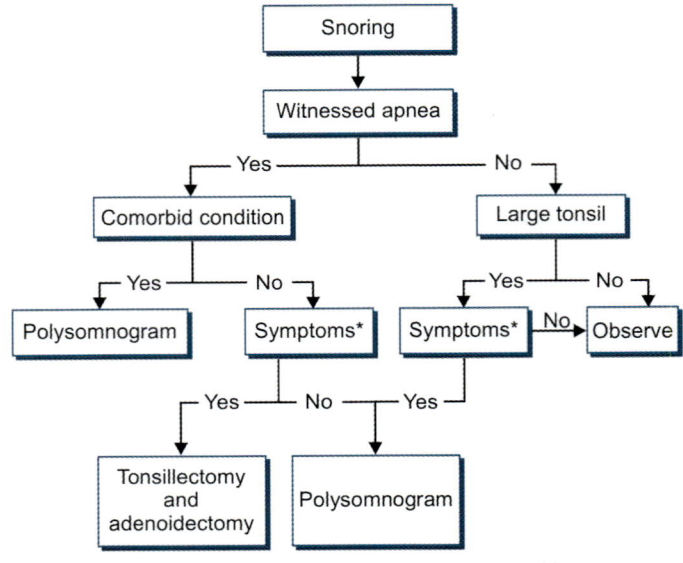

* = enuresis, behavioral problems, poor weight gain, or poor school performance

- Chest (Pectus excavatum?)
- Oropharyngeal examination (attention to oropharyngeal crowding and tonsil size)
- Poor muscle tone
- Cranial nerve examination
- Ancillary tools
  - Polysomnogram

REFERENCES

1. Dayyat E, Kheirandish-Goazl L, Gozal D. Childhood obstructive sleep apnea: one or two distinct disease entities? Sleep Med Clin. 2007;2(3):433-44.
2. Capdevila OS, Kheirandish-Gozal L, Dayyat E, et al. Pediatric obstructive sleep apnea. Proc Am Thorac Soc. 2008;5(2):274-82.

3. Roland PS, Rosenfeld RM, Brooks LJ, et al. Clinical practice guideline: polysomnography for sleep-disordered breathing prior to tonsillectomy in children. Otolaryngol Head Neck Surg. 2011; 145(S1):S1-15.

4. Baugh RF, Archer SM, Mitchell RB, et al. Clinical practice guideline: tonsillectomy in children. Otolaryngol Head Neck Surg. 2011;144(S1):S1-30.

5. Diaz RR, Picciafuoco S, Paraje MG, et al. Relevance of biofilms in pediatric tonsillar disease. Eur J Clin Microbiol Infect Dis. 2011;30(12):1503-09.

6. Tan J, Smith CH, Goldman RD. Pediatric autoimmune neuropsychiatric disorders associated with streptococcal infections. Can Fam Physicians. 2012;58(9):957-9.

7. Damesh D, Virbalas JM, Bent JP. The role of tonsillectomy in the treatment of pediatric autoimmune neuropsychiatric disorders associated with streptococcal infections (PANDAS). JAMA Otolaryngol Head Neck Surg. 2015;141(3):272-5.

8. Brambilla I, Pusateri A, Pagella F, et al. Adenoids in children: advances in immunology, diagnosis, and surgery. Clin Anat. 2014;27(3):346-52.

9. Brietzke SE, Shin JJ, Choi S, et al. Clinical consensus statement: pediatric chronic rhinosinusitis. Otolaryngol Head Neck Surg. 2014;151(4):542-53.

10. Guimarães AC, de Carvalho GM, Bento LR, et al. Clinical manifestations in children with tonsillar lymphoma: a systemic review. Crit Rev Oncol Hematol. 2014;90(2):146-51.

11. Jeyakumar A, Miller S, Mitchell RB. Adenotonsillar disease in children. In: Johnson JT, Rosen CA (Eds). Bailey's Head and Neck Surgery, 5th edition. Baltimore: Lippincott Williams and Wilkins; 2014.

Chapter 37

Neonatal Nasal Obstruction and Congenital Nasal Masses

Donald Solomon

OVERVIEW

Neonatal nasal patency is necessary for respiration and feeding. If the nasal cavities are not patent, the neonate experiences respiratory distress evidenced by stertor and retractions. Neonatal nasal obstruction frequently results in feeding difficulty. Depending on the degree of nasal obstruction, cyanosis and apnea may ensue. Respiratory distress related to neonatal nasal obstruction is often relieved by crying as the infant temporarily utilizes the oral airway for respiration. There are numerous causes of neonatal nasal obstruction, ranging from simple nasal debris occluding the nasal cavities to more complicated congenital malformations requiring surgical intervention. Clinicians should include the following entities in their differential diagnosis: nasal debris and crusts, pyriform aperture stenosis, septal deviation, congenital nasal masses, and choanal atresia. Direct examination via anterior rhinoscopy or nasal endoscopy may yield the diagnosis. Computed tomography (CT) scan or magnetic resonance imaging (MRI) may be necessary for definitive diagnosis and treatment planning. Conservative intervention such as McGovern nipple use or lavage feeding as well as frequent nasal irrigation or suction may fully alleviate feeding and breathing difficulty related to minor nasal obstruction. In the face of more significant nasal obstruction, temporizing measures such as placement of a nasal trumpet or endotracheal intubation may be necessary to allow time for planning more definitive surgical treatment.[1,9-12]

PYRIFORM APERTURE STENOSIS

Evaluation and Diagnosis

Pyriform aperture stenosis is a narrowing of the pyriform aperture such that it does not admit a standard flexible laryngoscope (3.5 mm) or a 10-French suction catheter. Computed tomography scan yields definitive diagnosis when revealing that the bony shelves of the lateral pyriform aperture encroach on the nasal vestibule (Fig. 37.1). One must evaluate for a single central incisor or mega-incisor when pyriform aperture stenosis is diagnosed as it is occasionally present and may indicate other congenital midline anomalies such as holoprosencephaly variants.[2,3,9-12]

Treatment

- *Conservative:* Lavage feeding or the use of a McGovern nipple with utilization of an apnea monitor as well as frequent nasal

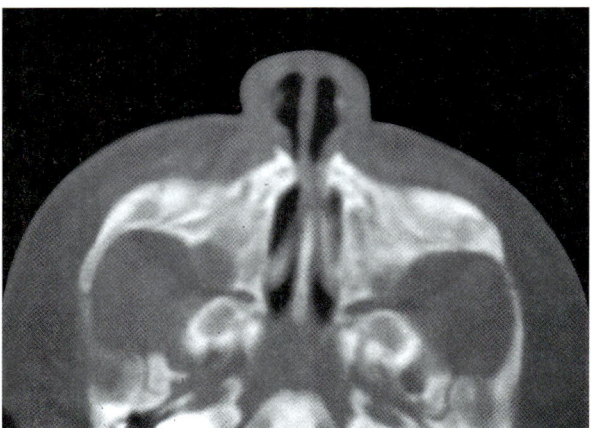

Fig. 37.1: Pyriform aperture stenosis, axial computed tomography scan.

suction may be enough to alleviate respiratory distress and feeding difficulty in mild cases.

- *Surgical:* A sublabial approach is utilized with elevation of the inferior nasal mucosa and curetting or drilling of the lateral pyriform bone to widen the aperture. One must proceed cautiously to avoid injuring the tooth buds. Postoperative nasal stenting is usually necessary.

DEVIATED NASAL SEPTUM

Evaluation and Diagnosis

Septal deviation in the newborn is most often the result of prolonged labor and associated nasal trauma within the birth canal leading to displacement of the nasal septal cartilage off the maxillary crest (Fig. 37.2). Nasal obstruction from septal deviation can range from mild to severe. The diagnosis is often made via anterior rhinoscopy utilizing a nasal speculum. Flexible or rigid nasal endoscopy may be necessary to make the diagnosis

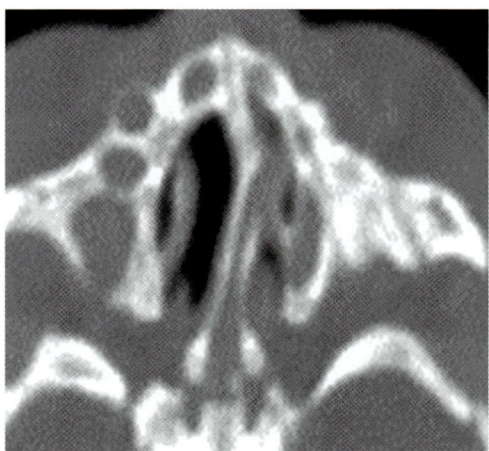

Fig. 37.2: Deviated nasal septum in a neonate, axial computed tomography scan.

when the neonatal nasal aperture is small or the septal deviation is posterior.[4,9-12]

Treatment

- *Conservative:* The vast majority of neonatal nasal septal deviation can be treated conservatively with frequent nasal irrigation and suction. Most neonates age out of the symptoms of nasal obstruction related to septal deviation within the first 6–12 months of life. Occasionally, an apnea monitor is necessary in the face of more severe obstruction.
- *Surgical:* A deviated appearance of the nasal dorsum or a severe degree of nasal obstruction secondary to septal deviation necessitates surgical intervention. Resetting the septal cartilage onto the maxillary crest via closed reduction is a simple and effective treatment.

NASAL MASSES

Evaluation and Diagnosis

Nasal masses that lead to neonatal nasal obstruction are varied and include nasal dermoids, gliomas, encephaloceles, hemangiomas, and nasolacrimal duct cysts. It is important not to biopsy a nasal mass in the neonate until one has established the absence of an intracranial connection or a high degree of vascularity.[5,6,9-12]

- *Nasal dermoids:* These congenital anomalies are the most common midline nasal masses. They often present in the neonatal period and contain both ectodermal and mesodermal components. They are theorized to arise from delayed closure of the fonticulus frontalis or foramen cecum, allowing dural and dermal elements to insinuate between the nasal bones and septal cartilage before they have fused. The most common presentation of a nasal dermoid is a midline nasal dorsal pit with a protruding hair (Fig. 37.3). In some cases, the connection with the skin may be lost during development, and a nasal dermoid may present as

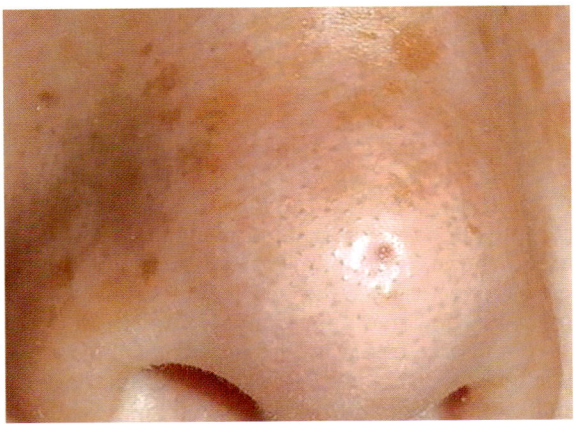

Fig. 37.3: Nasal dermoid pit at the nasal tip.

a subcutaneous mass along the path from the nasal tip to the foramen cecum. Nasal dermoids may also present intranasally or within the nasal septum. If a nasal dorsum mass, widened nasal septum, or intranasal mass suspicious for dermoid is noted, CT scan and MRI offer the best modalities for definitive diagnosis.

- *Glioma and encephaloceles:* These congenital anomalies arise when the foramen cecum undergoes delayed closure or fails to close at all, hence admitting and leaving intracranial tissue in the extracranial space. A glioma is a pinched-off remnant of glial tissue that loses its intracranial connection, whereas an encephalocele contains glial tissue (meninges, cerebrospinal fluid, and/or brain) that retains its connection with the intracranial space. Occasionally, a glioma will contain a dural or fibrous stalk with a connection to the intracranial space. A glioma or an encephalocele may present as a nasal dorsal mass or an intranasal mass, and should be further evaluated by CT or MRI before biopsy or planning treatment.

- *Hemangioma:* These highly vascular benign tumors arise in the first 2–6 weeks of life and may involve the nasal dorsum or the nasal mucosa. Soon after the onset, they enter a proliferative growth phase that lasts throughout the first year of life and may lead to nasal obstruction depending on location. Diagnosis is often made based on appearance and behavior alone. Presence of the glucose transporter protein-1 receptor noted on pathologic evaluation of tissue biopsy offers definitive diagnosis. Computed tomography or MRI may be necessary to assess the size and extent of an intranasal hemangioma.

- *Nasolacrimal duct cysts:* The nasolacrimal duct system may become occluded or fail to canalize both distally and proximally, leading to enlargement and cyst formation emanating from beneath the inferior turbinate, which can cause nasal obstruction. Diagnosis is made by direct visualization via anterior rhinoscopy followed by CT scan for confirmation of the diagnosis (Fig. 37.4).

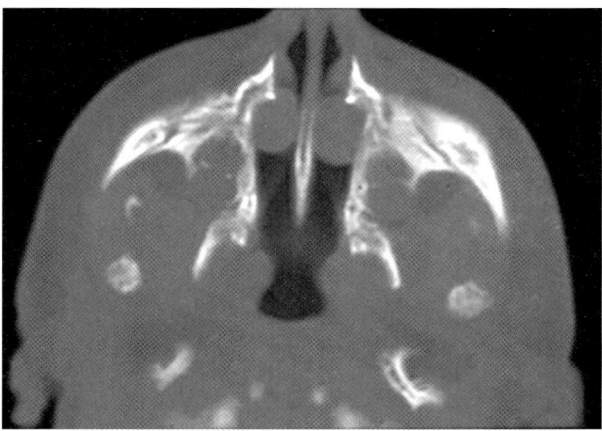

Fig. 37.4: Nasolacrimal duct cysts on axial computed tomography.

Treatment

Treatment of congenital nasal masses leading to nasal obstruction varies based on diagnosis and may include, for example, simple observation or propranolol therapy for hemangioma or complicated extranasal excision of a nasal dermoid or encephalocele with neurosurgical frontal craniotomy to address the intracranial component.

- *Nasal dermoid:* Complete surgical excision of the nasal dermoid including its stalk and intracranial component if one exists (30% of cases) will prevent recurrence and recurrent infection. Approaches include a vertical midline incision over the nasal dorsum or external rhinoplasty incision and dissection (Fig. 37.5). The intranasal component of the nasal dermoid may be addressed via both external and intranasal approaches. Neurosurgical co-management may be necessary in the face of an intracranial component, and frontal craniotomy is often performed as the first portion of the procedure.

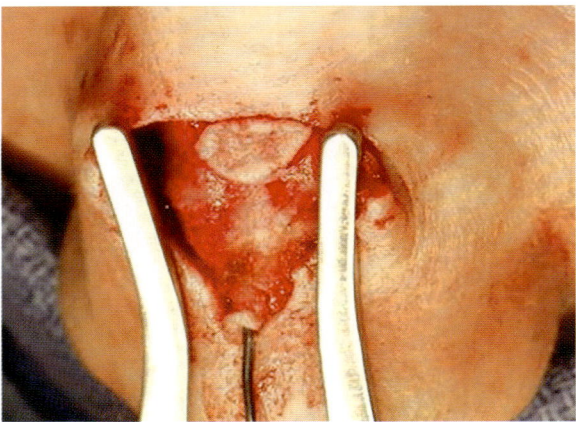

Fig. 37.5: External excision of a nasal dermoid pit and tract.

- *Glioma and encephalocele:* If the glioma does not have a stalk attaching it to the intracranial space, complete excision by the otolaryngologist may be performed via an external approach utilizing a vertical midline incision, external rhinoplasty incision, or lateral rhinotomy incision (Fig. 37.6). It is important to perform a complete dissection of the glioma, including occasional resection of involved skin, or recurrence is the rule. Encephaloceles are primarily treated by the neurosurgeon with secondary resection of any extracranial component.

- *Hemangioma:* Intra- and extranasal hemangiomas will grow for the first year of life and then involute for the next 3–5 years. If the hemangioma is large, pedunculated, ulcerated, bleeding, painful, significantly cosmetically deforming, or causing nasal obstruction, first-line treatment is oral propranolol with the hope of arresting, then reversing growth. Oral or intralesional steroids may be administered if propranolol therapy is unsuccessful. Surgical resection may be considered.

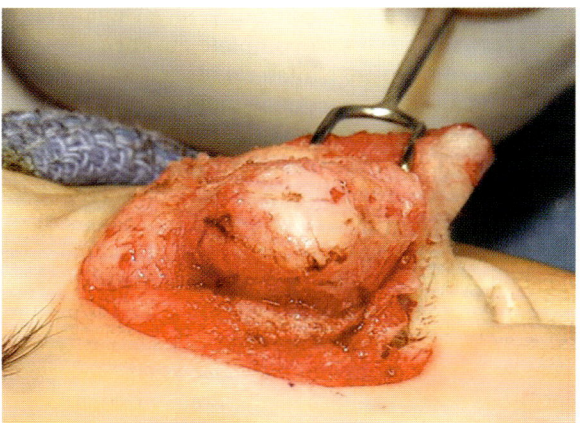

Fig. 37.6: Excision of a nasal mass via lateral rhinotomy incision.

- *Nasolacrimal duct cyst:* Surgery offers definitive treatment to relieve nasal obstruction and allow the nasolacrimal system to drain intranasally. An ophthalmologist cannulates the nasolacrimal duct system superiorly, allowing the otolaryngologist to unroof the nasolacrimal duct cyst intranasally via powered or nonpowered instrumentation. Nasolacrimal stents can be left in place thereafter to ensure that intranasal scarring and stenosis do not occur.

CHOANAL ATRESIA

Evaluation and Diagnosis

Choanal atresia is a rare entity occurring as infrequently as 1:10,000 live births. It is more often unilateral than bilateral. Most cases are a combination of both bony and membranous narrowings of the choana (70%) while the remainder occur secondary to bony narrowing alone. In the presence of bilateral choanal atresia, significant respiratory distress with associated desaturations and cyanosis, partially relieved by crying, will be present in the neonatal period. All neonates with bilateral choanal atresia will have significant feeding difficulty. Unilateral choanal atresia leads to less severe or complete absence of respiratory and feeding compromise. Unilateral atresia often presents as rhinorrhea and nasal obstruction without feeding or respiratory compromise. Diagnosis can be made by examination. When the choana is blocked, the nose fills with secretions that are unable to drain posteriorly. Attempted passage of a 6-French suction catheter will reveal that the nasopharynx is not patent. Placement of cotton Q-tip wisps under the nasal vestibule on the side of the blocked choana will reveal no air movement. Direct visualization with a nasal endoscope after suctioning secretions typically reveals an area of tapering in the posterior nasal cavity where the widened posterior septum and the mucosa-covered medialized pterygoid bone meet (Fig. 37.7). Computed tomography scan will offer definitive diagnosis of choanal atresia and characterize it as mixed bony and membranous or bony alone (Fig. 37.8). When

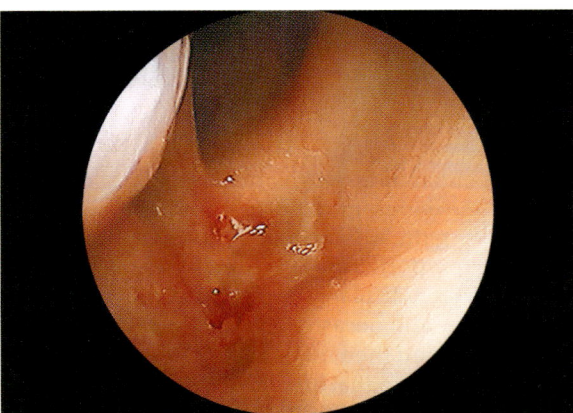

Fig. 37.7: Endoscopic view of right intranasal unilateral choanal atresia.

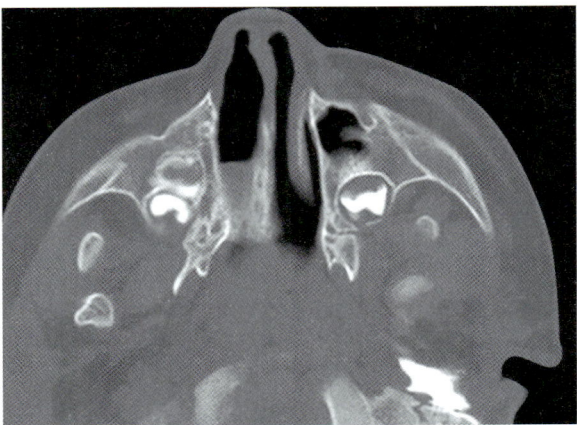

Fig. 37.8: Right unilateral choanal atresia axial computed tomography scan.

the diagnosis of choanal atresia is made, CHARGE association (coloboma, heart defects, atresia of the choana, retarded growth, genitourinary anomalies, and ear anomalies) and its inherent anomalies must be evaluated for. This association is present in up to 50% of neonates with bilateral choanal atresia.[7-12]

Treatment

Treatment of choanal atresia is primarily surgical, although temporizing measures may be instituted to allow time for the neonate to gain weight and mature prior to operative intervention. Temporizing measures in the face of bilateral choanal atresia include placement of an oral airway, placement of a feeding tube, and occasionally tracheotomy, if the patient is unable to learn and then maintain oral respiration. Timing of surgery in bilateral choanal atresia utilizes the same criteria as cleft lip repair or "the rule of 10s," in which the surgeon waits until the neonate is at least 10 weeks old, 10 pounds, and has a hemoglobin of 10. Surgery for unilateral atresia may be delayed significantly longer if the infant does not have substantial respiratory or feeding issues, although unilateral rhinorrhea and inability to clear secretions inevitably become problematic. Surgical approaches include the transpalatal, trans-septal, and endoscopic endonasal. The endoscopic endonasal approach has gained increasing favor. Posterior septal and lateral nasal wall mucosal flaps can be raised and the choana opened with a microdebrider, rongeur, or drill. A posterior septectomy creates a common cavity and decreases the risk of re-stenosis. The use of mitomycin C or nasal stents varies based on surgeon preference. Re-stenosis and the need for revision surgery are known risks.

REFERENCES

1. Olnes S, Schwartz RH, Bahadori RS, et al. Diagnosis and management of the newborn and young infant who have nasal obstruction. Pediatr Rev. 2000;21(12):416-20.
2. Visvanathan V, Wynne DM. Congenital nasal pyriform aperture stenosis: a case report of 10 cases and literature review. Int J Pediatr Otorhinolaryngol. 2012;76(1):28-30.

3. Shikowitz M. Congenital nasal pyriform aperture stenosis: diagnosis and treatment. Int J Pediatr Otorhinolaryngol. 2003;67:635-9.
4. Kent SE, Reid AP, Nairn ER, et al. Neonatal septal deviations. J R Soc Med. 1988;81:132-5.
5. Hedlund G. Congenital frontonasal masses: developmental anatomy, malformations and MR imaging. Pediatr Radiol. 2006;36(7):647-62.
6. Wang IJ. Congenital midline nasal mass: case series and review of the literature. Turk J Pediatr. 2010;52:520-4.
7. Kwong KM. Current updates on choanal atresia. Front Pediatr. 2015;3:52.
8. Kinis, V, Ozbay M, Akdag M, et al. Patients with congenital choanal atresia treated by transnasal endoscopic surgery. J Craniofac Surg. 2014;25(3):892-7.
9. Bluestone C, Casselbrant M, Stool S, et al. Pediatric Otolaryngology, 4th edition. Philadelphia: Elsevier;2003.
10. Wetmore R, Muntz H, McGill T. Pediatric Otolaryngology—Principles and Practice Pathways, 2nd edition. New York: Thieme; 2012.
11. Calhoun K, Healy G, Johnson J, et al. Byron Bailey Head and Neck Surgery, 3rd edition. Philadelphia: Lippincott Williams & Wilkins; 2001.
12. Cummings C, Flint P, Harker L, et al. Cummings Otolaryngology Head and Neck Surgery, 4th edition. Philadelphia: Mosby Elsevier;2005.

Chapter **38**

Pediatric Head and Neck Infections

Donald Solomon

OVERVIEW

The general and/or pediatric otolaryngologist is often the last line of defense in offering definitive treatment for complicated or recurrent infections of the ears, nose, throat, or cervical soft tissue. Whether the situation calls for antibiotic therapy alone, drainage of abscess, curettage of necrotic tissue in atypical mycobacteria infection, or more routine intervention such as myringotomy tube placement, pediatricians and family practitioners will often refer their patients when infectious processes extend outside of their clinical comfort zone. It behooves the otolaryngologist to be well versed in the symptoms, causes, complications, and treatment algorithms employed to address pediatric head and neck infections.

INFECTIONS OF THE EXTERNAL AND MIDDLE EAR

External Ear Canal

Bacterial Otitis Externa ("Swimmer's Ear")

Signs and symptoms: This type of infection follows head immersion in water leading to protective cerumen being washed away, an increase in ear canal pH, and introduction of bacterial pathogens into a warm, damp environment where they may thrive. The superficial layers of the ear canal skin become infected, evidenced by desquamation, edema, purulent otorrhea, and extreme pain. As the infection progresses, superficial cellulitis moves to the auricle, leading to edema, erythema, and a standing ear deformity (Fig. 38.1).[3,13,14]

Pathogens: *Pseudomonas aeruginosa* alone may cause infection, although concomitant *Staphylococcus aureus* or *Streptococcus pyogenes* growth is often present.

Treatments:

1. Debridement of the ear canal such that topical antibiotic/ steroid ear drops with *Pseudomonas* coverage (neomycin/ polymyxin/hydrocortisone or fluoroquinolone/ dexamethasone) may penetrate to the medial ear canal.

2. Ear canal stent (Otowick) placement when the ear canal skin is so edematous that adequate penetration of topical antibiotic/steroid ear drops is in question (Fig. 38.2).

3. Topical antibiotic/steroid ear drops may be adequate in early infection without significant ear canal edema or superficial auricular cellulitis. Oral antibiotics covering *S. aureus* and *S. pyogenes* should be administered when ear drop penetration is in question or when auricular cellulitis is present.

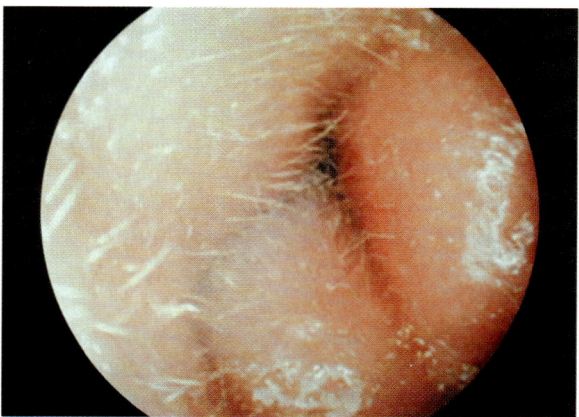

Fig. 38.1: Edematous ear canal in a patient with otitis externa.

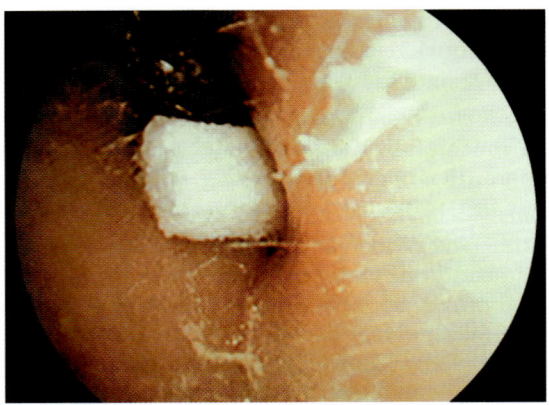

Fig. 38.2: Otowick placed to stent open the ear canal in otitis externa.

Complications:

Necrotizing Otitis Externa

Progression of otitis externa to involve the cartilage and bone surrounding the external auditory canal; more accurately described as skull base osteomyelitis. Infection spreads through the fissures of Santorini and is associated with granulation tissue at the bony cartilaginous junction in the ear canal (Fig. 38.3), purulent otorrhea and often facial nerve palsy. Magnetic resonance imaging readily shows soft tissue inflammation and marrow enhancement. Treatment involves intravenous (IV) antibiotics and debridement of necrotic soft tissue and/or bone when infection is progressing despite antibiotics. Correction of underlying causes, including diabetic hyperglycemia or immune compromise, is important.

Fungal Otitis Externa (Otomycosis)

Signs and symptoms: Fungal otitis externa may be caused by immersion in water, similar to bacterial otitis externa, or exposure to prolonged courses of antibiotic ear drops leading to removal of competitive bacterial skin flora. Symptoms typically include a

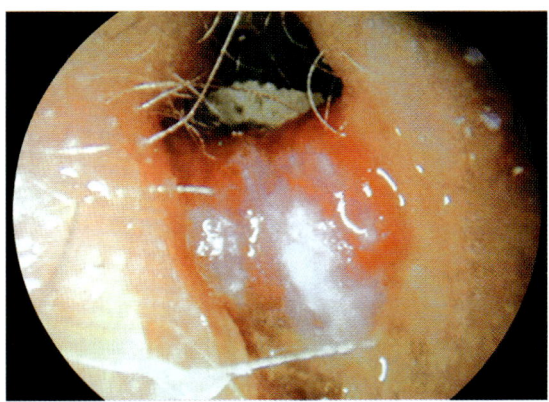

Fig. 38.3: Granulation tissue at the bony cartilaginous junction in the ear canal secondary to necrotizing otitis externa.

sensation of auricular fullness as "wet tissue paper" fungal debris fills the ear canal, ear canal pruritus, and occasionally pain. The ear canal skin tends to evidence mild superficial edema and erythema (Fig. 38.4).[3,13,14]

Pathogens: Most commonly *Aspergillus* or *Candida* species.

Treatments: Topical antifungal solutions or creams such as 1% clotrimazole for prolonged periods of ≥2 weeks are often effective. Oral antifungals such as fluconazole or itraconazole may be necessary in the face of nonresponsive or resistant infections.

Complications: Resistant infections causing prolonged symptoms necessitating culture-specific oral antifungal agents.

Middle Ear

Acute Otitis Media (AOM)

Signs and symptoms: Middle-ear infections most often occur several days after the onset of viral upper respiratory tract infection (URI) symptoms. Acute otitis media symptoms include

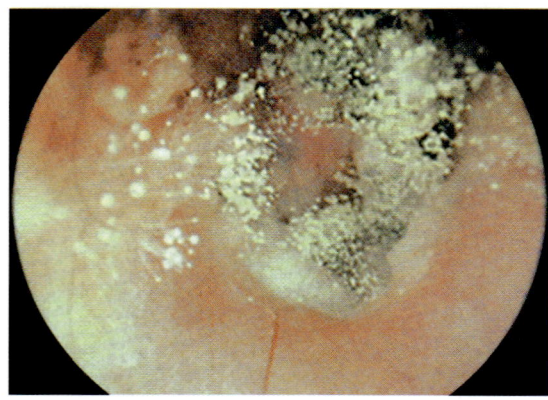

Fig. 38.4: Otomycosis/fungal otitis externa.

otalgia (variably evidenced by pulling at the ears), irritability (worse when lying flat), and fevers. Otoscopy reveals a bulging, erythematous tympanic membrane (TM) with hypervascularity (Fig. 38.5). The TM is not mobile on pneumatic otoscopy secondary to associated middle ear effusion. Risk factors include age <3 years, daycare attendance, secondhand smoke exposure, supine bottle feeding, a sibling with a history of recurrent AOM, craniofacial abnormalities, or immune deficiency. The incidence of recurrent AOM decreases after the age of 3 years.[1,2,13,14]

Pathogens: In decreasing order of incidence based on bacterial isolates obtained via tympanocentesis: *Streptococcus pneumoniae, Haemophilus influenzae, Moraxella catarrhalis*, and *S. pyogenes* [Group A strep (GAS) is more common in school-age children].

Treatment: First-line treatment for AOM is amoxicillin and should be given to patients < 23 months of age for unilateral or bilateral AOM with severe symptoms (otalgia for 48 hours or fever > 39°C) or for children >23 months of age with bilateral AOM without severe symptoms. Observation with follow-up evaluation

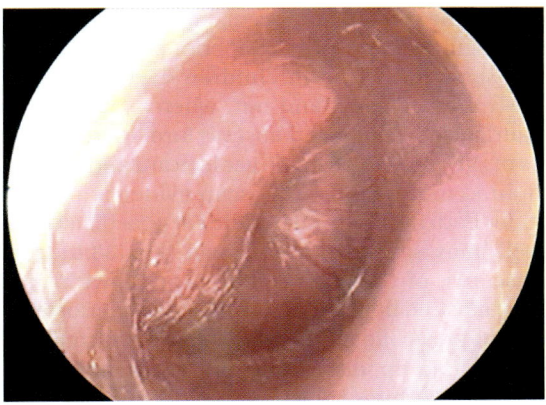

Fig. 38.5: Bulging tympanic membrane in acute otitis media.

can be instituted for children between 6 and 23 months of age with unilateral AOM and no severe symptoms or children >23 months of age with unilateral or bilateral AOM. An antibiotic with β-lactamase coverage is used when a child has received amoxicillin in the previous 30 days, or has concomitant purulent conjunctivitis or has a history of recurrent AOM unresponsive to amoxicillin.

Complications:

1. *Tympanic membrane perforation*: This is the most common complication of AOM and tends to occur more frequently in patients <1 year of age. Most perforations heal sponta-neously, although they will occasionally persist and require repair.

2. *Mastoiditis*: The incidence of mastoiditis has decreased markedly in the antibiotic era, though this complication of AOM still does occur. Hallmark symptoms include AOM with associated purulent middle ear effusion, standing ear deformity with postauricular edema, erythema, mastoid tenderness, fevers, and irritability. In mastoiditis, cortical

mastoid bone erosion may occur, leading to subperiosteal or frank subcutaneous abscess. Superior postauricular swelling and abscess formation in children < 2 years of age tends to push the ear down and out, whereas mid and inferior postauricular swelling and abscess formation in children >2 years of age tends to push the ear forward and up. Radiologic computed tomography (CT) scan evidence of mastoiditis includes both mastoid and middle ear opacification, mastoid air cell bony septation breakdown (Fig. 38.6) from acute coalescence of the suppurative process with or without cortical mastoid bone breakdown, and subperiosteal or frank subcutaneous collection. Rarely, abscess formation occurs at the mastoid tip, dissecting into the sternocleidomastoid (SCM) muscle; this is known as a Bezold's abscess. Treatment of acute mastoiditis includes hospital admission with IV antibiotics, myringotomy tube placement, and cortical mastoidectomy. Complications of untreated or aggressive mastoiditis include petrositis, meningitis, epidural, and/or brain abscess.[13,14]

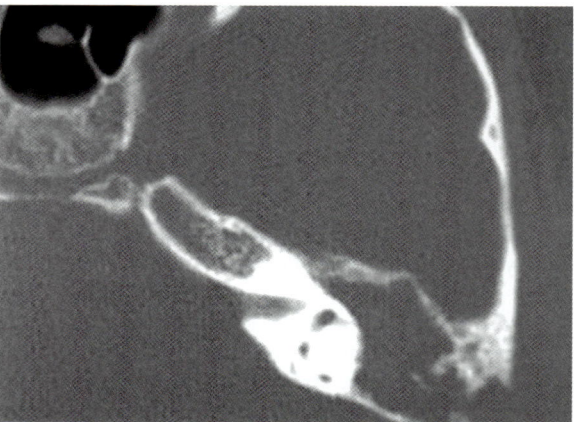

Fig. 38.6: Mastoiditis evidenced on axial computed tomography of the temporal bones with cortical erosion and mastoid air cell bony septation breakdown.

SINUSES/ADENOIDS

Sinusitis

Signs and Symptoms

1. Acute bacterial sinusitis usually occurs 10–30 days after the onset of a URI, evidenced by mucopurulent rhinorrhea, facial pressure, malaise, postnasal discharge, cough, and fevers.[4,5,13,14]
2. Subacute sinusitis persists for 30 days to 3 months.
3. Chronic sinusitis persists for >3 months. This is not simply an infectious process, but a multifactorial problem related to interplay between genetic, environmental, immunologic/ allergic, and anatomic factors. Obstructive anatomy and inflammation play a key role in allowing sinusitis to become chronic.

Pathogens

1. Acute and subacute sinusitis pathogens include, in order of prevalence, *S. pneumoniae*, *M. catarrhalis*, and *H. influenzae*. About 75% of *Moraxella* and 30% of *Haemophilus* are β-lactamase positive.
2. Chronic sinusitis pathogens include those above as well as *S. aureus*, *Corynebacterium*, *Bacteroides*, and *Fusobacterium*.

Treatment

1. *Acute sinusitis without fever >39°C or marked purulent rhinorrhea*: Amoxicillin (switch to augmentin if no improvement after 72 hours); treat for a 14-day duration. Oxymetazoline every 12 hours for 3 days beginning at the onset of antibiotic treatment and saline irrigations twice per day during the entire duration of antibiotic treatment.
2. *Acute sinusitis with fever >39°C or marked purulence*: Augmentin for 14 days without amoxicillin trial. Saline irrigations while on antibiotics and Afrin for 3 days only.
3. *Subacute sinusitis (symptoms for >30 days)*: Augmentin or second-generation cephalosporin for 20 days ± steroid taper.

Saline irrigations while on antibiotics and Afrin for 3 days only.

4. *Chronic sinusitis (symptoms for >3 months)*: Middle meatus culture directed or augmentin versus second-generation cephalosporin for 20 days + steroid taper. Saline irrigations while on antibiotics and Afrin for 3 days only.

Complications

1. *Preseptal cellulitis*: Extension of sinus infection to orbital and preseptal soft tissue without frank orbital collection. Treat with IV antibiotics (Unasyn or clindamycin + ceftriaxone). Saline irrigations while on antibiotics and Afrin for 3 days only.

2. *Subperiosteal or orbital abscess*: Extension of sinus infection to orbit with abscess formation (Fig. 38.7). Treat with hospital admission for IV antibiotics (Unasyn or clindamycin + ceftriaxone). Surgical approach to abscess—endoscopic sinus surgery versus external approach if no improvement occurs on 24 hours of antibiotics, if vision is threatened or if the abscess is large (>1 cm) to accelerate healing.

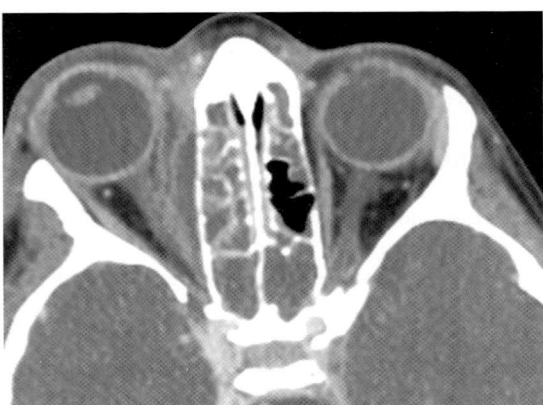

Fig. 38.7: Right subperiosteal orbital abscess.

3. *Pott's puffy tumor*: Osteitis of frontal bone with frontal soft tissue infection secondary to sinusitis. Treat with hospital admission for IV antibiotics (Unasyn or clindamycin + ceftriaxone). Saline irrigations while on antibiotics and Afrin for 3 days only. Surgical approach to abscess via external drainage and frontal sinus trephination or via endoscopic approach.

4. *Intracranial abscess*: Osteitis with intracranial extension of sinusitis. Treat with hospital admission for IV antibiotics (Unasyn or clindamycin + ceftriaxone). Saline irrigations while on antibiotics and Afrin for 3 days only. Neurosurgical consult and combined surgical management.

Adenoiditis

Signs and Symptoms

Adenoiditis is a chronic bacterial infection of the adenoid tissue for weeks to months, leading to thick mucopus overlying the adenoid tissue noted on endoscopy with associated symptoms of chronic nasal obstruction, rhinorrhea, postnasal discharge, and cough. Culture of the adenoid tissue may identify pathogens.[6,13,14]

Pathogens

Common adenoid pathogens include *S. pneumoniae*, *M. catarrhalis*, *H. influenza*, as well as *S. aureus*. Anaerobes may be present in infections lasting >30 days.

Treatment

Treatment is 20 days of culture-directed antibiotics on one or more occasions followed by adenoidectomy when antibiotic treatment alone fails to prevent persistence or recurrence of infection.

Complications

1. Episodes of AOM may be more frequent in children with adenoiditis.

2. Nasal obstruction with snoring and possibly obstructive sleep apnea may occur secondary to copious nasal secretions and inflamed, enlarged adenoids.

3. Postnasal discharge with chronic cough and asthma exacerbation may be present in children with chronic adenoiditis.

TONSILS/PHARYNX

Acute Pharyngitis (Tonsillitis)

Signs and Symptoms

Acute pharyngitis evidenced by complaint of sore throat and odynophagia with or without fever and generalized malaise. Tonsillitis is caused by viral or bacterial pathogens. It is more common in the colder months of the year and is often spread among school or daycare cohorts as well as among family members. Both viral and bacterial etiologies may be associated with fever, decreased oral intake, cervical lymphadenopathy, and exudative tonsillitis. Viral pharyngitis tends to be associated with cough, rhinorrhea, and conjunctivitis, whereas bacterial pharyngitis is not.[7,13,14]

Pathogens

Bacterial:

1. *Streptococcus pyogenes* (GAS) is the most common pathogen and may account for up to one third of cases in children. Group A strep infection leads to severe sore throat, fevers, headaches, and erythematous tonsillar mucosa. Rapid antigen detection test or rapid strep test has a high degree of specificity, while formal throat culture has high specificity and sensitivity.

2. Group C and G streptococci as well as mixed anaerobic bacteria may also cause pharyngitis. Symptoms are similar to GAS infection. Throat culture has varying degrees of sensitivity for positively identifying these infectious causes.

3. Mixed anaerobes or *Fusobacterium* species, *Bacteroides*, *Peptostreptococcus,* or *Prevotella* may also cause pharyngitis with associated exudative tonsillitis, significant odynophagia, and high fevers.

Viral:
1. Epstein–Barr virus (EBV) causes acute pharyngitis with marked tonsillar swelling in association with white exudative plaques over the tonsils. It is associated with diffuse cervical lymphadenopathy, including posterior chain adenopathy, distinguishing it from bacterial pharyngitis. Positive heterophile antibody or monospot test carries a high degree of specificity for acute EBV infection, while the presence of immunoglobulin M on serologic testing is both highly sensitive and specific in diagnosis.
2. Adenovirus causes acute pharyngitis and may be associated with concomitant conjunctivitis.
3. Coxsackievirus and enteroviruses cause acute pharyngitis associated with posterior oral cavity and pharyngeal ulcers and high fever.

Treatment

1. Group A strep pharyngitis remains sensitive to penicillin and amoxicillin as well as cephalosporins and clindamycin.
2. Group C and G streptococci first-line treatment is with penicillin and amoxicillin, similar to GAS.
3. Mixed anaerobe and *Fusobacterium* species may be treated with amoxicillin or clindamycin.
4. Viral pharyngitis treatment is directed at pain control and supportive measures. Steroid use is frequently employed when treating acute tonsillitis secondary to EBV infection that exhibits associated acute obstructive airway symptoms.

Complications

Peritonsillar abscess: Peritonsillar abscess (PTA) is the most common suppurative complication of bacterial pharyngitis/

tonsillitis. Peritonsillar abscess generally occurs several days after the onset of sore throat. It presents more often in teenagers and young adults than children. Hallmark symptoms and signs include acute worsening of odynophagia with associated decreased oral intake, fevers, muffled voice, leukocytosis, trismus, soft palate erythema/edema/asymmetry. Computed tomography scan (Fig. 38.8) is usually not necessary in diagnosis. Group C *Streptococcus* is the most commonly isolated organism. Treatment is drainage of abscesses >1 cm in diameter in concert with antibiotics (clindamycin or augmentin) and supportive care.

Parapharyngeal abscess: This infectious process presents with fevers, decreased neck range of motion, significant odynophagia and decreased oral intake, leukocytosis, neck swelling, and lateral pharyngeal wall deviation toward the midline on intraoral examination. Computed tomography scan with contrast offers definitive diagnosis. Bacterial isolates are similar to those noted in PTA. Treatment is surgical drainage via an external or intraoral approach and IV antibiotics (clindamycin or ampicillin-sulbactam).

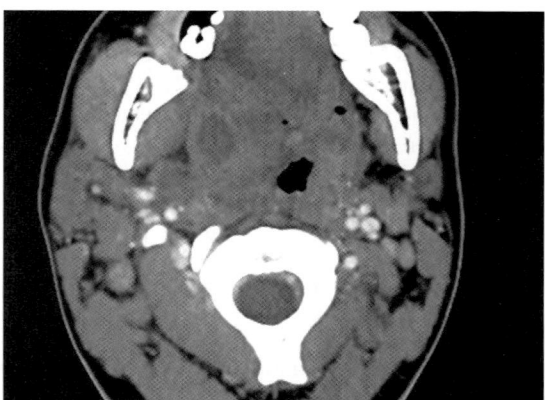

Fig. 38.8: Peritonsillar abscess on axial computed tomography.

Retropharyngeal abscess: This tends to present in younger children and is thought to arise when suppurative breakdown of the retropharyngeal lymph nodes occurs. It most often follows a pharyngeal or adenoid infection and symptoms are similar to those seen in parapharyngeal abscess, including odynophagia, decreased oral intake, decreased neck range of motion, fevers, and leukocytosis. Occasionally a posterior pharyngeal wall bulge is noted on intraoral examination.Computed tomography scan with contrast is helpful (Fig. 38.9), but not always definitive in diagnosis. Common intraoral aerobic and anaerobic bacteria are isolated from culture specimens, including GAS, group C *Streptococcus*, *S. aureus*, *Haemophilus* species, *Peptostreptococcus*, *Prevotella*, *Bacteroides,* and *Fusobacterium*. Treatment is intraoral surgical drainage and IV antibiotics (clindamycin or ampicillin–sulbactam).

LARYNGEAL AND TRACHEAL INFECTIONS

Viral Laryngotracheitis (Croup)

Signs and Symptoms

This infectious process presents most frequently in children from < 2 years of age as a barking cough progressing to biphasic stridor

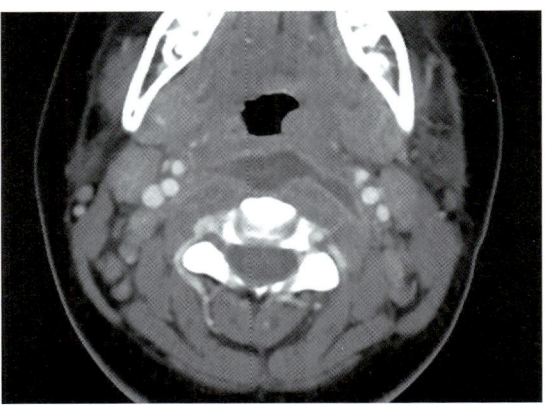

Fig. 38.9: Retropharyngeal abscess on axial computed tomography.

with associated inspiratory retractions. There is a continuum of symptom severity, and some cases do not progress past barking cough. Most cases are preceded by an upper respiratory viral syndrome. Diagnosis is based on clinical presentation, but lateral neck X-ray evidencing "steeple sign" or subglottic air space narrowing may be helpful.[8,13,14]

Pathogens

The most common etiologic agents are viral pathogens including the parainfluenza viruses, influenza A, influenza B, and respiratory syncytial virus.

Treatment

Mild cases of croup may be treated with humidification of air alone in the outpatient setting, whereas moderate cases require corticosteroids in either a single or 3- to 5-day dose regimen. Severe cases of croup associated with significant respiratory distress require hospitalization and treatment with racemic epinephrine as well as IV steroid.

Complications

Rarely, the respiratory distress associated with croup is not ameliorated by racemic epinephrine and IV steroid. Heliox may be used in these instances to avoid intubation, but if this fails intubation and mechanical ventilation are necessary.

Bacterial Supraglottitis (Epiglottitis)

Signs and Symptoms

This condition more frequently presents in older children and adults, although prior to the *Haemophilus* type b vaccine it more often presented in younger children. Classic signs and symptoms include sitting in the "tripod" or "sniffing" position with the child leaning forward and opening the hypopharynx via posturing as well as drooling, fevers, muffled voice, respiratory distress, and leukocytosis. Lateral neck X-ray may reveal a classic "thumbprint" sign or widened, blunted epiglottis that is strongly suggestive of epiglottitis (Fig. 38.10).[8,13,14]

Pathogens

Haemophilus influenzae type b previously accounted for the vast majority of infections, but the universal *H. influenzae* type b vaccine has virtually eliminated this bacterium as a causative organism and significantly reduced the incidence of this infection. Current causative organisms are those noted in pharyngeal soft tissue infection section and include GAS, *S. aureus*, nontypeable *H. influenza*, and *M. catarrhalis* among others.

Treatment

Airway management is the most pressing treatment need in patients with supraglottitis. Children who present with evidence of airway compromise should be treated rapidly in a setting where intubation and tracheostomy may be performed. These patients

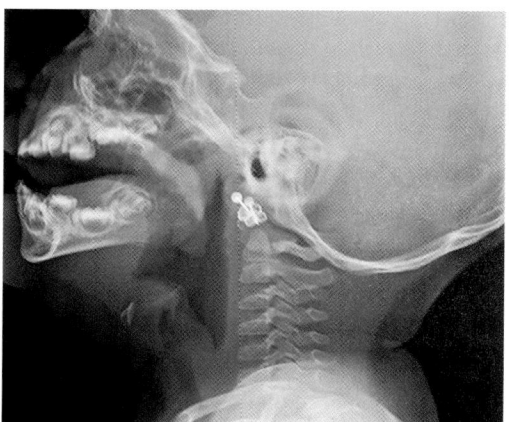

Fig. 38.10: Blunted epiglottis on lateral neck X-ray ("thumbprint sign").

should remain with familiar caregivers until mask induction of anesthesia, laryngoscopy, and subsequent intubation can be performed if necessary and/or tracheostomy. Intubation is usually not necessary for >48 hours. Broad-spectrum antibiotic coverage should be started after the airway is secured and includes third-generation cephalosporins, clindamycin, or Unasyn. Epiglottic swab cultures should be obtained during laryngoscopy, followed by blood cultures.

Complications

Tracheostomy may be necessary in the face of prolonged intubation or if initial intubation is unsuccessful. Epiglottic or deep neck abscesses may arise requiring incision and drainage. Sepsis may be present in severe cases.

Bacterial Tracheitis

Signs and Symptoms

This condition may follow a simple viral URI or other systemic infection such as measles. Children present with acute worsening of their underlying illness, respiratory distress including stridor and retractions, as well as productive cough and fevers. Flexible laryngoscopy commonly reveals a mildly inflamed larynx not accounting for the severity of presenting symptoms.[9,13,14]

Pathogens

Staphylococcus aureus is the most commonly isolated pathogen, although other classic upper respiratory bacterial pathogens including GAS, *H. influenzae*, *M. catarrhalis*, and *S. pneumoniae* have been isolated.

Treatment

Stabilizing and securing the distal airway is the most important primary treatment. Intubation may be complicated by significant narrowing secondary to crusts and debris as well as ulceration of the trachea. Frequently, a smaller than usual endotracheal tube is necessary. Meticulous endotracheal tube care to prevent obstruction is required during the course of intubation. Intravenous antistaphylococcal antibiotics are employed with consideration for methicillin-resistant *S. aureus* coverage.

Complications

Distal pulmonary infiltrates as well as significant pneumonia with attendant sequelae, including sepsis and respiratory distress syndrome, are possible. Post-tracheitis subglottic and/or tracheal stenosis have been reported.

SKIN/SOFT TISSUE OF NECK/REGIONAL NODES

Cervical Lymphadenitis

Signs and Symptoms

Cervical lymphadenitis presents with enlarged, tender or nontender cervical nodes that swell secondary to infectious etiology.[10-14]

1. A single unilateral, tender, enlarged lymph node with overlying skin erythema present for and progressing over hours to days is most often related to bacterial infection of the upper aerodigestive tract. Node tenderness, fevers, malaise, and leukocytosis are usually present.
2. Multiple unilateral, enlarged lymph nodes with overlying skin erythema or other discoloration, and potentially suppurative subcutaneous or superficial breakdown are often related to indolent bacterial or mycobacterial infection.
3. Multiple, bilateral, nontender enlarged lymph nodes present for and progressing over hours to days often follow a viral URI.

Pathogens

Bacterial pathogens:

1. *Staphylococcus aureus* and GAS are by far the most common causes of acute unilateral, suppurative cervical lymphadenitis. Children <6 of age are most often affected.

Suppuration occurs over a 2- to 3-day period from the onset of lymph node enlargement and may be diagnosed secondary to skin pointing and breakdown or via obtaining ultrasound, performing needle aspiration, or obtaining a contrast CT scan.

2. Anaerobic bacteria from dental caries can cause acute submental and submandibular lymphadenitis in older children, which may progress rapidly to complicated infection including Ludwig's angina, massive disseminated neck abscesses, and/or thrombophlebitis if not treated with antibiotics and drainage.

3. Tuberculosis mycobacteria (TB), nontuberculosis mycobacteria (NTM), actinomyces, and *Bartonella henselae* are the most common causes of subacute or chronic cervical lymphadenitis.

   a. Tuberculosis mycobacteria lymphadenitis usually occurs during active infection from spread to paratracheal nodes and can cause significant cervical adenopathy with or without suppuration progressing over weeks to months in children of any age group with a primary TB infection.

   b. Nontuberculosis mycobacteria presents most often with a unilateral submandibular or angle of mandible node with associated overlying violaceous skin changes that progress to suppuration over weeks to months with associated overlying skin breakdown and potential for sinus tract formation (Fig. 38.11). Nontuberculosis myco-bacteria infection is thought to arise from playing with or ingesting soil with NTM microbes and is usually seen in children <6 years of age.

   c. Actinomyces infection presents as unilateral cervical lymphadenitis along the body of the mandible progressing over weeks to months to a chronic, suppurative draining fistula if untreated and arises from an intraoral dental source.

   d. *Bartonella henselae* infection presents as a unilateral enlarged node or nodes weeks to months after inoculation

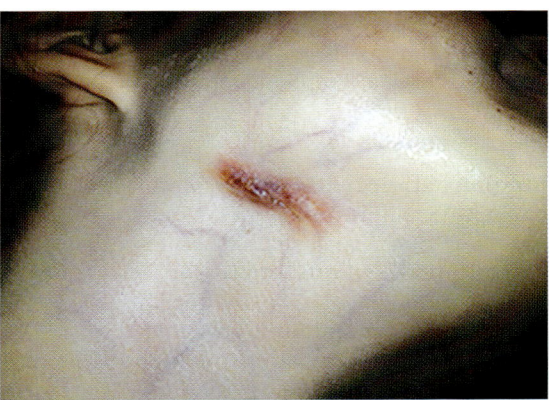

Fig. 38.11: Nontuberculosis mycobacterial infection.

from a feline source, most often infected kittens. Firm lymphadenopathy is noted initially, progressing to suppurative breakdown and potential chronic draining fistula.

Viral pathogens: Acute bilateral cervical lymphadenitis is often viral in origin. The lymphadenitis is most often nontender or only mildly tender.

1. Epstein–Barr virus causes acute bilateral posterior more often than anterior cervical lymphadenitis in concert with pharyngitis and exudative tonsillitis with tonsillar enlargement.

2. Herpes virus causes acute regional cervical lymphadenitis in association with ulcerative stomatitis of the oral mucosa or vermillion epidermis.

3. Cytomegalovirus may cause stomatitis or pharyngitis in association with cervical lymphadenitis in the anterior or posterior cervical distribution.

4. Enterovirus (coxsackievirus) may cause acute pharyngitis with associated malaise, fever, and cervical lymphadenitis.

5. Adenovirus causes pharyngoconjunctival fever with associated pharyngitis, conjunctivitis, fever, malaise, and generalized cervical lymphadenopathy.

Treatment

1. Acute unilateral cervical lymphadenitis secondary to *S. aureus* or GAS requires antibiotics. When suppuration occurs, incision and drainage hasten resolution and decrease risks of complication. Culture is necessary to rule out resistant bacteria, and consideration of methicillin-resistant *S. aureus* incidence in the community is important.

2. Acute unilateral cervical lymphadenitis secondary to anaerobic infection related to dental caries requires antibiotics with anaerobic coverage such as clindamycin or ampicillin–sulbactam. Extraction of the offending carious tooth and incision and drainage of suppurative lymphadenitis hasten infection resolution and decrease risk of complication.

3. Subacute or chronic lymphadenitis treatment:
   a. Tuberculosis mycobacteria should be treated with systemic antituberculosis antibiotics because needle or open incision and drainage can lead to chronic draining fistula.
   b. Nontuberculosis mycobacteria with suppuration may be treated with antituberculosis antibiotics or definitive curettage of necrotic skin and lymph tissue if the local nerves including the facial nerve are not at risk.
   c. *Bartonella henselae* infection may be treated with macrolides, Bactrim, rifampin, or later-generation cephalosporins. Suppurative nodes may be incised and drained or needle drained, but may recur several times before resolution over a 2–4-month period.
   d. *Actinomyces* infection may be treated with antibiotics alone. A prolonged course of 6–12 months may be necessary. *Actinomyces* remains sensitive to penicillin.

4. *Viral cervical lymphadenitis*: Treatment is aimed at support to address underlying symptoms related to viral sequelae, including tonsillar hypertrophy and pain, which may require steroids and pain medication to prevent obstructive symptoms and dehydration. It should be noted that splenomegaly occurs in more than half of EBV infections, so contact sports should be avoided for at least 6 weeks.

Complications

1. *Acute bacterial cervical lymphadenitis with suppuration*: Untreated or undertreated cervical abscesses may worsen to involve multiple deep neck spaces and progress to sepsis, mediastinitis, or thrombophlebitis.

2. *Subacute or chronic cervical lymphadenitis*: Even with treatment, bacterial infections leading to chronic cervical lymphadenopathy as listed above may cause prolonged and recurrent symptoms including resuppuration and/or chronic draining fistula tracts with associated disfiguring scars on eventual resolution of infection. Curative curettage risks injuring nerves, most commonly branches of the marginal mandibular nerve in NTM, or leaving a long-term scar.

3. *Viral lymphadenitis*:
   a. Epstein–Barr virus infection often leads to splenomegaly, which puts the individual at risk for splenic rupture. Obstructive upper airway symptoms may also arise, requiring hospitalization with varying degrees of airway support.
   b. It is necessary to rule out malignancy in the face of prolonged nonsuppurative lymphadenopathy. If viral titers are inconclusive, risk factors that may lead to biopsy include single enlarging node, posterior chain node, a child >13 years of age, presence of weight loss, fatigue, unexplained fevers, chills, or night sweats. Purified protein derivative placement and a chest X-ray will help diagnose TB and NTB.

INFECTED CONGENITAL NECK ANOMALIES

Acute Bacterial Infection of Congenital Neck Masses

Signs and Symptoms

Similar to symptoms present in acute unilateral cervical lymphadenitis, one notes rapid-onset swelling in the distribution of the congenital anomaly with associated tenderness, overlying skin erythema, fevers, malaise, and leukocytosis.[13,14]

Pathogens

Similar to acute unilateral cervical lymphadenitis; the most common organisms are *S. aureus* and GAS.

Treatment

Antibiotics and needle versus open incision and drainage. Given that these congenital anomalies need to be excised to prevent recurrent infection, judicious use of incision and drainage is utilized as scarred incision tracts make eventual excision more difficult.

Specific Infected Congenital Anomalies

1. *Infected thyroglossal duct cyst*: Mid-line erythematous, tender, swollen mass that elevates with swallowing; sometimes confused with a single, infected submental node that suppurates, but does not elevate with swallowing.
2. *Infected preauricular pit cyst and sinus*: Long-standing pit anterior to or above the root of the auricular helix that becomes associated with underlying swelling, tenderness, purulent pit drainage, and surrounding skin erythema (Fig. 38.12).
3. *Infected first branchial cleft anomaly*: Skin erythema, tenderness, and swelling in the area of a preauricular or infra-auricular pit anterior or inferior to the tragus or ear canal, which becomes associated with underlying

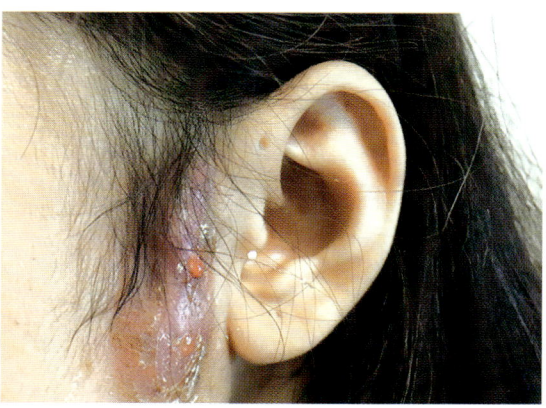

Fig. 38.12: Infected preauricular pit cyst and sinus.

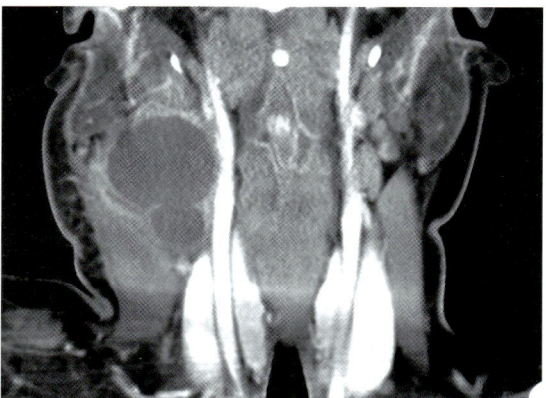

Fig. 38.13: Infected second branchial cleft anomaly.

swelling, tenderness, and purulent drainage in concert with surrounding skin erythema.

4. *Infected second branchial cleft anomaly*: Skin erythema, tenderness, and swelling anterior and deep to the SCM

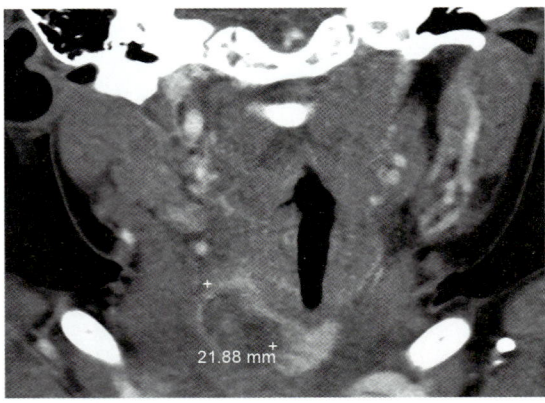

Fig. 38.14: Infected third branchial cleft cyst with thyroid abscess.

tracking below the angle of mandible toward the tonsillar fossa; variably associated with a superficial pit at the anterior border of the SCM (Fig. 38.13).

5. *Infected third branchial cleft anomaly*: Skin erythema, tenderness, and swelling at the level of the thyroid on one side (Fig. 38.14). This entity masquerades as an abscess of the thyroid gland's lateral lobe.

6. *Infected lymphatic malformation*: Rapid-onset swelling with associated skin erythema and tenderness in the region of a previously diagnosed lymphatic malformation, usually following a viral URI.

REFERENCES

1. Lieberthal A, Carroll AE, Chonmaitree T, et al. The diagnosis and management of acute otitis media. Pediatrics. 2013;131:964-99.
2. Venekamp RP. Antibiotics for acute otitis media in children. Cochrane Database Syst Rev. 2013;1:CD000219.
3. Jayakar R, Sanders J, Jones E, et al. A study of acute otitis externa at Wellington Hospital, 2007–2011. Australas Med J. 2014;7(10):392-9.

4. Ramadan HH. Surgical management of chronic sinusitis in children. Laryngoscope. 2004;114: 2103-09.

5. Clement PA, Bluestone CD, Gordts F, et al. Management of rhinosinusitis in children. Consensus Meeting, Brussels Belgium, September 13, 1996. Arch Otolaryngol Head Neck Surg. 1998;124:31-4.

6. Marzouk H, Aynehchi B, Thakkar P, et al. The utility of nasopharyngeal culture in the management of chronic adenoiditis. Int J Pediatr Otorhinolaryngol. 2012;76(10):1413-5.

7. Stelter K. Tonsillitis and sore throat in children. GMS Curr Top Otorhinolaryngol Head Neck Surg. 2014;13:Doc07.

8. Sobol SE, Zapata S. Epiglottitis and croup. Otolaryngol Clin North Am. 2008;41(3):551-66.

9. Shargorodsky J, Whittemore KR, Lee GS, et al. Bacterial tracheitis: a therapeutic approach. Laryngoscope. 2010;120(12):2498-501.

10. Block SL. Managing cervical lymphadenitis—a total pain in the neck. Pediatr Ann. 2014;43(10): 390-6.

11. Leung AK, Davies HD. Cervical lymphadenitis: etiology, diagnosis, and management. Curr Infect Dis Rep. 2009;11(3):183-9.

12. Walker PC, Karnell LH, Ziebold C, et al. Changing microbiology of pediatric neck abscesses in Iowa 2000–2010. Laryngoscope. 2013;123(1):249-52.

13. Long S, Pickering LK, Prober C. Principles and Practice of Pediatric Infectious Disease, 4th edition. Philadelphia:Elsevier; 2012.

14. Wetmore R, Muntz H, McGill T. Pediatric Otolaryngology— Principles and Practice Pathways, 2nd edition. New York: Thieme; 2012.

Chapter 39

Airway Foreign Bodies

Kristen Hurst

AIRWAY FOREIGN BODIES

Epidemiology

- Male predominance with male to female ratio of 2:1.[1-3]
- Around 75% of aerodigestive foreign bodies (FBs) are found in children < 3 years of age.[3,4]
- Aerodigestive FBs are the third most common cause of accidental death in pediatric population.[5]
- Annual incidence of death related to choking and aspiration of FB is ~3,000 children per year.
- Average interval from aspiration to intervention is ~2.5 weeks.

History

- Most reliable indicator:[2]
    - The higher the mass, the more the respiratory distress.[1]
    - Classic triad (cough, wheezing, and decreased air entry) is highly specific.[6,7]
- Around 50% can have a negative history.
- Three phases:
    - *Initial phase:* Choking, gagging, coughing spell/paroxysmal coughing event, and airway obstruction.
        - About 75% sensitivity and 92% specificity.

- Very sensitive in early (<2 weeks) presentation
- Very specific in late (>2 weeks) presentation[6,7]
  - *Asymptomatic phase:* Lag interval when FB becomes lodged, irritating sensation is dulled, and cough reflex fatigues.
  - *Complication phase:*
    - *Airway signs:* Stridor, hoarseness, and cyanosis
    - *Airway symptoms:* Cough, hemoptysis, fever, malaise, and respiratory arrest

Physical Examination

- Positive in ~60% patients.[3]
- Chest auscultation:
  - *Laryngeal obstruction:* Inspiratory as well as expiratory stridor
  - Tracheal obstruction
    - Object moving with cough or manipulation of trachea
    - "Asthmatic wheeze" present over trachea versus bilateral lung fields
    - Prolonged expiratory wheeze
  - *Bronchial obstruction:* Ipsilateral diminished breath sounds
- Perform flexible fiberoptic examination if suspicious for a supraglottic mass.
- Consider white blood cell count, which increases diagnostic specificity.[7]

Radiologic Evaluation

a. Chest X-ray (CXR):
   i. Motion artifact is challenged in young age group.[7]
   ii. Not sensitive, but helpful in the diagnosis of FB.
      1. It is used to predict the position of FB:
         a. Posterior–anterior view is necessary.
         b. Radiopaque FB is easily identifiable.

2. Findings:
   a. About 25–30% CXR may be normal.[2]
   b. Radiopaque FB: 5–15%.
   c. Indirect signs of FB:
      i. Atelectasis/collapse: 9–50%
      ii. Pneumonia: 2–4%
      iii. Air trapping/mediastinal shift: 30–60%
      iv. Direct identification of FB
3. *Biphasic films*—inspiratory/expiratory films:
   a. *Pros*: Only way to show mediastinal shift and air trapping.
   b. *Cons*: Child must be able to follow instructions and radiation is increased.
   c. *Normal*: Inspiratory hyperinflation and expiratory hypoinflation.
   d. *Abnormal*: Inspiratory hypoinflation and expiratory hyperinflation.
   e. *"Check valve"*: Obstructs on expiration, hyperinflation on the affected side and mediastinal shift away from the affected side.
   f. *"Ball valve"*: Obstructs on inspiration, atelectasis and mediastinal shift toward the affected side; expiration causes mediastinal shift away from the affected side.
   g. *"Stop valve"*: Complete obstruction of bronchus with consolidation of the affected lobe.
4. Lateral decubitus films:
   a. Useful in younger children.
   b. *Normal:* Dependent lung collapses.
   c. *Abnormal:* Dependent lung is inflated.
   d. Airway fluoroscopy:
      i. Alternative to inspiratory/expiratory films.
      ii. It does not require cooperation/coordination of patient.
      iii. Ten percent of cases with FB aspiration will be negative.

Preoperative Management and Surgical Decision Making

- Emergent endoscopy indications:
  - Respiratory distress.
  - Organic FB; tendency to swell with exposure to secretions.
  - Risk factors as predictors of FB:[7] immediate bronchoscopy recommended with more than two risk factors.
    - Witnessed choking crisis
    - Focal hyperinflation
    - Elevated white blood cell count
- "Three strikes" rule:
  - One positive from history/radiology/physical findings: "Think about taking a look."
  - Two positive from history/radiology/physical findings: "Talk about taking a look."
  - Three positive from history/radiology/physical findings: "Take a look!"
- Avoid delays in diagnosis by keeping low threshold for bronchoscopy:
  - History plus one positive from radiology/examination.
  - Negative history does not mean that there was no FB.
  - Never exclude on the basis of CXR alone.
  - Avoid misdiagnoses such as asthma, upper respiratory infection (URI), or pneumonia.
- Acute complete airway obstruction:
  - Back blows and chest thrusts for children <1 year of age.
  - Heimlich maneuver for those >1 year of age.
  - Intervention reserved for complete obstruction with inability to speak or cough due to risk of worsening incomplete obstruction.
  - Most FBs include hot dogs, nuts, grapes, and latex balloons.
- Informed consent:
  - *Complications secondary to FB:* Persistent cough, recurrent pneumonia, atelectasis, emphysema, laryngeal

edema, laryngeal trauma and swelling, bleeding, pneumomediastinum, pneumothorax, bronchiectasis, bronchial stenosis, persistence of cough, granulation tissue, strictures, and lung abscess.[8]

- *Complications secondary to endoscopy:* Hypoventilation, defective equipment, injury to mucosal surfaces, edema of mucosa due to manipulation, advancement of FB into distal airway, hypoxia and bradycardia/arrhythmia, pneumomediastinum, subcutaneous emphysema, laryngeal edema, and laryngeal spasm.
- *Alternatives:* Tracheostomy, thoracotomy, and bronchotomy and/or pulmonary resection.

Operative Technique

- Preparation:
  - "Failure for preparation is preparation for failure".
  - *Duration of case:* "2 hours or 2 minutes".
  - Identify defective equipment.
- Spontaneous respiration:
  - Avoid apneas and positive pressure ventilation.
  - Do not premedicate.
- Instrumentation should be assembled and ready for use.
  - Laryngoscope.
  - Ventilating rigid bronchoscope
    - *Benefits of rigid versus flexible bronchoscopy:* Ability to control the airway, larger caliber suction, wide working channel, ability to handle larger FB, excellent optical telescopic visualization, wide variety of extraction instruments to retrieve the FB, and range of various sizes
  - Complete set of FB optical forceps
  - Suction devices
  - Protective eyewear
- *Laryngospasm:* It is prevented by laryngotracheal anesthesia with local anesthetic (4 mg/kg of 1% plain lidocaine is

maximum dose; each 1 mL of 1% lidocaine solution has 10 mg of lidocaine).

- *Supraglottic FB:* Magill forceps should be nearby to remove FB.
- *Tracheal FB*: The FB may need to be pushed into main bronchus to establish an airway.
- *Multiple objects*: Around 5% incidence; look distal as well as on contralateral side for second FB.[3]
- *Sharp objects*: These are removed with pointed end within distal end of bronchoscope to protect; otherwise, have pointed end away from you as you pull out FB.
- *Large FB*: A large FB can be broken into smaller pieces or removed transcervically via tracheostomy.
- *Distal FB*: Be cognizant of ventilating contralateral lung when working distally in a bronchus with a rigid bronchoscope—pull back to trachea intermittently for right–left lung ventilation. Flexible bronchoscopes should be used for distal objects. You can use gastrointestinal instruments through a flexible bronchoscope. Consider a Foley catheter to retract object by inflating beyond the object and retracting.
- *Granulation tissue*: Balloon dilation to tapenade bleeding or microdebridement.
- *Plastic bronchitis:*[9] Obstruction of bronchi by mucous casts.
  - Inflammatory versus noninflammatory.
  - Consider in patients with comorbidities.
    - Asthma, cystic fibrosis, pulmonary infections, and even acute chest syndrome associated with sickle-cell disease.
    - High rate of mortality, especially if underlying cardiac disease.
    - Deoxyribonuclease and ribonuclease.
- *Surgical adjuncts*:
  - High-dose steroid for airway swelling.
    - Edema can be a limiting factor.
    - Elevate the head of the bed.

- Heliox for obstruction.
- Racemic epinephrine for hemorrhage or edema.
- *Failure*:
  - Abort if severely impacted/granulation tissue/edema.
  - *Previous instrumentation:* This contributes significantly to difficulty with procedure, concern about edema; it is reasonable to wait 24 hours, administer humidity, and antibiotics and steroids prior to second look.[2,10]
  - Extracorporeal membrane oxygenation (ECMO).[11]

Foreign Body Specifics

- *Location of FB*:[12]
  - *Glottic*: 1% FB, e.g. ring.
  - *Subglottic*: 1% FB, e.g. bead.
  - *Tracheal*: 10–17% FB, e.g. rock.
  - *Eighty to ninety percent found in bronchi*: e.g. crayon and sunflower seed.
    - Left-sided bronchus: 18–40%.
    - Right-sided bronchus: 45–55%.
- *Types of FB*:
  - *Food:* Most common, ~70%, carrot, popcorn, nuts/seeds, candies, and bones.
    - Above foods rule for age appropriateness—"You cannot eat unless you can spell them" foods.
  - *Toys*: 20% (balloons, balls, and marbles).
  - *Other*: 10% (pins, beads, and pen caps).

Postoperative Management

- Educate parents about prevention:
  - "Child-proofing" house
- Antibiotics for pneumonia.
- Steroids for edema.
- Postoperative CXR if concern for tracheal injury, pneumothorax, or pneumomediastinum.
- Consideration of second look if complications occur.

- Consideration of child abuse/neglect.
  - Higher incidence of aspirations/ingestions with "high family stress."
    - Marital conflict
    - Mental and physical illness
    - Loss of a family member
    - Unstable family relationships

NASAL FOREIGN BODIES

Epidemiology

- Children 2–4- years old and neurologically impaired.
- Males show predominance over females.
- Most commonly right-sided nose due to right-handed predominance.

History

- Unobserved events, resulting in delays in diagnosis.
- *Symptoms:* Halitosis, unilateral nasal obstruction, and nasal pain.
- *Signs:* Unilateral foul-smelling rhinorrhea or sinusitis, and epistaxis.
- *Differential diagnosis:* Polyposis, URI, sinusitis, nasal cavity or nasopharyngeal tumors, and choanal atresia.

Physical Examination

- Examine both sides of the nose; most likely to see with flexible scope.
- Take care to prevent aspiration event.
- Consideration of tumor/mass.
- Mucus, edema, granulations, and bony destruction occur with chronic FBs.[13]

Radiologic Evaluation if Poor Examination

Rule out radiopaque FBs and presence of multiple FBs.

Preoperative Management and Surgical Decision Making

- Emergent cases:
  - *Button battery:* Damage from leakage of the alkaline solution or by thermal burns from a generated current.
  - *Magnets:* Pressure necrosis.
- Nonsurgical technique:
  - Removal of nasal FBs by pediatric emergency department physicians has been reported to be successful in 92% and 98% of cases.[14]
  - Positive pressure expulsion while occluding nasal passage contralateral to FB.
    - Nose blowing, parents mouth to mouth, straw mouth to mouth (requires tight seal), Sorrell's technique (catheter into contralateral nostril with mouth occluded), nasal cannula/high-flow oxygen into contralateral nostril with mouth occluded and Ambu bag.
  - *Foley catheter:* 5–6 French.[13]
    - Pass distal to FB, inflate with air.
- Informed consent:
  - Bleeding is the most common complication of removal.
  - *Risk of FB in nose:* Pain, obstruction, rhinorrhea, epistaxis, infection, ulceration of mucosa, posterior dislodgement, aspiration, trauma caused by object, septal perforation, sinusitis, and acute otitis media.
  - *Risk of surgery:* Aspiration of nasal FB into airway, trauma from removal attempts, infection, and choanal stenosis.

Operative Technique

- Procedural sedation versus papoose if failed positive pressure, Foley or forceps technique:
  - Carefully select patients.
  - Aspiration risk is increased without secure airway.
- Vasoconstriction:

- – Avoid if possible; it may cause posterior displacement/aspiration of FB.
- – Most protective of airway if the patient is sitting up.
- Equipment depends on type, size, shape, and location of FB.
  - – Nasal speculum.
  - – *Forceps:* Straight, bayonet, mosquito, and alligator.
  - – *Hooks:* Spherical FB.
  - – Foley or Fogarty balloon-tip catheter.
  - – *Magnet:* Metallic FB.

Foreign Body Specifics

- Type:[14]
  - – Food: 12–27%.
  - – Toys: 23–46%.
  - – Other: 35–65%.
    - · Hair beads.
    - · Magnets.
    - · Disc battery:
      - a. Use magnet[15]
- *Risk factors for complications:* Length of time in nose; size, shape and consistency of FB; and clinician experience.

Postoperative Management

- Postoperative antibiotics for septal perforation or sign of secondary infection.
- Educate parents about prevention:
  - – "Child-proofing" house
- Consideration of child abuse/neglect.
  - – Higher incidence of aspirations/ingestions with "high family stress".

ESOPHAGEAL FOREIGN BODIES

Definition

Cricopharyngeus (CP) muscle: This is a true sphincter composed of striated muscle in tonic contraction. The CP is innervated by the vagus. It originates from the lateral borders of the cricoid cartilage and forms a sling around the wall of the superior aspect of the cervical esophagus. The CP is bordered superiorly by the inferior constrictor muscle and merges inferiorly with the muscular layers of the cervical esophagus.

Epidemiology

1,500 people die annually from complications related to esophageal FB ingestion; children are most commonly affected.[16]

History

- Signs and symptoms:
    - *Acute:* Odynophagia, globus, choking, drooling, oral irritation, tongue edema, dysphagia, stridor, wheezing, chest pain, emesis, and food refusal.
    - *Chronic:* Fever, emesis, hematemesis, abdominal pain, distention, hematochezia, failure to thrive, and mediastinal abscess.
- Prior esophageal FB is likely to have anomaly with or without a history of surgical correction of anomaly.
    - Consider eosinophilic esophagitis and stricture.

Physical Examination

- Patients is usually present with respiratory distress due to shared wall with trachea.
- Dysphagia and drooling may be delayed.

Radiologic Evaluation

- Rule out radiopaque FB and presence of multiple FBs.
- Two-view X-rays confirm location in airway or esophagus.
- Symptomatic patients with normal CXR:
    - Esophagram may outline object, rule out stenosis or stricture.
    - Consider endoscopy.

Preoperative Management and Surgical Decision Making

- Emergent cases:
  - Obstructive symptoms.
    - Airway compromise.
    - Total esophageal obstruction: drooling.
  - Sharp objects, e.g. pins and needles.
  - Caustic FB:
    - *Disc battery:* Double disc sign on X-ray differentiates from coin. Localize the battery, identify the type, and retrieve as soon as possible. Electric current results in liquefactive necrosis with devastating consequences to surrounding structures.
    - This injures mucosa immediately and is associated with esophageal perforation, stricture formation, and death.
    - Liquid within the battery has alkaline properties.
    - Leakage of liquid leads to alkali-induced liquefactive necrosis within ~4 hours: disintegration of mucosa with deep tissue penetration.
      a. Thermal injury from electric current
      b. Pressure necrosis possible as well
      c. Complications:
         i. Stricture, perforation, tracheoesophageal fistula (TEF), mediastinitis, aortoesophageal fistula.
            1. Patient must have computed tomography surgery involved, and consider thoracotomy and ECMO if concern for potential aortoesophageal fistula exists.
- Blunt, noncaustic, nonbattery FB without airway involvement, and time elapsed is <24 hours:
  - Observation without intervention, wait for passage, and follow with serial CXR.

- Consent:
  - *Complications of endoscopic procedure:* Laceration, bleeding, pyrexia, perforation, and failure to remove FB.

Operative Technique

- Most safely performed with airway secured.
  - Balloon removal without secured airway can lead to airway obstruction.
- Esophagoscopy with FB optical forceps.

Foreign Body Specifics

- Location:
  - At or below CP, level of sixth cervical vertebrae.
    - Narrowest portion of esophagus.
    - Consider anatomic anomaly/stricture if elsewhere.
      a. For example, TEF repair site
    - Mid-esophagus
    - At site of aortic arch crossover
    - Distal esophagus/lower esophageal sphincter
    - History of Nissen
  - *Stomach*:
    - An FB in the stomach should not be brought back into the esophagus unless there is concern about its passing (e.g. sharp object, large object).
    - An FB that has passed into the stomach should pass within 48 hours; if not, removal is necessary.
    - An FB < 15 mm generally passes.
- Type:
  - Most commonly coins, followed by food bolus, batteries, magnets, pins.
    - Treatment:
      a. Esophageal
        i. Consider barium swallow to rule out perforation if suspicion exists.

    ii. Endoscopy to assess injury
- 1. Within 48 hours due to friability of esophageal wall.
- 2. Sucralfate, proton pump inhibitors/antihistamines.
- 3. Antibiotics.
- 4. Steroid use is controversial.

  b. Stomach
- i. Observe up to 48 hours.
- ii. An FB <15 mm is likely to pass.
- iii. An FB >15 mm is unlikely to pass.

- Complications
- a. Stricture formation, esophageal perforation, TEF, gastric perforation, mediastinitis, peritonitis, and abscess.

– Safety pins
- Sheath sharp end in esophagoscope.
- Pass sharp into stomach, rotate, and pull out with sharp end trailing.

– Magnets
- Worrisome if more than one is ingested.

Postoperative Management

- NPO if concern for perforation.
- Barium swallow if concern for perforation.
- Educate parents about prevention.
  – "Child-proofing" house
- Consideration of child abuse/neglect.
  – Higher incidence of aspirations/ingestions with "high family stress."

REFERENCES

1. Friedman EM, Calzada G. Caustic ingestion and foreign bodies in the aerodigestive tract. In: Bailey BJ, Johnson JT, Newlands SD (Eds). Bailey Head and Neck Surgery Otolaryngology, 4th

edition. Philadelphia: Lippincott Williams & Wilkins; 2006. pp. 1069-73.

2. Strome M. Tracheobronchial foreign bodies: an updated approach. Ann Otol Rhinol Laryngol. 1977;86:649-54.

3. McGuirt WF, Holmes KD, Feehs R, et al. Tracheobronchial foreign bodies. Laryngoscope. 1988;98 (6 Pt 1):615-8.

4. Darrin DH, Holinger LD. Foreign body of the larynx, trachea and bronchi. In: Bluestone CD, Stool S, Kenna MA (Eds). Pediatric Otolaryngology, 3rd edition. Philadelphia: WB Saunders; 1995. p. 1390.

5. Friedman EM. Caustic ingestions and foreign body aspiration: an overlooked form of child abuse. Ann Otol Rhinol Laryngol. 1987;96(6):709-12.

6. Tomaske M, Gerber AC, Stocker S, et al. Tracheobronchial foreign body aspiration in children—diagnostic value of symptoms and signs. Swiss Med Wkly. 2006;136:533-8.

7. Heyer C, Bollmeier M, Rossler L, et al. Evaluation of clinical, radiologic, and laboratory prebronchoscopy findings in children with suspected foreign body aspiration. J Pediatr Surg. 2006;41: 1882-8.

8. Steen KH, Zimmermann T. Tracheobronchial aspiration of foreign bodies in children: a study of 94 cases. Laryngoscope. 1990;100:525-30.

9. Brogan TV, Finn LS, Pyskaty DJ Jr, et al. Plastic bronchitis in children: a case series and review of the medical literature. Pediatr Pulmonol. 2002;34(6):482-7.

10. Cohen SR, Herbert WI, Lewis GB Jr, et al. Foreign bodies in the airway. Five year retrospective study with special reference to management. Ann Otol Rhinol Laryngol. 1980;89:437-42.

11. Park AH, Tunkel DE, Park E, et al. Management of complicated airway foreign body aspiration using extracorporeal membrane oxygenation (ECMO). Int J Pediatr Otorhinolaryngol. 2014;78(12): 2319-21.

12. Singh H, Parakh A. Tracheobronchial foreign body aspiration in children. Clin Pediatr. 2014;53: 415-9.

13. Kadish H. Ear and nose foreign bodies. Clin Pediatr. 2005;44:665-70.

14. Kiger JR, Brenker TE, Losek JD. Nasal foreign body removal in children. Pediatr Emerg Care. 2008;24:785-9.

15. Alletag MJ, Jacobson D, Santucci K, et al. Nasal disc battery removal: a novel technique using a magnetic device. Pediatr Emerg Care. 2014;30(7):488-90.

16. Webb WA. Management of foreign bodies in the upper GI tract. Gastroenterology. 1988;94:204-16.

Chapter 40

Pediatric Airway Disorders

George Harris, Mariah Pate

ANATOMIC CONSIDERATIONS

- *Infant larynx:* Higher in neck than older children (at level C2–3), thyroid cartilage is broader, and cricoid cartilage is the most prominent palpable structure.
- Infants are obligate nasal breathers.
- Epiglottis in contact with soft palate at birth (resolves at 4–6 months).
- Subglottis is narrowest point in infant airway.
- Endotracheal (ET) tube size = (16 + age)/4.

EMBRYOLOGY

- *Fourth week of development:* Thickening of posterior wall of foregut (laryngotracheal groove) forms respiratory diverticulum.
- Respiratory diverticulum is located caudal to fourth brachial arch.
  - It divides and elongates to form the larynx, trachea, lungs (dorsal), and esophagus (ventral).
  - Esophagus and airway are separated by tracheoesophageal septum.
- Laryngeal recanalization (formation of lumen) occurs during 10th week.

- All laryngeal muscles are from the sixth branchial arch and supplied by recurrent laryngeal nerve except for cricothyroid (fourth arch and superior laryngeal nerve).
- Laryngeal cartilages are derived from fourth and sixth branchial arches.

LARYNGEAL ORIGIN

Laryngomalacia

Diagnosis

- Most common laryngeal anomaly.
- Most common cause of stridor in infants.
- Intermittent inspiratory stridor (high-pitched, wet).
  - Worse when crying, feeding or supine
- Normal cry.
- *Complications:* Poor weight gain, failure to thrive (FTT), apnea, and cyanosis.

Evaluation

- Flexible laryngoscopy.
- *Findings:* Obstruction of laryngeal inlet during inspiration by elongated tubular epiglottis, redundant and fore-shortened aryepiglottic (AE) folds and redundant arytenoid cartilages.

Treatment

- Observation in the absence of FTT, recurrent cyanosis, recurrent apnea; usually resolves by 12–24 months without intervention.
- Antireflux medication (H2 blocker vs proton pump inhibitor).
- Supraglottoplasty for FTT, recurrent cyanosis, recurrent apnea: transect shortened AE folds and remove excess arytenoid tissue; laser versus cold knife.

Laryngeal Cleft

Diagnosis

- Failure of airway to separate from esophagus during development.
- Presents with aspiration, cyanotic episodes during feeding, FTT, and recurrent pneumonia.
- Associated with Pallister-Hall, Smith-Lemli-Opitz (Opitz G), and VATER/VACTERL syndromes.

Evaluation

- Direct laryngoscopy and bronchoscopy with palpation of intra-arytenoid space.
- *Findings:* Cleft or deep space between arytenoids.
- Video swallow study to assess aspiration status.
- Benjamin-Inglis classification (Fig. 40.1)

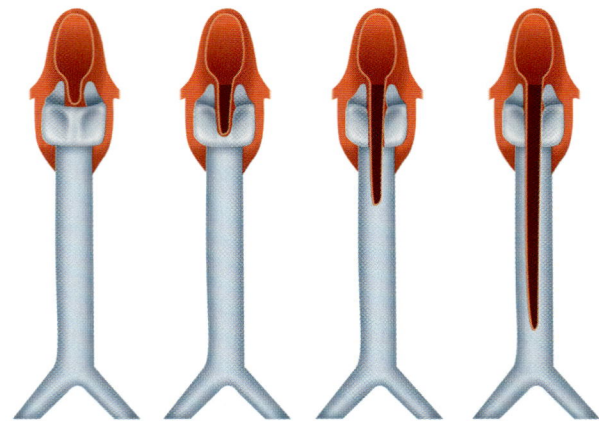

Fig. 40.1: Benjamin-Inglis classification of laryngeal cleft.
Source: Redrawn from Benjamin B, Inglis A. Minor congenital laryngeal clefts: diagnosis and classification. Ann Otol Rhinol Laryngol. 1989;98: 417-20.

- Deep intra-arytenoid notch without posterior cricoid involvement.
- Involves a portion of cricoid.
- Involves all the cricoid and into cervical trachea.
- Extends into thoracic trachea.

Treatment

- Observation in mild cases.
- Temporary control with gelfoam injection into cleft.
- Endoscopic repair is successful in most cases.
  - Contraindicated if subglottic stenosis (SGS)/other airway problems
- *Severe cases:* Open repair via laryngofissure or posterolateral approach.

Laryngeal Web

Diagnosis

- Most common location: Anterior (90%).
- It is due to incomplete recanalization of airway (10th week).
- Forty percent have associated anomalies or syndrome (velocardiofacial syndrome, 22q11 deletion).
- It presents with dyspnea and voice changes/abnormal cry (variable).

Evaluation

- Microlaryngoscopy reveals web with varied thickness and vibratory qualities.

Treatment

- Many thin webs are lysed at initial intubation.
- Ligation of a thick web, expect worse voice after treatment; ligation of a thin web, expect better voice after treatment.
- *Thicker webs:* Open reconstruction of anterior commissure or use of laryngeal keel.
- Tracheostomy.

Subglottic Hemangioma

Diagnosis

- Subglottis is the most common location in laryngotracheal airway.
- It presents within the first 6 months.
- Symptoms of progressive stridor and retractions, persistent "croup" symptoms, worse with crying.
- "Beard" hemangiomas (chin, jaw line, and preauricular) have high incidence of airway hemangiomas.
- About 50% of airway hemangiomas have associated cutaneous hemangiomas.

Evaluation

- Rigid bronchoscopy (avoid biopsy).
- *Findings:* Vascular lesion covered by normal smooth mucosa, usually asymmetric.
- Magnetic resonance imaging (MRI) with contrast to assess extent of lesion.

Treatment

- Propranolol has recently been advocated as primary treatment.
  - *Other treatments:* Systemic steroids, local steroids, prolonged intubation, CO_2/potassium titanyl phosphate laser ablation, microdebrider excision, and excision through vertical tracheotomy.
  - High rate of SGS postsurgical intervention.
  - Vincristine or interferon for refractory cases.

Recurrent Respiratory Papillomatosis (RRP)

Diagnosis

- Human papilloma virus (HPV-6 and HPV-11).
- Hoarseness with gradual onset of stridor (late).

Evaluation

- Flexible laryngoscopy.
- Sessile or pedunculated frond-like growths confined to larynx.

Treatment

- More severe than adult onset RRP.
- Microlaryngoscopy with lesion excision (frequent debridement).
- Cidofovir injections are of controversial benefit.
- Anterior papilloma should be treated with caution to prevent anterior webbing.
- *Histopathology:* Keratinized squamous epithelium around a fibrovascular core.

Inflammatory: Croup (Laryngotracheobronchitis) versus Epiglottitis (Supraglottitis)

Refer to Table 40.1.

Table 40.1: Croup versus epiglottitis.

	Croup	*Epiglottitis*
Onset	Rapid	Slow
Symptoms	Barking cough, stridor (early)	Odynophagia, drooling, fever, tripod position, muffled (hot potato) voice, stridor (late)
Age	6 months to 3 years	2–6 years
Origin	Viral (parainfluenza)	Bacterial (*Haemophilus influenzae* B)
Evaluation	Steeple sign on plain films	Thumbprint sign on lateral neck X-ray
Treatment	Humidified air, racemic epinephrine, inhaled and systemic steroids	Airway examination in operating room with intubation, intravenous antibiotics

Subglottic Stenosis

Diagnosis

- Subglottis is the narrowest point in pediatric airway; boundary is true vocal cords to inferior margin of cricoid cartilage.
- One millimeter of circumferential subglottic edema reduces airway by ~50% in a neonate.
- *Types:* Acquired and congenital
  - Acquired
    - Most common type of SGS
    - Intubation trauma responsible for majority of cases
    - Prolonged, repeated intubation
    - Inappropriately large ET tube
    - Infection during intubation
    - *Other causes:* blunt, caustic, and penetrating laryngeal trauma
  - Congenital
    - Failure of laryngeal recanalization during embryogenesis
    - *Membranous:* Circumferential thickening caused by increased fibrosis or submucosal gland hyperplasia
    - *Cartilaginous:* Thickening or scarring of cricoid, or rarely trapped first tracheal ring

Evaluation

- History of prematurity, prolonged intubation, and "noisy breathing."
- It presents with biphasic stridor, respiratory distress (if severe), recurrent "croup," and feeding difficulties.
- Flexible laryngoscopy is helpful but not definitive; microlaryngoscopy and bronchoscopy are required.
- Cotton–Myer grading system (Fig. 40.2):
  - Grade I: 50% obstruction.
  - Grade II: 51–70%.
  - Grade III: 71–99%.
  - No lumen is present (100%).

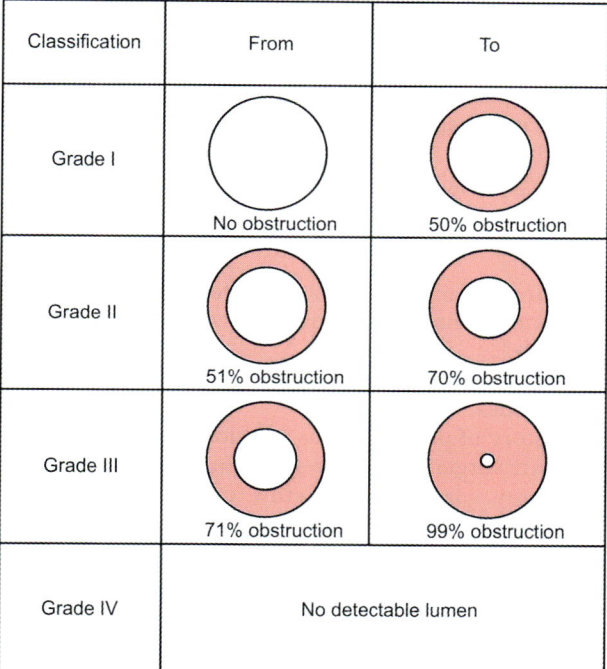

Fig. 40.2: Cotton-Myer grading system for subglottic stenosis.
Source: Redrawn from Myer CM, O'Connor DM, Cotton RT. Proposed grading system for subglottic stenosis based on endotracheal tube sizes. Ann Otol Rhinol Laryngol. 1994;103:319-23.

- Computed tomography (CT) or MRI to measure length of stenosis.

Treatment

- Gastroesophageal reflux disorder management.
- If asymptomatic, close observation in grade I/II.
- Surgical intervention for more severe cases.
  - Tracheotomy

- Endoscopic dilation
- Anterior cricoid split with possible anterior cartilage graft
- Posterior cricoid split (open or endoscopic)
- Laryngotracheoplasty
- Cricotracheal resection

Vocal Cord Paralysis

Diagnosis

- Unilateral
  - More common than bilateral; left dysfunction is more common than right (longer course of recurrent laryngeal nerve).
  - Weak/breathy voice, diplophonia, and aspiration episodes.
  - History of patent ductus arteriosus ligation/congenital heart surgery, anterior spine surgery, thyroid surgery, airway surgery, vincristine use, birth trauma, and idiopathic (viral neuritis and abnormal neural maturation).
- Bilateral
  - Inspiratory stridor, good voice/strong cry, aspiration, and airway obstruction.
  - Arnold–Chiari malformation/hydrocephalus and birth trauma.
  - It is difficult to distinguish from cricoarytenoid fixation, posterior glottis stenosis during awake examination.

Evaluation

- Flexible laryngoscopy with stroboscopy:
  - Position of vocal folds and arytenoids should be noted.
- Computed tomography or MRI from skull base to aorta for unknown etiology.
- Laryngeal electromyography is controversial in children.

Treatment

- Injection medialization laryngoplasty (Radiesse Voice gel, Restylane, and Cymetra).

- If good results, injection of Radiesse Voice or autologous fat for long-term results.
- Medialization laryngoplasty reserved for those who have gone through puberty.
- Bilateral paralysis:
  - Observation
  - Tracheotomy
  - Posterior cordotomy
  - Vocal fold lateralization
  - Posterior cricoid expansion

Congenital High Airway Obstruction Syndrome

Diagnosis

- Obstruction by mass (teratoma and lymphovascular malformation).
- Identified in utero during prenatal ultrasound, confirmed with MRI.
- Ex utero intrapartum procedure to secure airway during delivery.

Other Causes of Pediatric Stridor

Cricoarytenoid joint fixation, infectious, angioedema, rhabdomyosarcoma, lymphovascular malformation, airway burns/caustic ingestion, and neoplasm.

TRACHEAL CAUSES OF NEONATAL RESPIRATORY DISTRESS

Tracheomalacia

Intrinsic versus Extrinsic

- Intrinsic
  - Due to structural weakness of cartilage causing collapse during expiration.
  - *Risk factors:* Prematurity and tracheoesophageal fistulas.
  - Usually, it resolves by age 2.
  - *Treatment:* Observation (mild cases), tracheotomy, or airway stent.

- Extrinsic
  - *Vascular anomalies (see below):* Diagnose with rigid bronchoscopy and CT angiogram (CTA).
  - Head and neck masses (i.e. lymphovascular malformations).

Vascular Anomalies (Fig. 40.3)

Aberrant Right Subclavian

- Most common congenital vascular anomaly.
- Present with dysphagia lusoria with or without stridor.

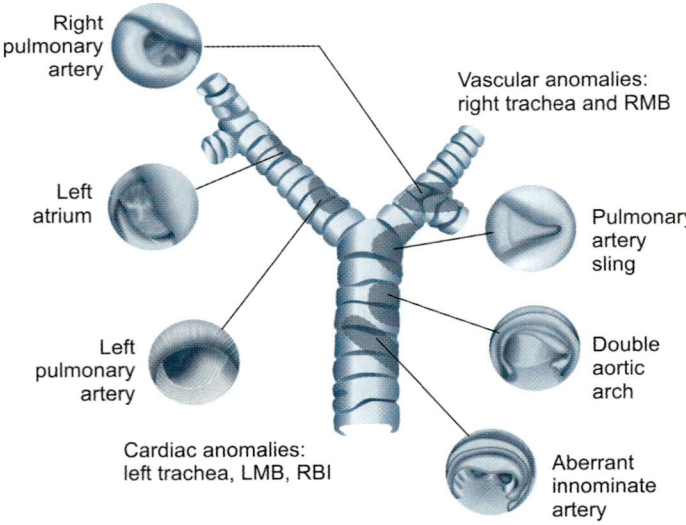

Fig. 40.3: Vascular anomalies causing tracheal compression. (LMB: Left main bronchus; RMB: Right main bronchus; RBI: Right bronchus intermedius)

Source: Redrawn from Rogers DJ, Cunnane MB, Hartnick CJ. Vascular compression of the airway: establishing a functional diagnosis algorithm. JAMA Otolaryngol Head Neck Surg. 2013;139(6):586-91.

- Barium esophagram shows esophageal filling defect.
- *Treatment:* Thoracotomy.

Aberrant Innominate Artery

- Present with biphasic stridor and recurrent croup/pneumonia episodes.
- Compression of anterior tracheal wall.
- *Evaluation:* Bronchoscopy, CTA, MRI/magnetic resonance angiogram.
- *Treatment:* Observation or arteriopexy, depending on symptom severity.

Double Aortic Arch

- Present with biphasic stridor, chronic cough, and dysphagia.
- Persistence of bilateral branchial arch vessels (fourth one).
- *Treatment:* Thoracotomy if symptomatic.

Pulmonary Artery Sling

- Present with biphasic stridor, chronic cough, cyanosis, and apneic episodes.
- Anomaly of sixth brachial arch.
- Associated with complete tracheal rings.
- *Treatment:* Thoracotomy if symptomatic.

Tracheal Stenosis

Diagnosis

- Acquired
  - *Most common cause:* Intubation trauma.
  - *Other causes:* Previous airway surgery (tracheotomy, cricothyroidotomy, and airway reconstruction).
- Congenital
  - *Most common cause:* Complete tracheal rings.
  - Presents with stridor, retractions, and recurrent upper respiratory symptoms.
  - "Wet" biphasic respiration (washing machine).

Evaluation

- Rigid bronchoscopy (with caution and small telescopes to avoid traumatic edema).
- Fifty percent have airway of <2 mm (smallest ET tube with outer diameter 2.9 mm).
- Computed tomography angiogram identifies length of segment and associated vascular anomalies.

Treatment

- When life threatening, extracorporeal membrane oxygenation until reconstruction is performed.
- Pericardial patch tracheoplasty, long-segment costal cartilage grafting, tracheal resection and anastomosis, and slide tracheoplasty (it results in trachea half the length, twice the diameter).

SUGGESTED READING

1. Benjamin B. Tracheomalacia in infants and children. Ann Otol Rhinol Laryngol. 1984;93(5): 438-42.
2. Benjamin B, Inglis A. Minor congenital laryngeal clefts: diagnosis and classification. Ann Otol Rhinol Laryngol. 1989;98:417-20.
3. Bitar MA, Moukarbel RV, Zalzal GH. Management of congenital subglottic hemangioma: trends and success over the past 17 years. Otolaryngol Head Neck Surg. 005;132(2):226-31.
4. Cooper T, Benoit M, Erickson B, El-Hakim H. Primary presentations of laryngomalacia. JAMA Otolaryngol Head Neck Surg. 2014;140(6):521-6.
5. Cotton RT. Management of subglottic stenosis. Otolaryngol Clin North Am. 2000;33(1): 111-30.
6. Cotton RT, Gray SD, Miller RP. Update of the Cincinnati experience in pediatric laryngotracheal reconstruction. Laryngoscope. 1989;99(11):1111-6.
7. Cressman WR, Myer CM III. Diagnosis and management of croup and epiglottitis. Pediatr Clin North Am. 1994;41(2):265-76.
8. Daya H, Hosnia A, Bejar-Solar I, et al. Pediatric vocal fold paralysis: a long-term retrospective study. Arch Otolaryngol Head Neck Surg. 2000;126(1):21-5.

9. Derkay CS, Wiatrak B. Recurrent respiratory papillomatosis: a review. Laryngoscope. 2008;118 (7):1236-47.
10. Hardingham M, Walsh-Waring GP. The treatment of a congenital laryngeal web. J Laryngol Otol. 1975;89(3):273-80.
11. Myer CM, O'Connor DM, Cotton RT. Proposed grading system for subglottic stenosis based on endotracheal tube sizes. Ann Otol Rhinol Laryngol. 1994;103:319-23.
12. Richter GT, Thompson DM. The surgical management of laryngomalacia. Otolaryngol Clin North Am. 2008;41(5):837–64.
13. Rogers DJ, Cunnane MB, Hartnick CJ. Vascular compression of the airway: establishing a functional diagnosis algorithm. JAMA Otolaryngol Head Neck Surg. 2013;139(6):586-91.

Chapter 41

Pediatric Balance and Vestibular Disorders

Katherine M McKee-Cole, Robert C O'Reilly

EMBRYOLOGY OF THE VESTIBULAR APPARATUS

- First sensory system to develop in humans.
  - Begins around the third week of gestation and completes at 25 weeks.
- Begins with formation of otic placode from surface ectoderm, which invaginates into the mesenchyme forming the otic pit.
- During the fourth week the otic pit becomes the otic vesicle.
- Neural crest migrates to the otic vesicle and forms the acousticofacial ganglion, which later differentiates into the geniculate, superior vestibular, inferior vestibular, and cochlear portions.
- Otic vesicle elongates, forming the endolymphatic diverticulum medially and utriculosaccular chamber laterally.
  - Endolymphatic sac and duct arise from the endolymphatic diverticulum.
  - The semicircular canals and utricle arise from the utricular portion of the utriculosaccular chamber and the saccule and cochlea from the saccular portion.
- Hair cells reach adult formation at different times by site.
  - Vestibular end organs at about 9 weeks.
  - Maculae at about 16 weeks.
  - Cristae at about 23 weeks.

- Mesoderm gives rise to the bony otic capsule, which contains perilymph while the membranous labyrinth is filled with endolymph.[1]

MATURATION OF BALANCE MECHANISMS

- Balance relies on vision, vestibular input and proprioception.
- Vestibular system functions
  - Maintain equilibrium, direct gaze of the eyes, and stabilize gaze during motion.
- Balance is also affected by cognitive processing of these sensory inputs and thus changes with neuromaturation and experience.
- Differences between adults and children
  - Somatosensory function is developed first in children, followed by visual function, which shows maturity at 14–15 years of age, and lastly vestibular function.
  - Adults rely mainly on somatosensory input, whereas children use mainly visual input for balance control and begin to integrate somatosensory input between the ages of 3 and 6 years.
    - Visual disorders may present as balance abnormalities in children.
  - Adults can also process misleading visual input using vestibular function, whereas children cannot until approximately 15 years.
- Gait pattern reaches maturity at around 7–10 years of age while coordination of balance responses continues development till age 10–15 years.[1]

HISTORY AND PHYSICAL EXAMINATION

- Typically children do not complain of vertigo or the sense of motion.
- Focused questions
  - "Can you tell me how it feels?"
    - Helps differentiate vertigo from presyncope.

- Peripheral vestibular disorders produce a true sense of spinning exacerbated by movement.
- Central vestibular disorders are typically not exacerbated by movement and have fewer vegetative symptoms.

  - "Is there anything that makes your symptoms better or worse or brings your symptoms on?"
    - Vertigo that worsens with straining or Valsalva can indicate perilymphatic fistula.
  - "How many episodes have you had, and how long do your symptoms last?"
    - Brief episodes of seconds to minutes may indicate benign paroxysmal vertigo of childhood (BPVC).
    - Vertigo lasting hours in children may be due to migraine.
    - One long episode may be associated with vestibular neuritis or labyrinthitis.
  - "Do you feel anything else with it, and what other medical problems do you have?"
    - Autoimmune disorders can have vestibular symptoms.
    - A personal history of otologic disease or surgery is important as well as a history of seizures, ophthalmologic disease, and vascular or cardiac disease.
    - Family history of malignancy, hearing loss, or migraine should be noted.
- Biggest risk factors for the development of vestibulopathy in children include sensory neural hearing loss (SNHL) and head trauma.
- Common symptoms
  - Ataxia, headache, visual disturbances, hearing loss, otalgia, otorrhea, oscillopsia, drop attacks without change in mental status, nausea, emesis, frequent falls, preference of the child to perform activities at high speed.
- Important to ask about delayed motor development.

- Examinations
    - Full neurotologic and cranial nerve examination as well as a complete head and neck examination.
    - Static and dynamic balance testing.
    - Visual testing and evaluation for nystagmus.
    - Developmental reflexes tested in infants.
    - Age-appropriate audiometric examination.
    - Head-thrust maneuver, head impulse test, Romberg or sharpened Romberg test, past pointing, and Fukuda stepping test.
        - Children may show alterations in the Fukuda stepping test late in the examination, so they should be observed for a minimum of 30 seconds.[1]

VESTIBULAR TESTING

- Vestibulo-ocular reflex (VOR)
    - Present at birth, absence by age of 10 months is abnormal.
    - Saccadic system continues development until 2 years of age.
    - Results measuring time of gain show a linear increase with age from 3 to 9 years, while phase remains stable.[2]
- Videonystagmography/electronystagmography
    - Short breaks between tests are often needed for children, so complete testing usually takes longer than in adults.
    - Baseline eye movement examination is done using toys before testing to allow accurate interpretation of testing results if baseline abnormalities are identified.
    - Strategies for success include doing a practice run prior to recorded testing and using rewards or making the test a game.
    - It is best to prioritize testing that provides the most useful information first as fatigue and test intolerance may make it impossible to complete all testing.
- Vestibular evoked myogenic potential (VEMP)
    - It can be completed as soon as the child can support his or her head, usually around 2 months of age.

- Middle ear effusion (MEE) can be a common cause for absent air conduction VEMPs with normal bone conduction VEMPs.
- Computerized dynamic posturography with sensory organization test (SOT)
  - Adapted SOT for pediatrics.
    - Toy fixed to the wall at appropriate height in order to keep attention.
    - Equilibrium score increases, meaning more stability, with age in both the eyes open and eyes closed stable platform condition as well as with the unstable platform.
    - Somesthetic score is stable from age 6 to 20 years.
    - Visual and vestibular scores progressively increase with age.
- Gait analysis[1]

PEDIATRIC VESTIBULAR DISORDERS

- Peripheral vestibular disorders
  - Balance dysfunction associated with MEE or otitis media with effusion (OME).
    - Likely the most common cause and risk factor for acquired balance disturbances in the pediatric population.
    - Effects of acute MEE have been well established; however, mechanism is yet to be determined.
    - Middle ear effusion with an impact on balance during a critical development time could result in balance delays beyond the resolution of MEE.[1]
    - Tympanostomy tube placement has been reported to improve balance dysfunction.[2]
  - Meningitis
    - Causes varying progressive ossification of inner ear structures.
    - Vestibular dysfunction occurs in a disproportionately larger degree of those affected, and the degree of

impact ranges from unilateral weakness to bilateral profound loss.

- Congenital cytomegalovirus (CMV) infection
  - Incidence of 0.4–2.3% of live births.
  - Symptomatic CMV leads to SNHL in 30–65%, and vestibular dysfunction can be seen in those severely affected.
  - One study showed vestibular dysfunction to be more common than hearing loss and perhaps a better marker.
- Abnormal cochleovestibular anatomy
  - Correlation between vestibular dysfunction and abnormal inner ear anatomy exists, but not all children show complete vestibular loss.
  - Pendred syndrome.
- Toxicity-induced vestibular dysfunction
  - Associated with several groups of antibiotics, chemotherapeutic agents, and diuretics.
    - Aminoglycosides are most common category of antibiotics leading to ototoxicity; rarely, patients can have a mitochondrial defect leading to susceptibility.
    - Also associated with vancomycin and viomycin.
    - Cisplatin is associated with ototoxicity, and monitoring is carried out using high-frequency audiometric testing at >8 kHz.
    - Monitoring typically by audiogram.
- Ménière's disease
  - Uncommon in children at <4% incidence.
  - Histopathologic correlate is endolymphatic hydrops.
  - Audiogram shows fluctuating, commonly low-frequency, SNHL.
  - Electrocochleography shows a summation potential to action potential ratio of > 0.4.
  - Significant weakness on caloric testing or head-thrust is present in 42–73%.

- Superior semicircular canal dehiscence syndrome
  - Well delineated in adult literature.
  - Pediatric literature shows only a few case reports and one series of seven patients.
  - Syndrome may be rare in pediatrics, unrecognized or not reported yet in the literature.
- Benign paroxysmal positional vertigo (BPPV)
  - While most commonly idiopathic in adults, often due to trauma in children.
    - Bilateral involvement more commonly seen in children.
  - Classic description includes the acute onset of vertigo lasting seconds to minutes, brought on by rotational head movements.
- Vestibular neuronitis
  - Extremely uncommon in children; incidence of < 5% of all pediatric presentations of vertigo.
  - Vertigo lasts for several days after acute onset and is associated with nausea and vomiting with an absence of hearing loss.
  - This is an idiopathic unilateral vestibular insult, possibly due to herpes simplex virus 1, and as such is a diagnosis of exclusion.
  - Magnetic resonance imaging for atypical, prolonged or uncompensated course.
  - Supportive management with antiemetics, hydration, vestibular suppressants, and early vestibular therapy.
  - Currently there is a lack of evidence to support the use of antivirals or steroids.[1]
  - Children compensate faster than adults, with resolution in days to weeks versus weeks to months.[2]
- Trauma-induced vascular dysfunction
  - Direct head trauma can result in temporal bone fractures, labyrinthine concussion, BPPV, and perilymphatic fistulas.
  - Barotrauma is associated with perilymphatic fistulas.[1]

VESTIBULAR MIGRAINE

- It has been shown to be the most common diagnosis in children referred for vertigo and balance disorders.
- Pediatric migraine is more commonly in the frontal or periorbital region, and headache is not usually throbbing and usually lasts <2 hours.
- Migraine can also be associated with cyclic vomiting, abdominal pain, and attacks of pallor or somnolence.
- Benign paroxysmal vertigo of childhood
  - Sudden brief attacks of vertigo lasting seconds to minutes.
  - Age of onset is 3–4 years, and spontaneous resolution occurs by 7–8 years.
  - Episodes usually occur at 4–6 weeks but range from weekly to every 6 months.
  - No associated change in position at onset, pain, headache, hearing loss, or change in mental status.
  - Pallor frequently observed during the episode and can be associated with sweating and vomiting.
  - Return to normal activity immediately after episode.
  - Diagnosis is based on strong family history of migraine, typical symptoms, and normal general physical, otologic and neurologic examination and testing.
  - If the diagnosis is in question, imaging can be obtained.
  - Entity recognized as a childhood periodic syndrome commonly a precursor to migraine.
- Benign paroxysmal torticollis of infancy
  - Self-limiting benign disorder of recurrent episodes of head tilting due to cervical dystonia.
  - Direction of head tilt can vary by episode.
  - Episodes begin at a few months of age and spontaneously resolve by age 3–4 years.
  - Half also show involvement of pelvic musculature with a bend of the trunk towards the cervical side affected.
  - Pallor, nausea, and vomiting may be associated.

- Duration shows a wide range from a few hours to up to a week, with resolution of symptoms during sleep in most cases.
- Episodes may occur every few days to months.
- Strong family history of migraine present in most, and family history of a similar childhood episodic syndrome can be seen.
- Normal general, otologic, and neurologic examination as well as radiographic studies.
- Reports of audiometric and vestibular testing results range from reduced caloric response to inconclusive or normal.

- Basilar migraine
  - Defined as two or more fully reversible neurologic symptoms/auras lasting > 5 minutes but <60 minutes, followed by a migraine headache.
  - Aura may consist of visual-field deficits, total loss of vision or diplopia, vertigo, ataxia, dysarthria, tinnitus, or hypoacusis.
  - The headache that follows the aura is typically described as throbbing, may be associated with nausea and vomiting and resolves with sleep.
  - Most often seen in adolescent girls related to menses.
  - Normal general, otologic, and neurologic examinations.

- Vestibular migraine
  - Symptoms similar to, but do not meet the criteria for, basilar migraine.
  - Most often seen in adolescent girls related to menses.
  - Episodes of vertigo associated with this diagnosis last for hours and are associated with nausea and vomiting with photophobia.
  - Family history of migraine and personal history of motion sickness are very common.
  - Normal general, otologic, and neurologic examinations between episodes.
  - Reduced unilateral caloric response in 20–30% of patients.

- – A trial of prophylactic migraine medication can be used diagnostically and therapeutically.
- Supportive treatment
  - – Stress reduction, sufficient sleep, and dietary restriction of food trigger.
- Medical treatment
  - – Analgesics such as acetaminophen or ibuprofen.
  - – Vestibular suppressants including meclizine.
  - – Prophylactic antimigraine medications for those with frequent, recurrent, and disabling attacks.[1]

STRUCTURAL LESIONS OF THE CENTRAL NERVOUS SYSTEM

- Rare cause of vertigo but important to diagnosis.
- Posterior fossa central nervous system lesions typically cause vertigo.
- Disequilibrium can be caused by a number of different pathways, including vestibular, visual, cerebellar, basal ganglia, or dorsal column.
- Posterior fossa neoplasms
  - – Symptoms due to obstructive hydrocephalus causing morning headaches and vomiting.
  - – Focal neurologic findings can show cranial nerve or brainstem dysfunction and include vertigo, nystagmus, and diplopia.
  - – Cerebellar tumors include juvenile pilocytic astrocytomas, ependymomas, and medulloblastomas.
  - – Brainstem tumors include astrocytomas and tectal plate gliomas.
  - – Cerebellar pontine angle tumors include nerve sheath tumors, especially vestibular schwannomas, glomus jugulare, and epidermoid cysts.
    - While common in adults, vestibular schwannomas are primarily seen in children with neurofibromatosis type 2.

- Cerebellar malformations
  - Chiari 1 malformation
    - Caudal descent of the cerebellar tonsil through the foramen magnum at least 5 mm.
    - Found incidentally in 0.3% of the general population.
    - Higher incidence in children with growth hormone deficiency or craniosynostosis.
    - Strong family history is generally present.
    - Symptoms include occipital headaches, swallowing dysfunction, central sleep apnea, and vertical nystagmus.
    - Asymptomatic patients do not require treatment.
    - Those with persistent symptoms, of whom 25% generally show vestibular dysfunction, require occipital craniectomy and C1 laminectomy.
  - Chiari 2 malformation
    - Open neural tube defects including caudal descent of the entire hindbrain with resultant changes in the fourth ventricle and cervicomedullary junction, a large massa intermedia, and interdigitation of the cerebral hemispheres with an incompetent falx.
    - Symptoms are generally due to hydrocephalus causing extensive lower cranial nerve dysfunction.
  - Arachnoid cyst
    - Generally forms at the same time as brain development and therefore changes the shape without causing dysfunction.
    - Become symptomatic with enlargement or rupture due to trauma, causing headaches and mass effect causing cranial nerve palsies based on the affected area.
    - Treatment is with fenestration into a normal cerebrospinal fluid cistern or cystoperitoneal shunt.
- Spinal disorders
  - Basilar invagination
    - When the cranial cervical spine, most often the odontoid tip, can ascend into the intracranial space.

- Most commonly seen in children with bony or connective tissue disorders, including osteogenesis imperfecta, spondyloepiphyseal dysplasia, and Ehlers-Danlos syndrome.
  - Direct compression of the brainstem causes change in balance and vertical down-beating nystagmus as well as headaches and lower cranial nerve dysfunction.
  - Treatment even for those who are asymptomatic due to slow progression of dysfunction.
  - Foramen magnum stenosis
    - Seen in children with skeletal dysplasia, especially achondroplasia.
    - Presenting symptoms include central sleep apnea, upper motor neuron dysfunction, and possibly profound brainstem dysfunction.
    - Change in gait and balance can be seen, but vestibular symptoms are rare.
    - Treatment is similar to Chiari 1 malformations.[1]

ACQUIRED BRAIN INJURY (ABI)

- Acquired brain injury occurs outside of the neonatal/perinatal period.
- Annual incidence is 150–250/100,000.
- Wide variety of causes including anoxia, infection causes, vascular causes, head trauma, and tumors.
- History
  - Mechanism and time of injury, studies and management undertaken after injury.
    - Perilymphatic fistulas occur shortly over injury.
    - Benign paroxysmal positional vertigo symptoms begin in a delayed fashion.
  - Characterize the balance complaint to delineate if it is true vertigo, lightheadedness, and motion sickness or disequilibrium.

- Determine if there is a certain trigger as well as length in duration of the symptomatic episodes and functional impact for the patient.
- Complete medication history as some can cause dizziness.
- Physical examination and testing
  - Complete examination to determine areas of weakness that can help determine location of the brain injury
  - Complete audiometrics
  - Vestibular system examination
    - Presence of nystagmus.
    - Vestibulo-ocular reflex alterations may generate head tilt suggesting unilateral vestibular loss.
    - Head-thrust testing can show a "catch-up" saccade when the head is facing the side of the injury.
    - Dynamic visual-acuity testing may be abnormal with a worsening of Snellen chart reading level by more than three lines during head turning.
  - Vestibular testing
    - Warm water irrigation or air for caloric testing can make the test more tolerable and can be performed in children 5 years or older.
  - Balance assessment
    - Patients with an ABI and normal examination may show balance dysfunction on more complex assessment.
    - Sensory organization test
      - Score based on the amount of sway exhibited.
      - Acquired brain injury patients with normal examination have been shown to have significantly decreased performance.
    - Functional reach test
      - Excellent reliability in pediatric ABI patients.
      - Patient stands perpendicular to the wall and baseline measurement of where the fifth finger on the preferred hand lies is taken; they then reach as far as possible with feet remaining planted with preferred and nonpreferred side, and the distance from baseline is measured.

- Community balance and mobility scale
  - Assessment of higher-order balance skills.
  - Shows excellent inter- and intrarater reliability in school-aged children and adolescents.[1]

VESTIBULAR COMPENSATION AND REHABILITATION

- The resting background activity in vestibular nuclear neurons is reweighted so that the resting discharge of the contralateral side is reduced, leading to a balanced level of activity from both sides.
- Vestibular rehabilitation exercises challenge the vestibular system, prompting the use of visual and proprioceptive cues to augment the now inadequate vestibular input.
- Rehabilitation also results in habituation to the mismatch of information.
- Exercises include those focused on gaze stabilization and balance.
- Although many studies have confirmed improvement in adult patients undergoing vestibular rehabilitation for unilateral vestibular defects, at this point only a small number of studies have been completed in the pediatric population.
  - These studies also showed improvement, but more research needs to be done.[1]

REFERENCES

1. Robert C O'Reilly TM, Cushing SL. Manual of Pediatric Balance Disorders. San Diego, CA: Plural Publishing; 2013.
2. Kesser BW, Gleason AT. Dizziness and vertigo across the lifespan. Otolaryngol Clin North Am. 2011;44(2):251-8.

Chapter 42

Vascular Anomalies

Katherine M McKee-Cole, Douglas R Johnston

VASCULAR SYSTEM DEVELOPMENT

Sequential phases[1]
- *Vasculogenesis*: A primitive vascular plexus is established from endothelial precursor.
  - Precursor cells form blood islands that coalesce to form the primary capillary plexus.
- *Angiogenesis*: New vessels arise from pre-existing vessels by migration and proliferation of endothelial cells.

Lymphatic development[1]
- Vessels develop as endothelial outgrowth from the venous system.

Regulators[1]
- *Positive*: Vascular endothelial growth factor (VEGF), fibronectin, transforming growth factor-1, and vascular endothelial cadherin.
- *Negative*: Angiostatin, endostatin, and thrombospondin.

CURRENT CLASSIFICATION

Published by Mulliken and Glowacki in March 1982[2]
- Based on histopathology features and clinical course[3]
  - Vascular malformations
    - Abnormal vessels present at birth that do not regress
    - Show normal endothelial mitotic activity

  – Vascular tumors/hemangiomas
    • Self-involuting tumors
    • Show increased mitotic activity/endothelial hyperplasia

Vascular Malformations

• Represent disordered vasculogenesis[4]
• Defined by vessel of origin[4]
  – *Single-vessel lesions*: Lymphatic, venous, and capillary
  – *Combination lesions*: Arteriovenous, venolymphatic, or other complex combined
• Present at birth, slow-growing/infiltrative, and do not regress (Tables 42.1 and 42.2)[4]

Lymphatic Malformations

• Most common pediatric head and neck vascular malformation: 1 per 2,000–4,000 births.[4]
• The hallmark of clinical presentation is local infection causing pain, swelling, and tongue protrusion.[4]
  – Most commonly involving the oral cavity, particularly tongue.

Table 42.1: Review of clinical presentation.

Type of lesion	Present at birth	Proportional growth	Involution phase	Episodes of infection
Hemangioma	–	–	+	+
Lymphatic	+	+	–	+
Venous	+	+	–	–
Arterial	+	+	–	–

Table 42.2: Review of physical exam findings.

Type of lesion	Skin color	Bruit	Dependent filling	Deflate	Refill
Hemangioma	Blue-red	–	–	+	Rapid
Lymphatic	No color (amber mucosal blebs)	–	–	–	Slow
Venous	Blue	–	+	+	Slow
Arterial	Blue-red	+	–	–	Rapid

- Clinical behavior by location[1]
  - Unilateral infrahyoid malformations of the posterior neck rarely spontaneously resolve (15%).
  - Unilateral suprahyoid malformations show increased involvement of the aerodigestive tract and more unpredictable behavior.
  - Bilateral suprahyoid malformations can cause facial skeletal deformation with bony overgrowth and show a poorer response to treatment.
  - Large bilateral supra- and infrahyoid malformations may cause lymphocytopenia by an unknown mechanism.
  - External appearance of the malformation is not indicator of degree of airway involvement.
  - Lesions may enlarge with hormonal changes in puberty or pregnancy.[4]
- Size classically defined by microcystic versus macrocystic.[4]
  - Microcystic < 2 cm, mixed, and macrocystic > 2 cm
- Imaging[1,4]
  - *Computed tomography (CT)*: Cystic fluid density and air-fluid levels
  - Magnetic resonance imaging (MRI)
    - *T1*: Well-defined low-signal cystic space
    - *T2*: High signal fluid without feeding/draining vessels
  - Cystic walls and interstitial areas can enhance
- Histology[1]
  - Enlarged lymphatic spaces lined by bland endothelial cells surrounded by smooth muscle cells.
  - Contains a proteinaceous fluid not contiguous with normal lymphatic channels.
- Treatment
  - Observation for a very select group with unilocular macrocystic posterolateral malformations.[4]
  - Antibiotics indicated for infectious episodes, and steroids may be added for aerodigestive dysfunction.[4]
  - Indications for intervention
    - Concern for airway obstruction; difficulty with feeding or speech.

- Detrimental effects on appearance.
- Recurrent infection.
– Sclerotherapy[4]
  - Malformation is outlined by injecting contrast into the lesion, after which sclerosant is administered with mix of contrast to allow early indication of extravasation.
  - Airway monitoring may be necessary; possible planned intubation.
  - *Agents*: Ethanol, sodium tetradecyl sulfate, doxycycline, OK-432 (pulled by Food and Drug Administration), and bleomycin.
  - Topical cautery/laser can be combined with sclerotherapy.
  - Complications can include local pain and perilesional tissue necrosis.
– Surgery[4]
  - Excision
    - *Favorable lesions*: Localized macrocystic lesions in posteroinferior neck, parotid, or submandibular regions.
    - Infiltrative lesions in the parotid may displace the facial nerve in an unpredictable fashion; preoperative superficial nerve mapping is helpful.
    - Bilateral suprahyoid lesions with mucosal involvement should undergo staged unilateral excision with contralateral excision at later date to reduce the potential for permanent tongue enlargement.
  - Topical cautery or coblation for mucosal surfaces.
  - Topical laser therapy with carbon dioxide (CO_2) or yttrium-aluminum-garnet (YAG) laser for interstitial lesions.[4]
  - Tracheotomy.
  - Complications
    - Most commonly recurrence due to incomplete excision (most common with microcystic lesions).[4]

- Large mixed suprahyoid lesions show a higher incidence of cranial nerve or great vessel injury or upper airway edema requiring a tracheotomy.

Venous Malformations

- Present in 1 per 10,000 births.[4]
- *Genetics*: Associated with loss-of-function mutation on angiopoietin receptor gene TIE2/TEK (tyrosine kinase): involved in endothelial-smooth muscle communication essential for venous morphogenesis in sporadic cases; attributed to mutations on chromosome 9p in inherited cases.
- Presentation[3]
  - Present at birth; slowly enlarge over time and with puberty or trauma.
  - Cause a blue hue under the skin or mucosa, compressible, and enlarge with Valsalva or dependent positioning.
- Imaging[3]
  - *Ultrasound*: Helpful in all vascular anomalies
  - *CT*: Calcified phleboliths
  - *MRI*: T2 bright signal without flow voids
- Histology[1]
  - Flat endothelium with dysplastic walls and thin basement membranes
  - No expression of VEGF or basic fibroblast growth factor
- Treatment[1,4]
  - Conservative measures for symptom control
    - Positioning and compression wraps to prevent dependent filling and expansion
  - Pharmaceuticals
    - Low-molecular-weight heparin for thrombosis of the lesion causing pain
    - Anti-inflammatory agents
  - Sclerotherapy[5]
    - May be used in isolation or preoperatively to decrease bleeding.

- Zygomatic/temporal branches of facial nerve most vulnerable to injury after ethanol sclerotherapy, and paralysis can occur.
  - Neodymium-doped yttrium-aluminum-garnet (ND:YAG) laser.
  - Topical cautery or coblation for mucosal surfaces.
  - Excision of favorable lesions that are small and localized.

Capillary Malformations

- Present in 1 per 300 children[4]
- *Genetics*: Attributed to mutations on chromosome 5q in inherited cases, but most are sporadic.
- Presentation[4]
  - Present at birth; progress with time to become darker and more raised.
  - Painless flat, red, or purple cutaneous patches with irregular borders.
  - "Port-wine stains" are capillary malformations that show a trigeminal nerve distribution.
- Histology shows dilated capillary-like channels in the reticular dermis.[1]
- Treatment mainstay is pulse dye laser, which shows significant skin lightening in 80% of patients.[1,4]
  - Absorption peak matches oxyhemoglobin; thermal damage is largely restricted to cutaneous blood vessels.

Arteriovenous Malformations (AVM)

- High-flow lesions with arterial feeding vessels and enlarged draining veins, which directly connect through micro- and macro-arteriovenous fistulas that create the epicenter of the arteriovenous malformation (AVM).[3]
- Presentation[3]
  - Can be present at birth, but some not prominent until third or fourth decade; enlarge over time; thrill and bruit often present.

- – Firm, pulsatile mass most commonly located on the cheek or auricle.
- – Clinical stages
  - · *Dormancy*: AVM may be mistaken for other vascular abnormalities at this stage.
  - · Expansion
  - · *Destruction*: AVM can behave like a neoplasm; advantageous to treat prior to this.
  - · Heart failure
- Histology shows variably enlarged hypertrophic arterial and venous spaces.[1]
- Imaging[4]
  - – Magnetic resonance angiography (MRA): Numerous hypolucent arterial flow voids
  - – Arteriogram: Definition of central nidus and early venous filling due to arterial connection
- Treatment[1]
  - – Indications for intervention
    - · Hemorrhage and ischemia
    - · Chronic venous insufficiency with venous hypertension
    - · Compromise of breathing, vision, hearing, and eating
    - · High-output cardiac failure
  - – Embolization can be used alone for lesions in bone or as preoperative adjunct.
  - – Excision after preoperative embolization, although heavy blood loss still common.[4]
  - – Recurrence is as high as 93% with excision of diffuse AVMs, so long-term follow-up is needed.

Vascular Tumors[4]

- Represent disordered angiogenesis.
- Benign lesions that can result in localized tissue distortion/destruction.
- Characterized by size, location, and blood flow (*see* Tables 42.1 and 42.2).

Hemangiomas of Infancy (HOI)

- Most common tumor in infancy: 1 per 10 children.[4]
- Risk factors include prematurity, chorionic villus sampling, and female gender.[3]
- Theories of pathogenesis[4]
  - Disrupted placental tissue embedded in developing fetus
    - Markers of hemangiomas of infancy (HOI) coincide with placental tissue.
    - HOI more common with chorionic villus sampling, placenta previa, and pre- eclampsia.
  - Arise from hematopoietic progenitor cells
    - Attributed to genetic errors in growth receptors in development
- Cellular components and mechanisms[6]
  - β-Adrenergic receptors and catecholaminergic nerve fibers found in all wall layers in normal vessels, but isolated to adventitia in hemangiomas.
  - β-Adrenergic receptors present at 30% of the level found in normal blood vessels.
  - Increased expression of the antiapoptotic gene BCL2 found in interstitial cells of proliferating hemangiomas; BCL2 expression is prolonged in highly vascularized hemangiomas.
- Presentation[4]
  - Absent at birth; grow rapidly for 6–9 months; period of quiescence from 9 to 12 months of age.
  - Involute over several years with 50%, 70%, and 90% involution by age 5, 7, and 9 years, respectively.
  - Soft, compressible mass that can affect cutaneous and mucosal surfaces.
    - Posterolateral subglottis is most common location for airway involvement.
    - 50% with laryngeal hemangiomas have a segmental lower facial hemangioma.
  - Superficial HOI are well-demarcated, flat, erythematous red patches, and deep HOI show overlying bluish tint.

- Types
  - Focal HOI follow embryonic fusion patterns.
    - Segmental HOI occur in prominences related to neural crest cells; greater associated morbidity.
- Location
  - Parapharyngeal HOI can cause compression, particularly during sleep, and may cause sleep-disordered breathing.
  - Laryngeal HOI can often mimic recurrent upper respiratory infection or croup.
  - Parotid hemangioma most common pediatric parotid mass.
- Histology[1]
  - Rapidly proliferating endothelial cells with frequent mitoses in the dermis.
  - Glucose transporter-1 (GLUT1) positivity is specific for HOI[3]
  - During involution endothelial cells flatten, vessel lumens dilate, and fibrous tissue is deposited.
- Treatment[1]
  - Goal is to stop angiogenesis in proliferating HOI.
    - Medical treatment is ineffective in nonproliferating HOI.
  - Propranolol (nonselective beta-antagonist)[4,7-9]—mainstay of medical treatment.
    - Proposed to decrease expression of VEGF/beta-FGF, trigger apoptosis of capillary endothelial cells.
    - Candidates must not have cardiac conditions, reactive airway disease, or other pulmonary conditions.
    - Approximately 90% show dramatic reduction in size in 1–2 weeks at doses below that used to treat cardiovascular disease.
    - *Regimen*: EKG, assess vitals, and continue therapy until plateau in improvement.
      - Wean is undertaken; regrowth prompts restarting propranolol.

- Complications can include hypotension, hypoglycemia, gastroesophageal reflux disease, and airway reactivity.
- Systemic corticosteroids[4]
  - Indicated for impending or present complications.
  - Prednisolone PO 1–5 mg/kg/day burst; 4–6 week taper.
- Intralesional corticosteroids[4]
  - Controversial in periorbital disease due to the risk of retinal artery thrombosis and blindness.
  - Can be considered for focal HOI of the airway; repeat injections common.
- Pulsed dye laser (PDL) treatment[4]
  - Removes redness while preserving epidermis.
  - Does not reduce HOI volume.
- Excision[1]
  - *Indications*: Functional compromise of vision/ breathing, facial involvement with large superficial component, scarring/ulceration, and abnormal fibrofatty skin changes after involution.[4]
  - Lack of response with medical therapy.
  - Advisable to wait until proliferation has ceased if possible.
  - Staged treatment with PDL induces dermal thickening, allowing excision with minimal skin loss.
  - Open laryngofissure with submucosal dissection for subglottic circumferential involvement.
- *Tracheotomy*: Another option for subglottic circumferential involvement.[1]
- Antiangiogenic chemotherapy[10]
  - Indicated for life-threatening or multifocal disease, visceral involvement, airway obstruction, and periorbital lesions.
  - Use is limited by significant side effects.
  - *Interferon*: Limited by spastic diplegia in up to 20%, especially in patients <1 year.
  - *Vincristine*: Limited by peripheral neuropathy.

Congenital Hemangioma

- High-flow vascular tumors present at birth that begin during pregnancy.[3]
- Types[4]
  - Rapidly involuting congenital hemangioma (RICH)
    - Involute more rapidly than HOI.
  - Noninvoluting congenital hemangioma (NICH).
  - Histology is identical to HOI except negative for GLU1.[1]
  - Treatment can include observation for RICH and laser or surgical therapy for NICH.[3]

Kaposiform Hemangioendothelioma

- Show significant lymphatic component in addition to blood vascular endothelium.[3]
- *Presentation*: Cutaneous violet nodule extending locally into deep tissues.[1]
- Imaging shows a diffuse infiltrative vascular process with impressive flow voids.[3]
- Treatment[1]
  - Excision is curative for localized tumors.
  - Antiangiogenic chemotherapy may be necessary for large lesions with pain, loss of function, or significant disfigurement.

Tufted Angioma

- Rare cutaneous lesion.[1]
- *Presentation*: Most commonly on the neck in children/young adults, with no tendency to regress.
- Histology shows vascular tufts of tightly packed capillaries in a cannonball pattern.[3]
- Treatment[1]
  - Excision is curative for localized tumors.
  - Antiangiogenic chemotherapy may be necessary for large lesions with pain, loss of function, or significant disfigurement.

Associated Syndromes and Conditions

- Kasabach-Merritt [1]
  - 1 per 300 hemangiomas.
  - Occurrence of profound thrombocytopenia with vascular tumors due to an unknown mechanism.[3]
  - *Complications*: Bleeding into pharynx, GI tract, or brain.
  - Treatment includes replacement therapy with platelets, fresh frozen plasma, and cryoprecipitate.
    - Extensive chemotherapy to try to reduce bleeding risk.
  - 30–40% mortality despite therapy.[3]
- PHACES syndrome[3]
  - Neurocutaneous syndrome that associates large, plaque-like, segmental hemangiomas of the face with one or more of the following:
    - Posterior fossa brain malformations
    - Arterial, cardiovascular, or eye anomalies
    - Ventral development defects such as sternal defects or supraumbilical raphe
  - 20% of infants with segmental facial hemangiomas meet criteria for PHACES syndrome.
  - Ophthalmology and cardiology consults and imaging of the head should be pursued.
  - Treatment includes antiplatelet therapy for abnormal cerebral vasculature to prevent stroke.
- Osler-Weber-Rendu syndrome [heredity hemorrhagic telangiectasia (HHT)][3]
  - Autosomal dominantly inherited syndrome of capillary malformations.
  - Commonly presents with spontaneous epistaxis.
  - Screening because catastrophic hemorrhage can occur in children with clinically silent disease; screening imaging for cerebral and pulmonary arterial malformations if a family history of HHT is present.
  - Treatment includes photocoagulation and cauterization of individual lesions.

- Sturge-Weber syndrome[4]
  - Capillary malformation over the distribution of the trigeminal nerve.
  - Associated with ipsilateral meningeal vascular malformations and may result in seizure disorder or mental retardation.
- Maffucci syndrome[1]
  - Multiple venous and lymphatic malformations.
  - Dyschondroplasia with shortening/deformity of involved bones and occasional visceral vascular lesions.
  - 25% incidence of chondrosarcoma.
- Von Hippel-Lindau disease[1]
  - Hemangiomas of the cerebellum and retina.
  - Cysts of the kidney and pancreas.

REFERENCES

1. Flint PW, Richardson MA, Haughey BH, et al. Cummings Otolaryngology: Head and Neck Surgery, 5th edition. Philadelphia, PA: Mosby Elsevier; 2010.
2. Mulliken JB, Glowacki J. Hemangiomas and vascular malformations in infants and children: a classification based on endothelial characteristics. Plast Reconstr Surg. 1982;69(3):412-22.
3. Lowe LH, Marchant TC, Rivard DC, et al. Vascular malformations: classification and terminology the radiologist needs to know. Semin Roentgenol. 2012;47(2):106-17.
4. Richter GT, Friedman AB. Hemangiomas and vascular malformations: current theory and management. Int J Pediatr. 2012;2012:645678.
5. Legiehn GM, Heran MK. Venous malformations: classification, development, diagnosis, and interventional radiologic management. Radiol Clin North Am. 2008;46(3):545-97.
6. Iannetti G, Torroni A, Chiummariello S, et al. Clinical and morphological characteristics of head-facial haemangiomas. Head Face Med. 2007;3:12.
7. Buckmiller LM, Munson PD, Dyamenahalli U, et al. Propranolol for infantile hemangiomas: early experience at a tertiary vascular anomalies center. Laryngoscope. 2010;120(4):676-81.

8. Leaute-Labreze C, Dumas de la Roque E, Hubiche T, et al. Propranolol for severe hemangiomas of infancy. N Engl J Med. 2008;358(24):2649-51.

9. Sans V, de la Roque ED, Berge J, et al. Propranolol for severe infantile hemangiomas: follow-up report. Pediatrics. 2009;124(3):e423-31.

10. Bischoff J. Progenitor cells in infantile hemangioma. J Craniofac Surg. 2009;20(Suppl 1):695-7.

Index

Page numbers followed by *f* refer to figure, *fc* refer to flowchart and *t* refer to table